Diagnosis of Sterility and its Traditional Chinese Medicine Treatment

Written by   Jin Weixin
Translated by   Nie Wenxin
                 Zhang Yu
Revised by   Bai Yongquan

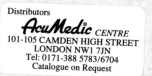
Shandong Science and Technology Press

First Edition 1999
ISBN 7 – 5331 – 2339 – 5

Diagnosis of Sterility and
its Traditional Chinese
Medicine Treatment

Written by   Jin Weixin
Translated by   Nie Wenxin   Zhang Yu
Revised by   Bai Yongquan
English Language Editor   Chen Ping

Published by Shandong Science and Technology Press
16 Yuhan Road, Jinan 250002, China

Printed in the People's Republic of China

Forward

This book is the results of my years of clinical experience and laboratory research as well as the combined experiences of many other colleagues in the field of TCM. In this text I will introduce in detail the methods of examination, diagnosis and TCM treatment of female and male sterility along with similar techniques in Western medicine. The book is divided into two parts, covering male and female sterility respectively. Each part is carefully referenced.

I hope this book may be a helpful reference for doctors working clinically on sterility.

Jin Weixin

Contents

PART ONE
MALE STERILITY

PART TWO
FEMALE STERILITY

2

PART ONE
MALE STERILITY

Chapter One
Diagnosis

If a male has got married for more than two years, no pregnancy occurs without taking any contraceptive measures, with his spouse's reproductive function being normal, he is considered to suffer from male sterility.

Diagnosis of sterility consists of two parts: diagnosis of TCM (Traditional Chinese Medicine) and diagnosis of modern medicine. In addition to inquiring the case history in detail and physical examinations, correct diagnosis is obtained according to Four Diagnostic Methods, Syndrome Differentiation in accordance with Eight Principals combined with various diagnostic and examining methods.

Diagnosis by Means of TCM

Four Diagnostic Methods

Like the diagnosis of the other diseases, TCM diagnostic methods of sterility includes inspection, auscultation and olfaction, interrogation, pulse-feeling and palpation, then TCM corresponding diagnosis can be achieved after comprehensively analysing symptoms and signs from Four Diagnostic Methods and Syndrome Differentiation in accordance with Eight Principals, together with Syndrome Differentiation in accordance with Zangfu.

• *Inspection*

As one of the diagnostic methods, inspection includes mainly observation of vitality, complexion, general appearance and observation of the changes of the volume, the color, the quality of seminal fluid.

Inspection of Vitality: Through this, the doctors can find

3

out the prosperity and the decline of Vital Essence and Energy of the body and the degree of the seriousness of the disease condition. In *Benshen*, a chapter in *Miraculous Pivot of the Yellow Emperor's Internal Classic* (*Ling Shu. Ben Shen Pian*), it is stated that "The combined condition of the Vital Essence and Energy is called vitality." The Vital Essence and Energy is the fundamental of the male, and the prosperity and decline of Vital Essence and Energy directly influence fertile ability of the male.

Inspection of Tongue: Tongue proper chiefly displays the prosperity and the decline of Qi, Blood and Zangfu. Tongue coating mainly reflects the location of the disease, the nature of pathologic changes, the ascending and descending of the pathogenic factor and the body's resistance and regenerative capacity. Inspection of the tongue has certain significance in the diagnosis of sterility in male.

Inspection of Tongue Proper: From the color of the tongue proper, Deficiency and Excess of Zangfu, the prosperity and the decline of Qi and Blood can be observed. For instance, Deficiency of Kidney Yang leads to decline of Fire from the Gate of Life, and pale tongue proper can be observed. Yin Deficiency brings about extreme Heat, bright red tongue with less fluid being observed. The Excess Heat from the Liver Channel causes the tongue proper to be red or crimson. The accumulation of Blood Stasis brings about livid or dark purple tongue proper.

Inspection of Tongue Coating: From the thinness and thickness of the tongue coating, the prosperity and decline of pathogenic Qi factors can be observed; from the color of the coating, Cold and Heat of pathologic changes; from the moisture and dry coating, insufficiency of the body fluids. Generally, yellow tongue coating denotes Heat Syndrome; white tongue coating, Cold Syndrome; thin and slightly yellowish coating, less seriousness of pathogenic Heat; thick and dark yellowish coating, the extreme Heat in the Interior; yellowish, thick and greasy coating, accumulation of Damp Heat; pale, moist and thick tongue coating, Cold and Damp in the Interior; gray, black and moist tongue coating, Deficiency Cold as well. Inspection of the tongue coating

4

and inspection of the tongue proper should be combined together with clinical symptoms to make comprehensive Syndrome Differentiation.

Inspection of Complexions: From this, the consistency and weakness of viscera, the prosperity and decline of Qi and Blood, the ascending and descending of pathogenic factor and Vital Qi can be detected and known. Especially, the inspection of male's genitals is very significant in the diagnosis of the diseases in male and sterility of male. Our forefathers said, "Five types of male sterility" can be diagnosed through inspection. If no testicle is found unilaterally or bilaterally on the scrotum, the patient suffers from eunuchism or cryptorchidism. If the testicles are smaller, and the glens penis is shorter, the patient suffers from dysplasia of external genital organ. This can be found in the cases with sterility without or with azoospermia.

Inspection of Seminal Fluid: From this, doctors can find out the conditions of seminal volume, seminal consistency, and seminal color. Together with considering the various examination results of the seminal fluid, doctors can judge whether seminal fluid is normal or not. This is quite crucial in the judgment of a male's fertility.

• *Auscultation and Olfaction*

In the diagnosis of the disorders in male and of sterility, differentiation of the odors of the patient's breath, physical body, excretion, seminal fluid offers one of the bases for Syndrome Differentiation. Seminal fluid smells slightly fishy. If it smells fetid or with smell of blood, it means the patient suffers from prostatitis, or seminal vesiculitis. After sexual maturity of the male, voices begin to change, becoming stronger. If the voices are like the ones of the child, it suggests hyperdysplasia of sexual development.

• *Interrogation*

Interrogation plays an important part among the four diagnostic methods of sterility. Correct diagnosis can be reached only through detailed inquiring because patients may feel embarrassed to confide his conditions completely to the doctor for it concerns marriage and reproduction.

Inquiry of Age: Age influences sterility greatly. According to TCM theories, a man enters his reproductive period at 16 when "his Kidney Qi is prosperous, his sexual function begins, and his sperm discharges." In reproductive period, men at different ages show different characteristics, and symptoms and signs in physiology and pathology. For instance, various mental disorders and sexual dysfunction happen easily in adolescence and middle-age period. With the growth of age, fertility decreases gradually.

Inquiry of History of Diseases: As various factors affect man's reproductive ability, the history of related diseases should be inquired in detail. When inquiring the past history of patient's diseases, special attention should be paid to the health conditions and diseases in his childhood. For example, whether the patient once suffered from parotitis complicated by testitis, tuberculosis, etc.; whether he once suffered from genital impairment or genital infection; whether he came into contact with radioactive rays, or toxic chemical substances; whether he always used cotton seed oil as edible oil; whether he is addicted to drinking or smoking; whether he has had a history of abnormal sexual life together with the inquiry of his overall health conditions. When getting to know the family case history, inquired are health conditions of the parents and the immediate relatives, whether they have suffered from any congenital diseases or genetic diseases. When inquiring the present history, the onset of the disease, self-feeling symptoms, diagnosis of the disease and methods of treatment should be chiefly inquired.

Inquiry of Seminal Signs: It has great significance as reference for the treatment of man sterile patients. Inquiry of seminal signs includes inquiry of seminal color, volume and quality; whether the patient suffers from nocturnal emission, spermatorrhea, prospermia, aspermatism. If the seminal fluid is watery, refrigerant and scanty, it is called "cold sperm," which results from Deficiency Cold. If the seminal fluid is sticky with flakes or balls, it is called "cloudy sperm," which results from Deficiency Heat. The color, the volume, and the quality of seminal fluid and ovulatory function, whether normal or not, directly influence the reproductive function of the male.

6

• *Pulse-feeling and Palpation*

Pulse-feeling: Male's pulse feels vigorous, but feels weak at Chi portion and feels more vigorous at Cun portion than Chi portion. In *19 Medical Problems*, a chapter of *Classic on Medical Problems* (*Nan Jing · Shi Jiu Nan*), it states: "Pulse in man is above the Guan portion, and that in woman is below the Guan portion; therefore, Pulse at Chi portion in male is constantly weak and female's is constantly vigorous. This is the usual condition···. If the male's pulse at Chi portion is vigorous, it indicates Deficiency; whereas, if female's is weak, it indicates Excess." So, when making diagnosis of the various diseases in male, pulse-feeling is needed to make pulse correspond with its syndromes, and correct diagnosis results.

Palpation: It is to approach such abnormalities as Cold and Heat, softness and hardness, tenderness, lumps by pressing and feeling the patient's such areas as muscles, hands and feet, abdomen, etc. In palpation of male's sterility, changes of the external genital organs should be observed, such as the appearance, size, tenderness, lumps and local temperature of testicles, epididymides, spermatic cord.

Syndrome Differentiation in Accordance with Eight Principals

Differentiation of diseases in male and male sterility is also related to Yin and Yang, Exterior and Interior, Deficiency and Excess, Cold and Heat. The nature of diseases is imbalance of Yin and Yang, and the property of diseases is manifested as in Cold or Heat attribute. The exterior and Interior refers to the location of the disease and the degree of seriousness of disease condition. Deficiency and Excess reflects Vital Qi being strong or weak, and the prosperity and decline of pathologic factor. Syndrome Differentiation in accordance with Eight Principals is also one of the important steps in the diagnosis of sterility. The specific methods of it are the same as those of diagnosing internal diseases, and see them in the book Diagnosis of TCM.

Syndrome Differentiation in Accordance with Zangfu

Zangfu Organs are places where Qi and Blood are produced. Among the five Zang Organs, the Heart governs the circulation of Blood, the Liver stores Blood, the Spleen controls the circulation of Blood. The Kidney stores Vital Essence and Energy, from which Blood is produced, and is transformed to Essence and Energy.

Vital Essence and Energy and Blood come from the same origin. The Kidney stores not only the congenital Essence and Energy, but also the acquired Essence and Energy which is a basis for genital development. The Kidney Qi contains Kidney Yin and Kidney Yang which should be not only profuse and prosperous but also balanced so that they can play their functions normally. The Liver stores Blood, governs its supply and regulates the flow of Qi, enjoys normal circulation of Blood and Qi, and has the functions of storing Blood and regulating the circulation of Blood. If Liver Qi flows normally, foodstuff can be digested, which offers a source for Blood and Vital Essence and Energy. Then the production of Vital Essence and Energy and transportation of it can be carried out normally. The Liver Channel directly runs around the genital organs. The pathology of the Liver can directly influence male fertility. The Spleen and the Stomach provide acquired Essence, and are the sources where Qi and Blood are produced. If the Spleen and the Stomach can normally play their functions, then Vital Essence and Energy has its source, and Blood in the Chong and Ren Channels is profuse. Because the Essence and Blood are profuse, they overflow outside. The Heart governs mental activities which have certain effects on fertility. The specific methods of Syndrome Differentiation according to pathologic changes of the viscera and their interrelations can be found in the book entitled Diagnostics of TCM. To make a summary of all what has been discussed above, in the diagnosis of sterility, four diagnostic methods must be all considered. Differentiating pathologic conditions in accordance with the eight principal syndromes must be applied in combination with Syndrome Differentiation according to pathologic changes of the viscera and their interrelations. Syndrome Differentiation must be

8

applied in combination with differentiation of diseases so that correct diagnosis can be gained.

Diagnosis by Means of Modern Medicine

Examination of Seminal Fluid

Seminal fluid consists of seminal serum and spermium. Spermium is produced in convoluted seminiferous tubule of the testicles, and seminal serum comes from the combined juice secreted by epididymides, seminal vesicle, prostate, bulbourethral gland, and paraurethral duct. Seminal serum is not only the essential transmitter for transporting spermia but also stimulates the mobility of spermia, and contains the essential stroma.

Analysis of seminal fluid is an important means to assay male's fertility. The result of the analysis is influenced by such factors as frequency of sperm ejection, atmospheric temperature, acid-base scale (pH), body conditions, technology conditions, etc. For better command of seminal analysis as a means of examination, several commonly-used indices of examination are analyzed and explained in the following.

• *Sperm Density and Total Sperm Count*

Sperm density refers to the number of spermia in a millilitre of seminal fluid. Total sperm count refers to the total number of spermia in the seminal fluid ejected each time (i. e., number of spermia/ml × volume of seminal fluid). Sperm density has greater influence on fertility. In the past, sperm density was generally considered to be 60,000,000-150,000,000/ml. Family Planning Laboratory of Renji Hospital Affiliated to Shanghai No. 2 Medical Institute compared the numbers of spermia of 365 male cases with fertility with 142 male cases with sterility. It was found that in the fertile group, sperm density of 95% of them was 10-180 millions/ml; that of 51% of them higher than 90 millions/ml; that of 9% of them, lower than 20 millions/ml; and that of 1% of them, lower than 10 millions/ml. In the sterile group, sperm

9

density of 30% of the patients was higher than 60 millions/ml; that of 34%, lower than 20 millions/ml; that of 16%, lower than 10 millions/ml. From the data of the two groups, a conclusion can be made that it is not all-sided to judge male's fertility only on the basis of sperm density, and that a comprehensive analysis of the various indices of sperm survival rate, sperm vitality, deformity rate of spermia should be made so that correct diagnosis can be obtained. According to the opinions of most scholars, it is appropriate to fix the normal number of sperm density to be above 20 millions/ml. The reasons are stated below: ① Renji Hospital Affiliated to Shanghai No. 2 Medical Institute passed scientific appraisal on 16th of August, 1983. Above 20 millions/ml was considered to be the normal value of sperm density. ② The statistic of fertile group shows that sperm density of 9% of the patients was lower than 20 millions/ml. In another word, sperm density of above 90% of the patients in fertile group was higher than 20 millions/ml. ③ When FSH value was within the normal value range in radioimmunoassay, the number of spermia was above 20 millions/ml. ④ From the experience of testicle biopsy, to those whose numbers of spermia were above 20 millions/ml, testicle biopsy will show that the spermatogenic function of most people is fine or good. ⑤ Blindly increasing sperm density and neglecting other items of examination, especially the sperm survival rate and sperm energy should be avoided. ⑥ Increasing the normal value too high that would lead to improper enlargement of incidence of sterility and should be avoided because it may cause the main attention to be placed on the male, and the search of infertile factors in female to be neglected and as a result the patients can not get correct diagnosis and treatment.

Sperm density is directly related to male fertility, but the diagnosis rate of sterility due to abnormal sperm density is not high, the parameters of the normal group and sterile group are distributed interlockingly. The borderline between them is sometimes hard to determine. The low line of sperm density of the Japanese male is 18 millions/ml. The sperm density of 95% of the specific patients is 24,900,000/ml.

There are no great differences between Europeans and Americans, and Japanese; therefore, the normal number of spermia reported in the document abroad is 20-200 millions/ml.

In addition, because of the influences of various objective factors, the same normal individual can show different results at different times and in different backgrounds. For instance, such factors as error rate of laboratory technology, ascetic period, body condition, mental factors, resting condition all can influence the results of test. The study abroad of the relation between sperm count and frequency of sperm ejection shows that if ascetic period is shorter than 12 hours, sperm volume and sperm concentration is 50% of the ones of the control group. The total sperm count decreases to 28% of that of the control group. When ascetic period is longer than 23-28 hours, seminal volume and sperm concentration increase to 70%, and total sperm count increases to 56%. In practical clinical work, we often find that after a patient gets high fever because of cold or other reasons, or after the patient drinks too much wine or after vigorous activities or frequent night-burning, sperm density and total sperm number decreases greatly. Therefore, this index should be obtained after more than 3 times of successive examinations when the patient is in healthy condition. The results of the examinations are averaged; therefore, reliable conclusion can be drawn.

• *Sperm Vitality*

Sperm vitality includes rate of sperm motility and sperm motility. The former refers to quantity analysis of the proportion of the immotile spermia and motile spermia, and the latter refers to quality grading of the motile spermia.

Analysis of rate of sperm motility: Generally, randomly select 10 different views of field, and count 100 spermia, both immotile and motile. The number of motile spermia forms rate of sperm motility. But in common smear examination, the non-moving motile spermia are often counted as immotile spermia. For correct quality analysis of dead and active spermia, sperm supravital staining technique can be used for confirmation. Usually, eosin stain is applied. Under the mirror, the immotile spermia appear to be red and

11

motile spermia appear to be colorless.

Sperm motility directly reflects sperm quality. Jenks divides sperm motility into 0-IV Grades.

Grade 0: The spermia are immotile.

Grade I: The spermia move around in the same place.

Grade II: The spermia move slowly with inconstant directions.

Grade III: The spermia move straight forward.

Grade IV: The spermia move rapidly and straight forward.

The sperm motility grading should be carried out in thermostat or under constant temperature. Choose 4-5 visual fields under 10×40 times cycloscope, count 100 spermia, observe their motile situation, and find out the percentage of the spermia of various motile grades according to motile grading standards. In normal condition, one hour after ejaculation, the number of spermia that move toward active line (Jenks III-IV) is more than 40%.

Sperm motile rate and motility symbolize the survival ability of the spermia in vitro after they are ejaculated. Duration of survival time, the condition of motility suggest the quality condition of the spermia. Sperm motile rate and motility of most of clinical observation are below: One hour after ejaculation, normal rate of sperm motility was $\geqslant 60\%$; 3 hours, $\geqslant 40$-50%; 6 hours, $\geqslant 20$-30%. The sperm motility one hour later and sperm mobility 3 hours later after ejaculation are almost equal. Motile spermia of Grade III take up 50-40%. 6 hours later, motile spermia of Grade III take up only 15-10%. If no motile spermia can be observed 6 hours later, or spermia of Grade III decrease to 5%, it may affect reproductive ability.

For correct estimate of sperm motility, recently, rate of sperm motilityscoring has been suggested. If the percentage of straightforward moving spermia is 40% among the total number of spermia, and the rate of sperm motility is 50%, then, that the score of rate of sperm motility is more than 150 is considered to be normal on the whole.

Examples of Rate of Sperm Motility Scoring

Way of Sperm Movement	Sperm Mobility Grade	Percentage	Score
Straight forward rapidly	IV	10 (5)	40 (20)
Straight forward	III	30 (30)	90 (90)
Uncertain direction	II	10 (10)	20 (20)
No motion forward	I	0 (5)	0 (5)
No motion at all	0	50 (50)	0 (0)

Note: The numbers in the brackets stand for values of normality.

Capillary penetrating test is a special method of evaluating sperm motility. By using different sperm penetrating transmitters, forward penetrating power of spermia in them can be observed more objectively in vitro. This can not only help observe the the quality of the spermia themselves but also the interaction of sperm juice, cervical mucus, and spermia. For instance, there are pathologic changes in the male's seminal fluid or the wife's cervical mucus, the changes of this kind may decrease or restrain sperm forward movement and sperm penetrating power. The penetrating test in vitro can help diagnose the reasons of sterility. This test is carried out like this. A specially-made glass capillary is applied, in which different sperm transmitters (liquescent sperm juice) are kept. In fixed period of time (30 minutes), observe the distance of forward movement in the transmitters, by which sperm moving ability can be judged. The normal value should be lower than 20mm/30 minutes.

The determination of sperm velocity is carried out according to the following procedure. The liquescent seminal fluid in vitro is injected into a specially-made counting board. Under a microscope, observe the motor ability of 100 active spermia by themselves, the duration of time for going through the fixed distance (50μm). Then through calculation, the averaged velocity of spermia tested can be obtained (When carrying out the determination test, preheat the seminal fluid and the counting board is needed). The normal value should be above 20μm/s.

13

According to a penetrating test of 10,000 person-times of Shandong Institute of TCM, the normal value was 23.5±11.6mm/30 minutes. The normal value of averaged velocity of spermia was 22.62 ± 7.5μm/s. From sperm penetrating and velocity tests, it can be concluded that to those whose sperm motility is poor, the values obtained are lower than the normal ones; to those with general sperm motility, most of the values obtained are normal or near to normal, but many were below normal value; to those with fine sperm motility, most of the values obtained are in normal range, and a few are above the normal value or slightly lower than the normal value; to those with excellent sperm motility, the values obtained are far higher than the normal value. Comparing the sperm penetration and velocity, it can be seen that the sensitivity and authenticity of the latter are better than the former. The two tests greatly improve the rate of correct diagnosis of sperm mobility, and offer the reliable indices of quantity dynamic observation.

• *Sperm Morphology Examination*

Sperm morphology examination is to find out the proportion of the spermia with variation in physiology and pathology among the normal spermia. The proportion is an important index in finding out reproductive ability. Staining is an important means in analyzing sperm morphology, and normal spermia and the spermia with variation in physiology and pathology can be analyzed through staining. The common method is smear technique, such as H. E staining method (hematoxylin staining, eosin staining), or Giemsa staining method. But Papanicolaou's vaginal smear technique can help observe and differentiate the special appearances of the spermia. The appearances of the spermia in the human body are not the same. The appearances of common abnormal spermia include macrocephaly, microcephaly, amorphous head, bicephalus, bicaudal, rounded tail, etc. The appearances of the variant spermia are often related to infection, injuries, the condition of local body temperature and blood circulation, androgen level, medicines and genetic factors. Analysis of the appearances of spermia is indispensable in distinguishing the germ cells and spermia of dif-

14

ferent kinds, and in judging the functions of testicles and e-
pididymides.

Differentiation of sperm appearances can be carried out at
the same time when sperm motility observation is being
held, and the percentage of the spermia with normal appearances can be reported. If necessary, seminal fluid is made
into thin piece. By using methylene blue-eosin staining
method or Papanicolaou's vaginal smear technique, appearances of 200 spermia were observed under oil immersion objective. Generally, the percentage of the spermia with normal appearances is $\geqslant 70\%$. There were people who compared a fertile group of 136 people and a sterile group of 137
cases. They found that the abnormal rate of 88% of the people in fertile group was within 20%, and that of 20%
reached 40%. In sterile group, abnormal rate of 25% of the
cases was 20%, and that of 46% reached 40%.

• *Liquefaction of Seminal Fluid and Examination of Seminal Viscosity*

Seminal viscosity and liquefying time are also one of the
indices reflecting normality or abnormality of seminal fluid.
These indices are determined by the activity of proteolytic
enzyme in male's genital canal. Normal seminal fluid is in
liquid state when it is ejected out, then it becomes tremel-
lose or grumose, and liquescent again in 10-30 minutes. Liquefying time refers to the time from ejaculation to seminal
fluid becoming homogenous and liquescent. If seminal fluid
is not liquefied in one hour at room temperature 25-37℃, it
is considered to be abnormal. So far, clinically, observation
and standards for determination of seminal viscosity and liquefying time are quite different, only depending on personal
judgment, and having no objective determining indices.
Therefore, diagnostic rate of non-liquefaction of all the
places are greatly different. The Central Laboratory of the
Affiliated Hospital of Shandong Institute of TCM carefully
observed the liquefying time of 260 sterile patients by fixing
temperature and regular time. Non-liquefying rate was
31%, and during the same period, seminal non-liquefying
rate was 60% when they were examined in the laboratory.
Seminal liquefaction is directly related to sperm motility,

15

and at the same time, reflects the function condition of accessory sexual glands. Being divided according to time, generally, seminal non-liquefaction can be divided into 1 hour non-liquefaction, 2-hour non-liquefaction, ⋯ 24-hour non-liquefaction. To divide according to viscosity, seminal fluid can be divided into thready mucus filament, coarse mucus filament, claviform or patchy mucus ball or flocculent ball. For better observation of seminal liquefying time, seminal viscosimeter examination is added clinically, i. e. put 0.5ml of liquescent seminal fluid into the funnel above the viscosimeter, and work out the time of all the seminal fluid passing through the tube of the viscosimeter. In the case of a capillary, 93mm long, diameter being 0.725mm, the normal averaged time is $36.6 \pm 13.4s$ (Beijing). If a capillary, 93mm long and diameter being 0.798mm, the normal averaged time is $17 \pm 4.7s$ (Shanghai).

• *Seminal Quantity*

Usually, graduated centrifuge tube (10ml) is used to measure seminal whole quantity. The normal value is 2-6ml. If it is lower than 1.5ml, but higher than 8ml, it is considered to be abnormal. Less seminal quantity leads to fewer spermia and less total number of spermia. Excessive seminal quantity always comparatively dilute sperm density. Seminal quantity is closely related to ascetic period of time, ways in obtaining seminal fluid and conditions of the body and mental condition as well.

• *Acid-base Scale of Seminal Fluid*

Normal seminal fluid appears to be basic, and pH is 7.0-8.0, in average 7.4. When pH is inclined to be acid, sperm activity and metabolism appear to decrease sharply. In summary, if seminal fluid ejected out is kept too long, it is inclined to be acid easily. Therefore, seminal fluid should be sent for test in time. If pH is lower than 7 or higher than 9, sperm activity decreases greatly.

• *Seminal Biochemical Examination*

Over 95% of seminal fluid is seminal pulp. Seminal pulp determines the biochemistry and physiology properties of seminal fluid. Seminal pulp contains many elements of plasma, and some "special elements," which exert great influ-

16

ence on sperm activity and fertilization ability. Generally, seminal samples are put into water bather at 35-37℃, and 1. 2-1.5ml of it is put into a centrifugal separator after it gets liquefied (3000 revolutions/minute, altogether 15 minutes). The upper seminal pulp is taken for biochemical determination.

Fructose Determination: Fructose is produced mainly from seminal vesicles, is the main source of sperm energy metabolism, related to rate of sperm motility and sperm activity, and is not necessarily related to sperm count. Decrease do the fructose contentsof the people with vesiculitis, hypoleydigism, and of the aged people. This determination can help distinguish simple spermatic duct-obstructed azoospermia and vasovesicula defective azoospermatism. The former's fructose content is normal but the latter has no or little fructose. Fructose determination is an index of judging vesicula function, and indirectly judging testosterone. Fructose content of diabetic patients may increase. Method of determination is generally m-dihydroxybenzene method, and the normal value is 256 ± 104mg/dl. If it is lower than 120mg/dl, then it is abnormal.

Citric Acid: It comes mainly from prostate. It affects seminal coagulation and the process of liquefaction after ejaculation after it gets combined with calcium ion. It maintains the balance of osmosis in seminal fluid, and plays an important role in maintaining sperm activity and hyaluronidase activity. The content of testosterone in blood and citric acid in seminal fluid are in positive proportion. So, determination of citric acid content in seminal fluid can help to learn indirectly secretory situation of male hormone in the body. If a patient suffers from prostatitis, citric acid content in seminal fluid decreases markedly. Determination of citric acid content can serve as one of the parameters for judging prostate function. Through Furth-Herrmann Response Assay, the normal content of citric acid is 5.6±2.0mg/dl.

Acid Phosphatase: It mainly comes from the prostate. It's physiological function is to hydrolyze such substances as phosphocholine, phosphoglycerol, and nucleotide in seminal fluid through phosphorylation process. It is related to sperm

17

activity and metabolism. If a patient suffers from chronic prostatitis, the content of acid phosphatase decreases. Acid phosphatase activity is also affected by androgen in the body. Clinically, glycerophosphate method is used to determine the content of acid phosphatase. To a normal person, the content of it is 882 ± 412 Broder's indices/ml.

Trace Elements Zinc, Copper and Iron: The trace elements in seminal fluid are significant to male reproductive power and reproductive endocrine function. Through determination of atomic absorption spectrometry, in seminal fluid, the normal value of zinc is $130 \pm 5.6mg/ml$; that of copper is $1.84 \pm 0.158\mu g/ml$; and that of iron is $0.801 \pm 0.104\mu g/ml$.

Sperm Specific Enzyme-lactic dehydrogenase x (LDHx): LDH and work enzyme have comparative tissue-specificity. LDHx zone is related to the number of spermia and enzyme activity. Therefore, clinically, there are cases of sterility though seminal test of some men is normal and examinations of the women are also normal, the reason of which might be because of the decrease of LDHx activity. This may be required as an objective index to evaluate male's reproductive ability. Methods of determination are polyacrylamide gel densitrophoresis enzyme-linked staining and light densitometer scanning, from which 6 stripes of zone can be observed, and one LDHx zone can also be seen between LDH3 and LDH4.

• *Seminal Microbiological Examination*

It includes two ways: Smear examination and common bacterial cultivation. The former refers to smearing the seminal fluid well-distributedly on the slide, and fixing it by slightly heating. Then Gram's staining, acid-fast staining, and microscopy are carried out respectively. The latter refers to vaccinating the sample to various plates and glucose bouillon enriched medium by means of aseptic technique, and to observing colony growth through incubator's culture. According to the appearances from smear, staining and microscopy, and colony properties, biochemical test and determination of bacterial species are carried out. Besides, there are also anaerobic bacteria culture, mycobacterium tubercu-

18

losis culture, fungus culture, etc. Invasions of microorganism all can make seminal fluid infected. The common diseases include prostatitis, seminal vesiculitis, epididymitis, urethritis, all of which can lead to the changes of seminal quality and the decrease of reproductive ability.

Testicle Biopsy

With the development of male reproductive pathology and the application of quantity method of spermatogenic state, a further emphasis on and practice of testicle biopsy are quite necessary.

Testicle biopsy can help distinguish obstructive azoospermia and testicular azoospermia can help observe states of germ cells and interstitial cells of Leydig in convoluted seminiferous tubule, and can help learn the degree of change between convoluted seminiferous tubule and spermiduct. How to correctly estimate testicle biopsy is a key in the diagnosis of sterility.

• *Indications of Testicle Biopsy*

After examinations of seminal fluid, the number of spermia is below 10 millions/ml, the sizes of testicles are normal, hypospermia or azoospermia but FSH value is within the normal range.

With a combination of testicle biopsy and endocrine examination, it can be determined whether hypofunction of testicles are primary or secondary.

Hypospermia due to spermophlebectasia. Biopsy can help diagnose the degree of influence of spermophlebectasia on spermatogenic function of the testicles.

Vasography shows obstructed spermiduct, and the conditions of sperm producing function of testicles are needed.

• *Contraindications of Testicle Biopsy*

Testicle volume shows smaller than 10ml, primary testicle withering with marked increase of FSH in blood.

Azoospermia or hypospermia accompanied by reduced or softened testicles and increase of FSH.

Klinefelters' syndrome due to abnormal chromosome, and biopsy is unnecessary.

• *Pathological Types of Testicle Biopsy*

19

Testicle biopsy of healthy people: In testicular convoluted seminiferous tubule of healthy people, spermatogenic cells of various grades can be observed, which are arranged in the direction from basement membrane to lumen: Spermatogonia, first spermatocyte, secondary spermatocyte, spermatid and spermia. Besides these spermatogenic cells, there are also supporting cells with large volume. Because all those spermatogenic cells are formed at different times, spermatids of different periods can be seen in the cross-section of testicular convoluted seminiferous tubule.

Hypospermatogenesis: Hypospermatogenesis can be divided into three types: Mild, moderate and severe. All these cases of hypospermatogenesis have the phenomenon of the decrease of cell layers, disorder of cell arrangement and cell exfoliation. Among mild hypospermatogenesis cases, 45% have pathologic changes in canaliculi; 45-75% of the moderate cases have the problem of the decrease or exfoliation of spermatogenic cells; over 75% of the severe cases not only have pathologic changes in canaliculi, but have the problem of increased limiting membrane fibers or hyaline degeneration, which leads to severely damaged spermatogenesis, and thus irreversible pathologic changes are resulted in.

Maturity-Disturbed or Obstructed Type: Disturbance to the maturity of testicular spermatogenesis happens in spermatogenic cells of different periods, and most commonly ends during the period of spermatocyte. No spermia are formed in canaliculi.

Simple Supporting Cell and Mixed Supporting Cell: There are only supporting cells but not spermatogenic cells in convoluted seminiferous tubule, and increase of limiting membrane as well. This is congenital abnormality. Mixed supporting cells' picture shows that there are few spermatogenic cells in canaliculi, in which there are mainly supporting cells.

Hyaline Degeneration of Convoluted Seminiferous Tubule: It is manifested as hyaline degeneration of basement membrane and epithelial fibrous tissues of convoluted seminiferous tubule, accompanied by spermatogenic disturbance to the varying degree, and the disappearance of spermato-

20

genic cells and supporting cells in canaliculi with severe pathologic changes.

Klinefelters' Syndrome: Testicle biopsy shows that the diameter of convoluted seminiferous tubule is smaller than normal, and there are only supporting cells in the canaliculi or complete hyaline degeneration happens to the canaliculi, in which there are no spermatogenic cells.

Spermophlebectasia: Because testicular blood circulation is affected, spermatogenic cells of various stages can be observed in the convoluted seminiferous tubule, but which are arranged in disorder, and some of which exfoliate in the lumen, and fibrous hyperplasia or hyaline degeneration of limiting membrane can be observed.

Mixed Pathologic Changes: There are more than one types of pathologic changes, such as hypospermatogenesis and hyperplasia of limiting membrane or hyaline degeneration exists at the same time. Pathologic changes of this kind are largely irreversible.

• *Diagnostic Method of Testicular Tissue Biopsy*

Quantity Analysis Method of Spermatid of Convoluted Seminiferous Tubule: Serial section of testicular biopsy tissues is carried out, and observe 10 cross-sections of convoluted seminiferous tubule of unilateral testicle, and 20 or more canalicular cross-sections by adding together those of the two testicles, count only the mature spermia on each canalicular cross-section but not spermatogonia, spermatocytes, and supporting cells. See the following table:

Siber's Spermatid Evaluation of Convoluted Seminiferous Tubule

Number of Mature Spermia in Canaliculi Bilaterally	Sperm Count ($\times 10^6$ml)
6-10	3-7
10-25	10-15
40-42	40-60
45-80	85-100

21

Comprehensive Scoring Method to Record Testicular Function State: It is recommended by Pesce. It comprehensively uses Johnsen's Meinhard's and Honores's Scoring Methods together with 5 such indices as diameter of convoluted seminiferous tubule, changing or not of basement membrane, etc. in order to record testicular function state. This recording method compensates the one-sidedness of each individual scoring record.

Johnsen's, Meinhard's, Honore's Scoring Standards

Johnsen's	Meinhard's	Honore's
Normal formation of spermia 10	Normal Spermatogenic function 1	Difference between biopsy and sperm count 1
Disordered spermtogenic cells 9	Convoluted seminiferous tubule obstruction 2	Infrequent or irregular formation of spermia 2
Few spermia in convoluted seminiferous tubule 8	Decrease of seminferous epithelium 3	Supporting cells only 3
No spermia 7	End-up of spermatogenic cells 4	Abnormal development of testicles 4
Fewer spermatid 6	Supporting cells only 5	
No spermatid 5	Hyaline degeneration of convoluted seminiferous tubule 6	
Fewer spermatocytes 4		
Spermatogonia only 3		
Supporting cells only 2		
No cells in convoluted seminiferous tubule 1		

Double Diagnostic Method of Testicular Pathologic Changes and Disturbance of Sperm Formation: As diagnosis of testicular pathologic changes in male, disturbance of sperm formation is graded according to testicular sperm formation states. 5 grades are made:

Grading Standards for Disturbance of Sperm Formation

Grades	Standards
Normal or Normal on the whole	Formation of 75% of spermia in convoluted seminiferous tubule is good
Mild Spermatogenic disturbance	Less than 45% of convoluted seminiferous tubule has problem of spermatogenic disturbance
Moderate Spermatogenic Disturbance	45-75% of convoluted seminiferous tubule has problem of spermatogenic disturbance
Severe Spermatogenic Disturbance	More than 75% of Convoluted seminiferous tubule has problem of spermatogenic disturbance
Irreversible Spermatogenic disturbance	No or fewer spermatogenic cells in convoluted seminiferous tubule, and pathologic change is severe

Penetrating Test of Sperm in Vitro

Human's Sperm in vitro Penetrating Apellucid Zone of Hamster ovum Assay (SPA), established in 1970's, is a new technique to evaluate fertilization ability. Yanagimachi and others were the first to confirm that hamster ovum with pellucid zone being removed penetrated by human's spermia can be an effective mold for predicting male fertility. This method comparatively reflects completely such biological phenomena of sperm functions as sperm capacitation, acrosomal response, flagellum movement like fertilization membrane-egg membrane fusion and coordination. Sperm Penetrating test, that is, observation of the ability of whether human's spermia in vitro can successfully penetrate animal ovum, overmatches routine sperma analysis, and practical clinical application in evaluating fertility potential of human's sperm samples. It has been confirmed that SPA test is well related to the ability of sperm fertilization. SPA greatly

23

improves correctness in diagnosis of sterility. Research has shown that SPA is markedly superior to SFA (SP erma Assay) in determining whether fertility is possessed or not. Some people hold that in the diagnosis of sterility, sensitivity of SPA is 100%, but that of SFA is 47%. Pseudopositive of SPA is 0, but that of SFA is 53%. Pseudonegative of SPA is 0, but that of SFA is 16%. Many people point out that between sterility and fertility, there is no inter-overlapping in SPA fertility percentage, and the border of each is clear. Therefore, at present, SPA is regarded as the best method in determining male's fertility potential. In clinical practice, this effective assay can be used in the following aspects: ① Evaluate the correctness of SFA in determining male fertility. ② Examine and determine the sperm function of the patients with sterility due to unknown causes. ③ Evaluate the seriousness of the indices of abnormal sperma of the sterile patients and the effects after treatment. ④ Before fertilization in vitro, determine sperm quality of the husband or spermia provider. ⑤ Predict the fertility of the patients with immunosterility. ⑥ SPA is also used to study the mechanism and curative effects of TCM drugs in treating sterility. ⑦ SPA is used as a mold to study male contraceptives with potential.

The instruments and equipment of SPA are expensive, and operations of them are complicated. The process involves sperma collection, processing, incubation, the drawing of ovum, removal of pellucid zone, incubation of sperm-ovum and penetration of them, etc. If enlarged sperm head or sperm pronucleus can be observed in ovum serum, then record, "penetrated ovum." Penetrating rate stands for fertility index, which is expressed as: The numbers of penetrated ova by spermia/total numbers of ova $\times$ 100%. Generally, the penetrating rate, 10% of hamster ova, is used as the lowest value of sperm fertilization ability of normal people. If it is lower than 10%, a person can be considered to have no fertility; between 11-14%, it is doubtable values; over 15%, it is normal. Department of Gynecology and Obstetrics of Hongkong University reported that the penetrating rate of SPA of fertile group was $31.9 \pm 3.2\%$; that of sterile group,

24

$4.6 \pm 0.7\%$; and that of the patients, not married, and having no child-bearing history, $29.5 \pm 3.0\%$.

Recently, some hospitals improved Yanagimachi's method slightly by common incubator in place of CO_2 incubator, BSA in place of HSA. The male's pronucleus becoming enlarged sperm head is regarded as an index to indicate that the ova are penetrated by spermia. Besides, some researchers applied direct ovum-impacting technology. Using the index of stiff sperm tail to help find out and distinguish fertilized ovum, using common microscope in place of different microscope, and this technique is used to study curative effects of TCM drugs.

Diagnosis of Immunosterility

According to statistical data, 10-20% of the sterile cases are caused by immune factors. These married couples suffer from no organic diseases in reproductive system. The male can produce antibodies to their own spermia, i. e., self-immunity. The female also can produce antibodies to the spermia which lose mobility or the ability to penetrate uterine neck in vagina.

Clinically, blood serum of some sterile patients are found to have special antibodies counteracting against spermia. These special antibodies may exist in blood and as well as in genital duct of both the male and the female. The antibodies in blood serum mainly are IgG, and IgM; and in genital duct, IgA. Titers of the antibodies in genital duct and blood serum are quite different. The antibodies in seminal juice are only 1-2% of those in plasma. In male reproductive system, blood-testicle barrier prevents antigen substances in sperma from entering blood circulation. In normal occasions, no immune reaction happens. In the cases of injuries, operation, or inflammation, this barrier will be destroyed and immune reaction takes place, from which antibodies counteracting against spermia will be produced. Such infections in male genital duct and urinary tract as prostatitis, seminal vesiculitis, epididymitis, etc. are the common etiological factors that cause self-immunity.

The antisperm antibodies of this kind can act on spermia

25

whose survival rate will decrease and whose mobility will also decrease. The seminal fluid will not be liquefied either. These antibodies also can obstruct the formation of normal spermia or destroy reproductive cells, thus leading to the decrease of sperm numbers or to azoospermia. According to Fattam's and other's reports, among 115 cases of sterile male, the positive rate of male antisperm antibodies of the patients with circulating antibodies was 28%. Hargreave examined 300 male cases diagnosed to suffer from sterility, and found that 30.3% of them had agglutination-braking antibodies. Hendry believed that 1/3 of the oligospermia cases were caused by self-immunity.

Immunosterility has not clinically drawn people's enough attention, and other factors that cause sterility should be excluded before confirmed diagnosis of the disease. The common immunological examination methods of antisperm immunity include:

Huhner's Test and Sperm-Cervical Mucus Penetrating or Contacting Test: Huhner's test is one of the effective indirect means of determining sperm antibodies, but the date of this test, mental state during sexual intercourse, physiochemical property of cervical mucus, ways and technology of obtaining samples, etc., all may affect the results of the test. However, sperm-cervical mucus penetrating or contacting test shows ignorance to these factors, and can not only precisely reflect the effects of immune factors upon the penetration of spermia through cervical mucus, but also determine whether etiological factors come from the male of the female by a cross test by comparing the normal ones and the diseased patients.

Complement-Dependent Sperm Braking or Cytotoxic Assay: Sperm antigens and antibody molecules interact, complement system is activated, and the permeability and the integrity of sperm cytomembrane are damaged. Therefore, it results in the loss of mobility of spermia and in the staining of spermia by some days. That is to say, after the surface of spermia combines the sperm antibodies that can fix complement, with the cooperation of the complement, spermia are braked or die. Under a microscope, it can be observed that spermia are braked or staining is positive. This method can only determine the sperm antibodies in sperm tail shaft, but the antibodies located at antisperm head can only interfere with the combination of sperm and ovum, but show ignorance to sperm activity. The tests of this kind include sperm braking test, sperm cytotoxic test. These tests can be used to determine the antisperm antibodies in blood serum and spermia serum of the infertile women, and in blood serum and cervical-vagina secretion of the existence and titer of cytotoxic antibodies have no obvious relation with sterility both in male and the female. The blood serum that has sperm braking and cell toxicity often show coagulation activity, especially tail-tail or mixed coagulation types. The spermia used in these experiments should be obtained in high-quality seminal fluid, and blood serum used as a source of complement should be fresh. Blood serum of the people with AB blood types, guinea pigs, and rabbits are better source of complement. The dependent methods of the complement of this kind commonly include sperm braking experiment, and sperm braking and cytotoxic microdetermination.

Spermagglutination Test: The test is based on the principle that antibodies and antigen molecules interact and agglutination happens. This is a traditional and sensitive method. Sperm antibodies can make spermia agglutinate, and agglutination manners can be observed through microscope or with eyes. The methods of determination include gelatin agglutination, tube-plate agglutination, disc agglutination, capillary agglutination, and plate agglutination. Gelatin agglutination is reliable, and capillary agglutination requires fewer spermia and is simple to carry out. Because such non-immune factors like bacteria, some non-crystal substances in seminal fluid, and steroid-globulin compounds, etc., can also cause spermia to agglutinate; therefore, this method is poorly specific, and can only be used for preliminary screening. Recently, Haas and others used indirect Coobs' Quantity Determination after the improvement of it to determine antisperm antibodies. This method, compared with routine sperm agglutination and braking determination, is greatly

27

specific and sensitive.

Immunolabeled Assay

Indirect Immunofluorescence Test (Coon's Test): The second antibody labeled with fluorescein acts with the sperm combined with sperm antibody. Under fluorescent microscope, fluorescent light can be observed, but only pseudopositive is higher during the process of the assay.

Enzyme Linked Immunosorbent Assay (ELISA): Enzyme linked second antibody acts with sperm antibody combined on the surface of antigen of sperm membrane. After zymolyte is added, determine the result according to the change of color of zymolyte (This method can directly use the objective recording results of enzyme labeling meter, and can determine the types of antibodies. In another word, ELISA is to make blood serum for determination and the corresponding solid antigens form immunocompound, and is determined by the second antibody. For quantifying the latter reaction, the second antibody is labelled with enzyme. This combined enzyme can make stroma change to chromogen. The color reaction can be observed with eyes or through spectrophotometer. Enzyme labeling efficiency is not so high as isotope labeling of RIA, but because enzyme transformation rate is very high, the sensitivity of ELISA can be compatible to that of RIA; what's more, this method is advantageous for it requires no fresh spermia, and is appropriate to a large number of samples determination.

Radio-labelled Anti-immunoglobulin or A Albumen: Radio-labelled anti-immunoglobulin or staphylococcic A albumen combined with the sperm antibody combined on the surface of the spermia, and R-counter is used to determine radioactivity of sperm surface. But because each time, antigens are different, repetition is poor, and the results of different laboratories can not be compared; what's more, the equipment is expensive, and the operators are easily damaged by radioactivity, and ordinary hospitals can not bear the expenses.

Besides the above methods of tests, there are also mixed antiglobulin reaction and immunoglobin combination.

28

To summarize the above test methods, spermagglutination and braking assay are traditional means of studying sperm antibodies, but sensitivity and specificity are poor. At present, it is generally held that enzyme-linked immunosorbent assay has the advantages of sensitivity, objectivity, quantity and of requiring no special equipment. Therefore, it is easy to popularize the technique.

The sperm antibodies in the local areas of reproduction duct greatly, directly, and effectively influence human's fertility compared with those in blood serum, especially the sperm antibodies in female cervical mucus. Because there is complement in the cervical mucus, uterine neck is the place where local immunity is likely to produce in female reproductive duct. Besides, in cervical mucus, of many patients, sexual intercourse positive, antisperm antibodies also exist. This indicates that determination of antisperm antibodies in cervical mucus is also very important to the diagnosis of the causes of sterility. Before determination, cervical mucus should be liquefied, usually with bromelain liquefaction. What is more, antisperm antibodies in cervical mucus, immunoglobin in sperm serum should be paid attention and stressed. In sperm serum are mainly IgG and IgA, which take up 1-2% of blood serum concentration, but there is little IgM.

For improving diagnostic rate of immunosterility, a better command of the indices and signs of antisperm antibodies determination: ① Those with sterility due to unknown causes, and various examinations of female fertility and examination of the male sperm are normal. ② Huhner's test abnormal, the mobile spermia under each high multiple perimeter are fewer than 5, or the spermia turn round in the same place or agglutinate in cervical mucus; ③ After many times of examination, rate of sperm motilitys are lower than 20-30%. No spermia moves forward; ④ SPA abnormal; ⑤ Many times of seminal examination show agglutination of motile spermia.

Examination of Endocrine Function
Examination of endocrine function plays an important part

in the diagnosis of sterility in male. It is closely related to the activities of hypothalamus-hypophysistesticular axis. The convoluted seminiferous tubule of the testicles is the place where spermia are formed, and is constituted by Sertoli's cells with supporting and nourishing function, and spermatogenic cells of various grades in Sertoli's cells. For male, FSH mainly acts at spermatogenic cells and supporting cells, and LH mainly acts at Leydig's cells. FSH mainly combines with specific FSH receptor in Sertoli's cells, and androgen-binding protein (ABP) is produced through cAMP system. ABP may get conjugated with testosterone, and more into lumen of the convoluted seminiferous tubule through the lymphatic system of the testicles, and androgen concentration in the lumen increases sharply which enhances and improves the spermatogenic process of the convoluted seminiferous tubule. The main cells of interstitial tissue of testis are Leydig's cells, and there are LH receptors on cell membrane. LH secreted by hyophysis conjugates with LH-receptors and therefore adenylate cyclase is activated and combines with ATP, which results in cAMP. Under catalysis of cAMP, phosphorylating process of protein is speeded, and various kinds of phosphorylated proteins are formed. They are helpful for cholesterol to enter the mitochondrion; therefore, the cleavage of cholesterol is enhanced, and biological combination of testosterone is speeded. Under the effect of LH, testosterone produced by Leydig's cells of testis is released into blood stream, and then combines with sex hormones-binded globulin (SHBG) and with other plasma proteins. Then, they are transported to the target cells, or directly combines with testosterone receptors, or are transformed to dihydrotestosterone with the effect of α-reducing enzyme; or are transformed to estradiol with the effect of aromatized enzyme, then plays their parts. To make a sum-up about what has been discussed above, FSH and LH play an important role in regulating spermatogenic process. Spermia get mature after spermatogonia undergo 6 growing stages with a period of time of 74 days. Spermatogenic process is actually controlled by testosterone and FSH.

Radioimmunoassay technique offers a promising future for

reproductive endocrine function determination. radioimmunoassay (RIA) is a supermicroanalysis combining high specificity of antigen-antibody reaction with high sensitivity of radioisotope. Using it to determine the fundamental values of various hormones is quite reliable for clinical diagnosis and the judgment of sexual gland-axis function state. Male's blood serum sex hormones basal values determined by WHO's paired medical design are listed in the following table:

Blood Serum Sex Hormones Basal Values of Grown-up Male

Name of Hormone	National (5) Averaged	National (5) ± SD	WHO (11) (Range)
FSH (Iu/L)	2.42*	1.56-3.75	1.2-5.0
LH (Iu/L)	2.64*	3.23-6.67	2.5-9.8
PRL (mIu/L)	360.2	207-513.4	110-510
T (nmol/L)	22.7*	19.0-27.0	13.0-33.0
T/LH	5.72	4.05-8.08	
E_2(pmol/L)	212.3	95.6-329	70-190
P. S. Cortisol (F) (nmol/L)	422.5	316.4-528.6	160-660

    * Geometrical mean

The determined hormones basal values should be considered in accordance with clinical symptoms and signs and other various examinations for overall analysis.

If basal values of FSH, LH, T and E_2 are all normal, then, reproductive endocrine diseases can on the whole be excluded, but disorders in convoluted seminiferous tubule and subordinate sexual glands can not be wholly excluded. In the light of sperm analysis, if the patient has no spermia or low fructose in seminal serum or no fructose in sperma serum, this suggests obstructive azoospermia or congenital absence of vas deferens.

Values of FSH, LH, and T are all low. The reasons of low gonad stimulating hormone of low gonadotropic hormone type are generally considered to be the hypofunction of hypothalamus, and hypophysis, and secondary hypofunction of the testicles. Commonly seen is hyposexual function of spe-

31

cific low gonadotropic hormone type, including Kallmann's syndrome and acquired organic diseases or injuries in hypophysis and hypothalamus. Values of FSH and LH increase, and the proportion of T and T/LH decrease. This sex hypofunction of high gonadotropic hormone type suggests primary exhaustion of testicle function, such as azoospermia, or haperazoospermia caused by Klinefelter's syndrome, severe spermophlebectasia, radioactive rays and damages from drugs.

Values of PRL markedly increases, and the values of FSH and LH are low at normal border, accompanied by hypofunction of sexuality, impotence, aspermia, etc., indicating hyperprolac-tinemia, and suggesting the possibility of hypophysoma or pituitary microadenoma.

Vasography and Seminal Vesiculography

It refers to injecting contrast agent into vas deferens through scrotum, and to making spermatic duct and scrotum and ejaculatory duct developed and displayed in x-ray photos. The newest method is to directly puncture spermatic duct through the skin of scrotum and contrast technique is carried out. This technique is simple and easy to carry out with less pain and therefore easy to be popularized. 50-60% meglucamine diatrizonate is selected as contrast agent for the development, the photos from which are clear, reliable. Generally, each side is injected 2.5ml contrast agent so that the whole sperm duct can be filled up. Injection should be carried out slowly, and each side needs about 1-2 minutes. The patient feels a sense of urination. This suggests that the contrast agent reaches the far part of spermatic duct. Conway reported that obstruction azoospermia takes up 4-12% among sterility. Obstruction takes place in groin of spermatic duct, ampullae or ejaculatory duct, which may be unobstructed or obstructed completely. Vasography not only judges whether spermatic duct is obstructed and congenital abnormalities exist, but is also significant in the diagnosis of organic damages caused by inflammation, tuberculosis. But some scholars hold that cases should be carefully chosen; otherwise, it will impose unnecessary pain on the patients.

32

Only those patients, whose testicle biopsy is normal or the reasons are unknown, and who need to exclude sperm duct abnormality, need vasography.

Chapter Two
Treatment Methods

Treatment Principles

In TCM, treatment based on Syndrome Differentiation is the essential principle of diagnosis and treatment of the disease. The following are the methods of treatment of sterility in male.

Restoring the Kidney and Nourishing Yin

In the theory of TCM, the Kidney is divided into Kidney Yang and Kidney Yin which are the essential substances for male's growth, development, and functions of reproduction. Kidney Yin and Kidney Yang should be not only plentiful and prosperous, but also balanced relatively in order to maintain the normal activities of the body. Deficiency and Decline of Kidney Yang, or the excessive consumption and impairment of Kidney Yin, or Deficiency of both Kidney Yang and Kidney Yin result in Deficiency and Decline of Kidney Qi, the consumption and impairment of Essence and Blood which result in sterility and sexual disorders. Therefore, the method that restores the Kidney and nourishes Yin is the commonest way to treat sterility. For sterile patients with Deficiency of Kidney Yang, and decline of Fire in the Gate of Life, warming and reinforcing Kidney Yang, tonifying and benefiting the Gate of Life are needed if impotence, thinness of seminal fluid, Cold of seminal fluid occur every time because of the spread of pathogenic Cold, and the decline of Kidney Yang as what is called, "benefiting the source of Fire to remove pathogenic Cold." The commonly used herbal drugs include aconite root (Radix Aconiti Praeparata), cinnamon bark (Cortex Cinnamoni), pilose antler (Cornu Cervi Pantotrichum), morinda root (Radix Morindae Officinalis), Epimedium (Herba Epimedii), curculigo (Rhizoma Curculiginis), dodder seed (Semen Cuscutae), fenugreek seed (Semen Trigonellae), Chinese chive seed (Semen Allii Tuberosi), silk moth (Bombyx Mori), cynomorium (Herba Cynomorri), desertliving cistanche (Herba Cistachis), psoralea fruit (Fructs Psoraleae), etc. The common prescriptions include Yougui Yin (the Kidney Yang-Reinforcing Decoction), Shenqi Wan (Bolus for Restoring Kidney Qi), Er Xian Tang (Epimedium and Curculigo Decoction), etc. In this way, Kidney Yang is supported by Kidney Yin, which in turn is warmed by Kidney Yang which has the source to rely on. As a result, Kidney Yang and Kidney Yin are well balanced and the disease is cured. For sterile patients with impairment and Deficiency of Kidney Yin, various kinds of Essence and reproduction diseases occur because of Deficiency of Essence and Blood. The principle of treatment should be nourishing Kidney Yin and replenishing Essence to benefit Marrow. The commonly used herbal drugs include dried rehmannia root (Radix Rehmanniae), dogwood fruit (Fructus Corni), wolfberry fruit (Fructus Lycii), mulberry (Folium Mori), siberian solomonseal rhizome (Rhizoma Polygonati), glossy privet fruit (Fructus Ligustri Lucidi), eclipta (Herba Ecliptae), tortoise-plastron (Plastrum Testudinis), fresh-water turtle-shell (Carapax Trionycis), donkey-hide gelatin (Colla Corii Asini), etc. The prescriptions commonly used are Liuwei Dihuang Wan (Bolus of Six Drugs Including Rehmannia), Zuogui Yin (Kidney-Yin-Tonifying Decoction), Zuogui Wan (Bolus as Kidney-Yin Tonics), etc. , and Yin and Yang in equilibrium will be achieved, and the disease will be cured. For sterile patients with impairment and Deficiency of Kidney Essence, because of which the formation of Kidney Qi will not happen, then impotence, spermatorrhea, premature ejaculation, and various kinds of Essence diseases will appear for Deficiency of Kidney Qi. Principles of treatment should be to reinforce Kidney Qi with usually both Kidney Yin and Kidney Yang being restored and regulated. The drugs commonly used are the same as what has been listed above. The commonly used prescriptions are Shenqi Wan (Bolus for Restoring Kidney Qi), and Shengui Wan (Bolus as the Kidney Yin-tonic), etc. As what was said in the ancient China, "A good way to replenish Yin is through Yang; a good way to reinforce Yang is through Yin."

Therefore, Yang-invigorating should not be neglected while Yin is replenished and Yin nourishment should not be neglected while Yang is nourished. Because most drugs that nourish Yin are greasy and wet, the prescriptions of nourishing Yin should be added with the drugs that warm Yang and regulate Qi-circulation. Most drugs that tonify Yang are warm and dry; therefore, the prescriptions for reinforcing Yang should be added up with the drugs that replenish Yin. These can prevent reinforcing Yang from impairing Yin, nourishing Yin from damaging Yang.

Promoting Blood Circulation and Removing Blood Stasis
Essence and Blood enjoy movement but not stagnation. They should move and circulate endlessly so that they can perform normal biological functions. The pathological disorders due to seven emotional conditions (joy, anger, melancholy, anxiety, grief, fear and terror). six climatic conditions (Wind, Cold, Summer-Heat, Damp, Dryness and Fire), injuries from fall, excessive sexual activities, improper use of drugs—all can lead to Blood Stasis. Therefore, Blood Stasis accumulates. As a result, pathogenic change of sperma and disorder of sexual function can be resulted in. Clinical experience has illustrated that Blood Stasis widely exists in sterile patients, so promoting the circulation of Blood and removing Blood Stasis should be an important principle of treatment for sterility. Some call it the principle of treatment of andrological disease in the second place.

Li Laitian (1990), having carried out a laboratory study of the cases with Blood Stasis by means of blood rheology and examination of nail fold microcirculation, put forward that the selection of the drugs that promote the circulation of Blood should be made not only on the basis of Syndrome Differentiation but also in accordance with the result of whether Blood Stasis exists after blood rheological examination and examination of nail fold microcirculation. It has been confirmed clinically that for those whose examination results suggest that the whole blood viscosity or plasma specific viscosity, packed cell volume are higher than normal levels, and whose nail fold microcirculation examination suggests abnormality, appropriate drugs that promote the circulation of Blood and remove Blood Stasis should be used as well even though there are no symptoms and signs of Blood Stasis clinically and in tongue, thus satisfactory clinical results can be obtained. After the treatment, the whole blood viscosity and plasma specific viscosity and packed cell volume of these patients return to normal values. Compared with the condition before drug application, there's marked statistical significance. Compared with the treatment solely by drugs restoring the Kidney to support Yang, nourishing Yin to reduce Fire. This method brings an earlier effect and curative effects show more quickly. Li's experience is consistent with the statistic result of Syndrome Differentiation and signs in treating sterility at home in recent 10 years and with the experience "Don't Forget to Treat Blood Stasis" of the medical workers of all the dynasties of China. Therefore, promoting blood circulation and removing Blood Stasis should be popularized as an important principle of treatment of sterility. Restoring the Kidney and promoting the circulation of Blood should be both stressed, which is better than solely strengthening the Kidney.

Regulating and Replenishing the Spleen and Stomach
　The Spleen and Stomach are the source of acquired substance and the places where Qi and Blood are generated, and are what Five Zang and Six Fu Organs, limbs and skeleton rely on for nourishment. If the Spleen and Stomach are healthy and prosperous and foodstuff is profuse, then, Qi and Blood will be prosperous, from which Vital Essence and Energy are supplied. If the Spleen and Stomach are weak or poorly regulated, then, they are weak as well in food digestion, absorption and nutrient transportation; therefore, it is hard to form refined nutritious substances, and the Kidney has nothing to store, and there will be no essential sub-

stances for reproduction.

What's more, because of dysfunction of the Spleen's absorption of watery fluid, water runs wild until it reaches the Lower Jiao and Kidney Yang is checked and reproduction is impossible. Therefore, regulating and nourishing the Spleen and Stomach should also be a commonly used method for curing sterility. The commonly used drugs that tonify Qi and strengthen the Spleen, and regulate the Spleen and Stomach include ginseng (Radix Ginseng), dangshen (Radix Codonopsis Pilosulae), white atractylodes rhizome (Rhizoma Atractylodis Macrocephalae), poria (Poria), Chinese yam (Rhizoma Dioscoreae), licorice (Radix Glycyrrhizae), Chinese-date (Fructus Ziziphi Jujubae), etc. The commonly used prescriptions are Si Junzi Tang (Decoction of Four Noble Drugs) and Shenling Baifu San (Powder of Ginseng, Poria, and Bighead Atractylodes), etc. For the cases complicated by Spleen Deficiency, the following drugs are usually used: Tangerine peel (Pericarpium Citri Reticulatae), pinellia tuber (Rhizoma Pinelliae), amomum fruit Fructus Amomi), chicken's gizzard-skin (Endothelium Corneum Gigeriae Galli), parched germinated barley (Fructus Hordei Germinatus) and parched hawthorn fruit (Fructus Crataegi), etc. The prescriptions are Xiang Sha Liu Junzi Tang (Decoction of Costus and Amomum with Six Noble Ingredients), etc. What attention should be paid to when clinically the drugs are chosen in accordance with the method of regulating and tonifying the Spleen and Stomach is that drugs for tonifying should not be too greasy; drugs for warming the Spleen should not be too hot and dry; and the drugs for checking should be especially avoided in order not to damage Qi in the Middle Jiao and affect the function of digestion, absorption, and nutrients transportation.

Regulating Coordination between the Heart and the Kidney

Normally, Heart Yang goes down to warm Kidney Yin, and Kidney Yin goes up to nourish Heart Yang. When they are balanced, the normal physiological coordination between the Heart and the Kidney is maintained. If Kidney Yin is deficient, and only Heart Fire is excessive or Heart Fire reaches up but not coordinates down with the Kidney, then, Heart Yang and the Kidney Yin can not be assisted. This is breakdown of the normal physiological coordination between the Heart and the Kidney, marked clinically by spermatorrhea, premature ejaculation, etc. It is appropriate to use method of restoring normal coordination between the Heart and the Kidney. To use this method, it mainly uses the drugs aiming at the treatment of the Heart and the Kidney, such as the drugs that nourish the Kidney like dried rehmannia root (Radix Rehmanniae), dogwood fruit (Fructus Corni), lucid asparagus root (Radix Asparagi), wolfberry fruit (Fructus Lycii), and the drugs that clear up Fire like coptis root (Rhizoma Coptidis), capejasmine (Fructus Gardeniae), lotus plumule (Plumula Nelumbinis), lophatherum (Herba Lopatheri); mind-easing and sedative drugs like ginseng (Radix Ginseng), poria with hostwood (Poria cum Ligno Hospite), polygla root (Radix Polygalae) and longan aril (Arillus Longan). The commonly used prescription is Jiaotai Wan (Bolus for Easing Mental Stress and Restoring Coordination between the Heart and the Kidney.

Removing Toxicity to Increase Spermia
This method refers to increasing the number of, and improving the quality of spermia by clearing Heat and removing Toxins. It is referred to the patients with spermacrasia, low rate of sperm motility and asthenospermia due to accumulation and obstruction of Damp Heat in the Lower Jiao, such as sterility caused by prostatitis, seminal vesiculitis and epididymitis.

The symptoms and signs of the disease include dark urine, stabbing and itching urethra, burning sensation during urination, stranguria, uncomfortable feeling in perineum, sharply decrease in lecithin corpusole of succus prostaticus, pus cells and erythrocytes, etc., and sperm count decreased, sperm activity reduced, pyocyte cells, white cells and erythrocytes in seminal fluid determination. Because the disease is caused by accumulation and obstruction of Damp Heat inside the uterus, it is appropriate to use the method of reducing Heat and causing diuresis, removing Toxins and increasing sperm count and improving sperm quality. The following drugs are commonly used: Honeysuckle flower (Flos Lonicerae), forsythia fruit (Fructus Forsythiae), dandelion herb (Herba Taraxaci), patrinia (Herba Patriniae), oldenlandia (Herba Hydyotis Diffusae), wolly yam (Rhizoma Dioscoreae Septemlobae), coix seed (Semen Coicis), rhizome of wind-weed (Rhizoma Anemarrhenae), phellodendron bark (Cortex Phellodendri), gentian root (Radix Gentianae), dried rehmannia root (Radix Rehmanniae), moutan bark (Cortex Moutan Radicis), red peony root (Radix Paeoniae Rubra), etc. The prescriptions commonly used include Wuwei Xiaodou Yin (Decoction of Five Ingredients for Removing Toxins), Zhibo Dihuang Tang (Decoction of Anemarrhena, Phellodendron and Rehmannia) and Longdan Xiegan Wan (Bolus of Gentiana for Purging the Liver Fire). After the application of the above drugs, clearing away of Damp Heat and removing of pathogenic Toxins and improving of seminal fluid are taking place concurrently.

Consolidating the Kidney to Control Seminal Emission
Qi, Blood, Vital Essence and Energy and body fluids are the refined nutrients to nourish the human body. Excess and Deficiency, prosperity and decline go around again and again. If they are excessively consumed, the normal activities of life will break down. It is appropriate to use the method of reinforcing the Kidney and controlling nocturnal emission, which is referred to spermatorrhea, premature ejaculation caused by Kidney Deficiency, which makes it unable to store reproductive Essence and foodstuff, and by the dysfunction of the Gate of Life. The actual application of the method should be based on the clinical symptoms and signs of Deficiency of Kidney Yin or Deficiency of Kidney Yang to nourish and reinforce Kidney Yin or to warm and strengthen Kidney Yang together with such drugs that reinforce the Kidney and control nocturnal emission as dragon's bone (Os Draconis Fossilia Ossis), oyster shell (Concha Ostreae), cherokee rose-hip (Fructus Rosae Laevigatae), gordon euryale seed (Semen Euryales), raspberry (Fructus Rubi),

40

flatstem milkvetch seed (Semen Astragali Complanati), dogwood fruit (Fructus Corni), mantis egg-case (Ootheca Mantidis), etc. The prescription commonly used is Jinsuo Gujing Wan (Golden Lock Bolus for Checking Spermatorrhea).

The above mentioned methods should be used simply or combined comprehensively according to the condition of the individual patient. Clinically, a combined method of promoting the circulation of Blood, clearing Heat, and tonifying can bring better results in treating the comparatively complicated cases of sterility.

Treatment by Differentiating the Conditions of Seminal Fluid

Better curative results can be obtained to treat cases of sterility, caused by seminal fluid abnormality, which is the main proof of differentiation, in accordance with the general clinical manifestations.

Seminal fluid is made up by succus prostaticus, seminal vesicle fluid, epididymis fluid, bulbourethral gland fluid, and paraurethral Gueris's glands fluid. According to Yin and Yang theory, that Vital Essence and Energy which is natured Fire belongs to Yang; that seminal fluid, which is water-natured belongs to Yin; seminal fluid is considered to be Yin in Yang and spermia are considered to be Yang in Yin. Spermia themselves can be divided into two aspects: The sperm-Yin and and the sperm-Yang. The body of sperm is Yin in Yang. Sperm survival rate and sperm activity are Yang in Yang. According to theory that Yang resolves Qi and Yin, the number of spermia depends on Excess or Deficiency of Kidney Yin, the sperm activity depends on the prosperity or decline of Kidney Yang. Therefore, to treat azoospermia, it is mainly to reinforce Kidney Yin, to treat low sperm survival rate and poor sperm activity, invigorating Kidney Yang should be the main thing. Also, because Yin and Yang rely on each other and restrain each other, very often, Deficiency of Yin affects Yang, and excessive consumption of Yang af-

41

fects Yin with a manifestation of Deficiency of both Yin and Yang, i.e. azoospermia accompanied by low sperm survival rate, poor sperm activity. Then reinforcing both Yin and Yang are needed. In sum, to treat cases of sterility caused by abnormality of seminal fluid, treatment by differentiation of seminal fluid should be the main thing. However, it will bring better results if combined with treatment based on Syndrome Differentiation.

Treatment by Differentiating Constitutional Types

Treatment based on differentiation of individual conditions means that suitable method of treatment is worked out through correctly distinguishing the characteristics of each constitution in accordance with specific characteristics of different constitutions, i.e. types of constitution. Because of the differences in congenital Essence of life, acquired nourishment, living environment, and surroundings, and living habits, there must be great differences among individuals in constitution. These differences will make different types of physique. To carefully distinguish the differences in physique among the individuals will be helpful to make up the shortcomings in Syndrome Differentiation. What's more, many patients have no syndromes for differentiation. Treatment depends on differentiation of constitutional conditions.

The commonly seen Syndromes include Deficiency of Kidney Yang, Deficiency of Kidney Yin which produce Deficiency Heat, Deficiency of both Qi and Blood, Blood Stasis and Damp Heat in the Lower Jiao, etc. Clinically, different ways of treatment are applied according to Syndrome Differentiation. To find out the type of constitution has practical significance in correctly using drugs clinically, and avoiding using drugs wrongly. For example, for constitution of Kidney Yin, the following drugs that aim at warming should not be used, or used with caution: Aconite root (Radix Aconiti Praeparata), cinnamon bark (Cortex Cinnamoni), curculigo

42

rhizome (Rhizoma Curculiginis), epimedium (Herba Epimedii), pilose deer horn (Cornu Cervi Pantotrichum), psoralea fruit (Fructus Psoraleae), etc. For constitution of Deficiency of Kidney Yang, such drugs as rhizome of windweed (Rhizoma Anemarrhenae), phellodendron bark (Cortex Phellodendri), gentian root (Radix Gentianae), and the drugs, bitter in taste and cold in nature, that clear Heat and remove Toxins should not be used or used with caution.

In sum, differentiation of constitution, in the diagnosis of sterility, has certain significance of guidance in enriching and replenishing contents of differentiation of symptoms and signs, determining etiopathogenesis, and appropriately selecting and using prescriptions and drugs.

The Natures and Tastes of the Herbal Drugs and the Selection of Channel Tropism

Herbal drugs have certain natures and tastes which are important signs of drug functions and characters. Four natures refers to the cold, hot, warm and cool properties of a drug, among which drugs of hot and warm nature, and drugs of cold and cool nature are of opposite properties. A warm-natured drug and hot-natured drug have common characters, so do a cold-natured drug and a cool-natured drug. For instance, the warm and hot-natured drugs are different in degree and so are cool and cold-natured drugs besides their common properties.

Five tastes refer to pungent, sweet, sour, bitter and salty. Five tastes are also the flavors of drugs which are related to their functions, each of which has different effects. Because every drug has its own natures and tastes, the two aspects should be considered in combination. A drug can be used correctly if only a doctor learns and masters the whole properties and characteristics, and the specific differences of the drugs with the same natures and tastes. Channel tropism refers to a drug's selective therapeutic effects on a certain part of the body, i. e., a drug mainly exerts its effect on a

43

certain channel or channels. The channel tropism theory should be associated with theories of the four natures and five tastes so that it can play its clinical role to a larger degree.

The success in the treatment of sterility is closely related to the selection of four natures, five tastes and channel tropism of herbal drugs. Sperma abnormality in sterility is mainly manifested as azoospermia, low sperm survival rate and poor sperm activity. According to theory "Kidney Yang produces vital energy, and Kidney Yin helps the formation of the sperm body," azoospermia is mainly because of Deficiency of Kidney Yin. The principle of the treatment should be to invigorate the Kidney to enrich spermia. The drugs, sweet in taste and neutral in nature and invigorating the Kidney Channel, should be selected, such as wolfberry fruit, prepared siberian solomonseal rhizome, etc. Low sperm survival rate, poor sperm activity are mainly due to Deficiency of Kidney Yang. The treatment principle is to warm and restore Kidney Yang. The drugs, pungent in taste and warm in nature and invigorating the Kidney Channel, should be selected, such as morinda root (Radix Morindae Officinalis), epimedium (Herba Epimedii), etc. Also, according to the principle of treating Yin to treat Yang and treating Yang to treat Yin, replenishing both Yin and Yang should be paid special attention, i. e., according to Deficiency of one side, properly invigorating the other side will very often bring better results. Besides, while restoring the Kidney, nourishing Qi and Blood will further improve curative results.

In sterile cases, another case with sperma abnormality is sperm non-liquefaction. This disease is mostly caused by impairment and Deficiency of Kidney Yin. Body fluids are burned by Heat, which leads to sticky sperma, and even non-liquefaction. The disease may also be caused by Damp Heat, Blood Stasis and Phlegm obstruction. In order to treat the disease, the drugs, cold and cool in nature or drugs that promote Blood circulation and remove Blood Stasis, Damp Heat and Phlegm, are often used. The protracted cases which are manifested by azoospermia, low sperm survival rate, poor sperm activity complicated with non-liquefying sperma, are generally treated by the drugs that increase sperm count, and rate of sperm motility and improve sperm activity, then the problem of non-liquefaction of sperma can be solved. However, the course of treatment is much longer than usual and the patients can not bear it sometimes. To use the drugs warm and hot in nature too much and too long a time sometimes worsens the degree of sperm non-liquefaction. On the other hand, if treating sperma non-liquefaction first, then because of using the drugs cold and cool in nature too long, or because of poor tolerance of the patient to the drugs cold and cool in nature, the sperm quality will go worse further, or it will result in sexual hypofunction. To solve this hard problem, a method of treating the disease with the drugs both cold and warm in nature, i. e., for the patient whose sperm weight is light with mediate abnormality complicated with sperm non-liquefaction, drugs warm and hot in nature and drugs cold and cool in nature are used at the same time, but drugs warm in nature and invigorating Kidney Yin should be sweet in taste and neutral or slightly warm in nature should not be too hot, drugs cold and cool in nature should be cool sweet in taste but should not be too cold; and use drugs sweet in taste and cold in nature, but not the drugs bitter in taste and cold in nature. Using the drugs bitter in taste and cold in nature in great quantity can directly affect the Gate of Life and result in the decrease of sperm quality.

In treating sterility, besides mastering four natures and five tastes of herbal drugs, attention should also be given to channel tropism. The commonly used herbal drugs mostly invigorate the Liver Channel and the Kidney Channel. This shows that the Liver and the Kidney directly influence reproductive function. While the Kidney is replenished, the Spleen is also reinforced. Because congenital Essence depends on the replenishing of the acquired Essence, drugs that tonify the Spleen should be used to enrich the source of acquired Essence. To sum up, during the treatment, reinforcing Deficiency, but not removing Excess should be born in mind. The drugs chosen should not be too dry and greasy to avoid damaging Yin while Yang is tonified, and to avoid

45

consuming Yang excessively while Yin is nourished. The drugs should not be too cold in nature and too bitter in taste to avoid the decline of Fire from the Gate of Life which leads to Cold Uterus. If the natures of the drugs are well selected, and the drugs are well prescribed, and the doses are well made, the drugs are taken according to the requirement, good result can be resulted in. The sperm quality is improved and sperm liquefaction is normal, too. For the patients with azoospermia, dead spermia and severely poor sperm activity, in principle, first of all, replenishing the Kidney to nourish Blood is needed. After sperm quality is improved, try to solve the problem sperm non-liquefaction. When actually using the drugs, if the patients had the problem of non-liquefaction or the inclination of it in the past, a doctor should slightly improve sperm quality, avoid using or use with caution such drugs warm and hot in nature as aconite root (Radix Aconiti Praeparata), cinnamon bark (Cortex Cinnamoni), fenugreek seed (Semen Trigonellae), curculigo rhizome (Rhizoma Curculiginis), psoralea fruit (Fructus Psoraleae), etc. The dose of epimedium (Herba Epimedii) is generally under 15g. On condition that the sperm quality is low, the purpose is to treat sperm non-liquefaction, a doctor should avoid using or use wind-weed rhizome (Rhizoma Anemarrhenae), phellodendron bark (Cortex Phellodendri), capejasmine (Fructus Gardeniae), scutellaria (Radix Scutellariae), gentian root (Radix Gentianae), and such Heat and Toxins removing drugs bitter in taste and cold in nature. Especially, a doctor should avoid using these drugs in great quantity and for a long time.

Other Therapeutic Methods

Acupuncture Therapy
Acupuncture therapy has positive curative effects in treating sperm abnormality and sexual dysfunction. Most cases of sperm abnormality are caused by Kidney Deficiency, and differentiated to be Deficiency of Kidney Essence, and decline of Fire from the Gate of Life. It is closely related to the

Du Channel and the Ren Channel. Ginger (Rhizoma Zingiberis Recens) and argyi leaf (Folium Artemisiae Argyi), warm in nature, can replenish Kidney Essence and strength-·en Fire from the Gate of Life. So, better curative results can be obtained by using acupuncture combined with ginger moxibustion. The commonly used acupuncture points include Dahe (KID 12), Qugu (REN 2), Sanyinjiao (SP 6), Baliao, Shenshu (BL 23), etc. The acupoints for ginger moxibustion include Guanyuan (REN 4), Zhongji (REN 3), and Mingmen (DU 4), etc. According to actual conditions, several supplementary points Taixi (KID 3), Zhaohai (KID 6) are selected to regulate and replenish Kidney Qi to reinforce congenital Essence. Qihaishu (BL 24), Guanyuan (REN 4) are selected to strengthen Qi of the Kidney Yang, and thus Kidney Qi is replenished. Sanyinjiao (SP 6), Diji (SP 8), Yinlingquan (SP 9) are selected to regulate and tonify Qi of Sanyin Channel, and nourish and reinforce the acquired Essence together with Shenshu (BL 23), Zhishi (BL 52), Fuliu (KID 7) being selected so that Kidney Qi can circulate and be transported. The final aims will be realized: Nourishing and replenishing Kidney Yin, warming and strengthening Kidney Yang, transporting Kidney Qi, increasing sperm count, and improving sperm activity. Better medical results were gained in treating sperma abnormality by point-injection therapy in placenta tissue fluid and catgut implantation at acupoints. The method is carried out as stated in the following: Selected are Sanyinjiao (SP 6), Zusanli (ST 36), Guanyuan (REN 4), Zhongji (REN 3), Qihaishu (BL 24), and 2-4ml of placenta tissue fluid is injected to each point and one time every other day. The above acupoints are applied alternately. Or used is a styled need together with No. 0 surgical catgut, about 1-2cm to push down for about 1 *cun* at Sanyinjiao (SP 6), and buried there is the catgut after De Qi (De Qi refers to the needling sensation which follows insertion, a hollow sensation, initially experienced by the practitioner, that gradually develops into a tight and heavy feeling upon twiling and vertical lifting and thrusting). This is done one time monthly. After the treatment described above, the condition of the disease is improved to a certain degree.

Acupuncture therapy shows remarkable curative effects in treating dysfunctional impotence. The acupoints selected are Guanyuan (REN 4), Qihaishu (BL 24), Zhongji (REN 3) and Qugu (REN 2) of the Ren Channel; Shenshu (BL 23) and Ciliao (BL 32) of the Bladder Channel; Sanyinjiao (SP 6) and other impotance acupoints of the Spleen Channel. Impotence has three locations: The first one is located at 2.5 *cun* up Shenshu (BL 23), 1 *cun* outward the Du Channel; the second is located at the hollow between Yaoshu (DU 2) and Changqing (DU 1); the third one refers to a group of acupoints: On the line from navel (Shenque, REN 8) to pubis (Qugu, REN 2), one acupoint is located at upper 1/3 of the line, and another at middle 1/3 of the line, and the last at lower 1/3 of the line. At the middle acupoint, 1 *cun* on both sides, two other acupoints are located. The 5 acupoints together are called impotence acupoint. The manipulation stresses that it is finest that the sensation of Ren Channel radiates to penis. The manners of needling are from needling and ginger moxibustion to point-injection and catgut implantation at acupoint. It was reported that the total effective rate was 70-90%. According to "A Clinical Observation of 41 Cases of Impotence Treated With Acupuncture Therapy," the following acupoints were selected: Shenshu (BL 23), Mingmen (DU 4), Sanyinjiao (SP 6), Zusanli (ST 36), Neiguan (PC 6), Guanyuan (REN 4), Zhaohai (KID 6), Yinlingquan (SP 9), Qihaishu (BL 24) and Shenmen (HT 7). Twirling reinforcing method was applied to them all together with the alternative application of moxa cone for moxibustion. 23 of 41 cases were cured and 8 of them obtained effect. The whole effective rate was 87.8% (Li Shijie, 1989).

To treat dysfunctional aspermtism, it is regarded as a main thing to soothe the Liver to relieve stagnation of Liver Qi. Selected are Zuwuli (LIV 10) of the Liver Channel of Foot Jueyin (to regulate the flow of Liver Qi and remove Blood Stasis), Qugu (REN 2) (the crossing point of the Ren Channel and the Liver Channel of Foot Jueyin), Zuwuli (LIV 10). Use the method of lifting and thrusting and twirling the needle and the needling sensation spreads to perineum.

48

Twirling method is applied to Qugu (REN 2). Manipulation is stopped after the lower abdomen and vulva area feel sore, numbness and distension. The needles are retained there for 30 minutes, and therapy is carried out one time daily. 10 times make one course of treatment. In recent years, there have been researches about aspermatism treated through acupuncture together with digital pressuren points. The following points are selected: Dahe (KID 12), Zhongji (REN 3), Ligou (LIV 5), Taichong (LIV 3), Sanyinjiao (SP 6) and Yonquan (KID 1). These points are used alternately, one time daily. The points in the legs are needled with strong stimulation. 60 cases were treated with this method, among whom, 55 were cured, with a curative rate of 91.6% (Shui Houdi, 1990). Also, according to a report of 110 cases of aspermatism treated through acupuncture, the following points were selected: Qugu (REN 2) (acupunctured), Yinlian (LIV 11) (acupunctured) and Dadun (LIV 1) (moxibusted for 5 minutes each time). For those also with weakness, poor appetite and dyschesia, Zusanli (ST 36) was added. For the cases also with wakeful sleep, Baihui (DU 20) and Neiguan (PC 6) were added. For the cases also with impotence, Ciliao (BL 32) was added and Shenque (REN 8) was moxibusted. The treatment was carried out one time every 2-3 days, and 10 times accounted for one course of treatment. The needling sensation should be that at Qugu (REN 2), electrical sensation appears and that sensation radiates to bottom area of urethra and at Yinlian (LIV 11), sore, distending and heavy feelings occur. 94 of them were able to ejaculate with a curative rate of 85.5% (Zhang Qin, 1984).

Most cases with spermatorrhea were caused by consumption of Essence and Blood, Yin Deficiency involving Yang, Excess Fire produced by Yin Deficiency—all of this interferes with the sperm system. According to a clinical report of 60 cases with spermatorrhea treated through the application of Huiyin (REN 1) and Baihui (DU 20) as master acupoints. A large-gauge rounded sharp needle (with the tip being ground blunt) was pushed against but not into Huiyin (REN 1) handle-scrapping method was used for 3-5 minutes (150-200 times). In sitting position, needling first then moxibustion was applied to Baihui (DU 20). The needling was inserted down about 1-1.5 *cun* by lifting and thrusting and twirling the needle over 2-3 minutes. Then the needle was retained there over 10 minutes, and moxibustion was applied for 2-3 minutes. The treatment was carried out one time daily, and 10 times accounted for one course of treatment. Among the 60 cases treated, 54 were cured (Wang Zhongmin, 1990).

Dietary Therapy

Dietary therapy, having certain supplementary values in the treatment of sterility, is divided into two types: Type of animal visceras, type of vegetables and fruits.

Type of animal visceras include animal kidneys and testes. The former exert their effects on the Kidney Channel and can replenish Kidney Qi, enrich Essence, remove obstruction in bladder, and treat weakness and exhaustion. The latter can strongly restore the Kidney and replenish spermia (including sheep's and dog's penis and testicles). Dog's meat exerts its effects on the Stomach channel and the Kidney Channel, ease five organs and replenish Kidney Yang, tonify the Stomach and the Kidney, warms lumbar area to reduce soreness, invigorates five kinds of strain and seven kinds of impairment to strengthen the bady. Sparrow reinforces the Kidney and replenishes Yang, but its meat is hot in nature, so those with Interior Heat should avoid eating it. Holothurian reinforces the Kidney and Essence, nourishes Blood and moist Dryness, remove Damp to induce diuresis. Shrimp meat, warm in nature, restores the Kidney and replenishes Essence. Dried human placenta can exert its effects on the Liver Channel, the Spleen Channel and the Kidney Channel—nourishing the Kidney and replenishing Essence, promoting Qi and nourishing Blood. It is a great tonic which has better curative results in the treatment of a sterile patient with problem of azoospermia due to insufficiency of Essence.

Vegetables and fruits, Chinese chives seed, having the function of tonifying the Liver and the Kidney, reinforcing waist and knees and replenishing Yang, are commonly used to treat impotence. Chinese yam, sweet in taste and neutral in nature, replenishes the Spleen and benefits the Stomach, invigorates the Kidney and benefits the Lung is effective for cases with abnormal seminal fluids. The Peach kernel, sweet in taste and warm in nature, can astringe the Lung and reinforce the Kidney. It has curative effects on sterility caused by sperma abnormality.

Chapter Three
Treatment of
Common Diseases

Impotence

Impotence, a male sexual disorder, refers to that a male has sexuality, but erection of penis is hard, or though erection is possible, the penis is not hard enough, and thus it is impossible to perform sexual activities. Most of impotence cases result from relaxed penis caused by impairment and Deficiency of Kidney Essence, stagnation of Liver Qi, Damp Heat in the Liver and the Gallbladder, etc. It is one of the common male sexual disorders, and is one of the reasons of sterility.

In *Complete Works of Zhang Jingyue* (*Jing Yue Quan Shu*), Zhang Jingyue (Ming Dynasty) was the first to name the sexual disorder as impotence, and said, "Male's impotence is mostly caused by decline of Fire from the Gate of Life, Deficiency Cold of Vital Essence and Energy; or by excessive exhaustion of seven emotions (joy, anger, melancholy, anxiety, grief, fear and terror) which impairs Qi to form Yang ··· also by Damp Heat—all this leads to relaxed penis and thus impotence results from it." "Excessive work and mental depression will also lead to impotence." "If fear and terror can not be relieved, impotence will also be resulted in ··· while Yang is prosperous, fear and terror attack, then impotence happens." According to Zhang's statements, the etiopathogenesis of the disease is of decline of Fire from the Gate of Life, stagnation of Liver Qi, Damp Heat and sudden fear and terror, etc. In treatment, it is suggested to warm and reinforce the Gate of Life, to soothe the Liver to

52

regulate stagnation of Liver Qi, to normalize functioning of the Gallbladder by purging Liver Fire, replenishing the Kidney and relieving mental stress.

Etiology and Pathogenesis
• *Stagnation of Liver Qi*

Emotional stress and stagnated anger impair the Liver, so it results in stagnation of Liver Qi, thus Liver Qi is unable to flow smoothly and dysfunction of penis thus happens. Thus impotence occurs. *Sharp Explanations to the Causes of Miscellaneous Diseases* (*Za Bing Yuan Liu Xi Zhu*) says, "Again, some people suffer from mental stress, and the depression impairs the Liver. Then, Liver Qi can not circulate smoothly. As a result, impotence happens." Flaccidity of external genitals means impotence. The Liver governs the penis and links to external genitals. Because stagnated anger impairs the Liver, which therefore loses smooth circulation of Liver Qi; then, the dysfunction of the external genitals will be resulted in because of the flaccidity.

• *Decline of Fire from the Gate of Life*

The Kidney is the source of congenital Essence, the origin of Kidney Yang and Yin, Five Zang Organs, and the place for primary Yin and Yang. Congenital defect or excessive sexual activities will lead to Deficiency of Kidney Essence, which in turn leads to Kidney Yang syndrome. As a result, decline of Fire from the Gate of Life, Deficiency Cold of Vital Essence and Energy, male sexuality being not active—all this leads to impotence. As *Complete Works of Zhang Jinyue* (*Jing Yue Quan Shu*) holds, "Male's impotence is mostly caused by decline of Fire from the Gate of Life, and Deficiency Cold of Vital Essence and Energy." "Seven or eight out of 10 cases of impotence are caused by decline of Fire." *Collection of Additional Works on Diagnosis and Treatment* (*Zheng Zhi Hui Bu*) says, "The reason that excessive sexual activities and flaccidity of penis lead to impotence is of decline of Fire from the Gate of Life, just as in winter, all kinds of the flowers will wither and fall."

• *Damp Heat of the Liver and the Gallbladder*

Excessive consumption of the fat food sweet in taste, or

53

excessive drinking, or the attack of pathogenic Damp Heat will stagnate in the Middle Jiao. The stagnated Fire will burn the Liver and the Gallbladder, and penis is impaired; therefore, flaccidity of penis appears and impotence happens. Or Damp Heat runs downward, and will soak the Liver and the Kidney which therefore are not able to control the external genitals, and flaccidity of penis results from it, and impotence happens. In *Channels and Tendons*, a chapter of *Miraculous Pivot* (*Ling Shu·Jingjin*), it says, "Heat results in flaccidity of tendons, and it in turn results in impotence."

• *Deficiency of Both the Heart and the Spleen*

Excessive worries will impair the Heart and the Spleen, so Deficiency of both Qi and Blood appears; therefore, male sexuality can not be encouraged and as time passes, impotence happens. As is said in *On Impotence*, a chapter of *Complete Works of Zhang Jingyue* (*Jing Yue Quan Shu*), "Excessive worries will probably cause impotence. Because the Yangming Channel governs confluence of tendons··· if a patient worries excessively, it will depress and impair the Heart and the Spleen. Then, the pathogenic factors will spread to the Yangming Channel and the Chong Channel, and this will lead to Deficiency of Qi and Blood. This in turn discourages the male sexuality."

• *Impairment of the Kidney due to Fear and Terror*

Mental fear and terror due to unexpectation, or sudden attack of fear and terror in the course of sexual intercourse lead to palpitation, timidness, lassitude, low male sexuality. Thus impotence is caused. Zhang Jingyue says, "While Yang is prosperous, sudden attack of fear and terror will cause Yang duct to be flaccid immediately. This is also the reason of impotence." *Explanations of Phenomena of Yin and Yang*, a chapter of *Plain Questions* (*Su Wen·Yin Yang Yin Xiang Da Lun*), says, "Terror impairs the Kidney." *On Complete Cases of Pain*, a chapter of *Plain Questions*, too says, "Terror leads to no seminal fluid." Terror disturbs the normal flow of Qi and internalr activities. Therefore, restlessness will be caused. Terror causes Qi to go downward and impairs Kidney Qi. The impairment and Deficiency of Kidney Qi cause poor nourishment to urogenital region, and

54

impotence is caused finally.

Contemporary medical workers think that Stomach Qi is the source for sexual life. Tendons are gathered to the Yangming Channel which moist tendons in turn. The Yangming Channel is selected to treat flaccidity and impotence is included, as well. The Stomach is the Sea of five Zang Organ and six Fu Organs. The living things live on food which provides foodstuff, from which vital energy comes. If the Spleen and the Stomach suffer from diseases, it will affect the other organs; or if other organs suffer from diseases, it will affect the Spleen and the Stomach. Then, male sexual disorder will be caused. Therefore, during the treatment of impotence, Spleen Qi and Stomach Qi should be taken care. Normal functioning of the Spleen and the Stomach will lead to active penis (Xu Fusong, 1990).

Main Points of Diagnosis

The important bases in the diagnosis of this male disease are: Flaccidity of genitals, astysia, or not-hard-enough erection, which disturb normal sexual activities. When diagnosing, what should be differentiated clearly is the location of the affected area. For the cases with stagnation of Liver Qi, the Liver is the affected area; for the cases of decline of Fire from the Gate of Life, the Kidney; for the cases with Damp Heat in the Liver and Gallbladder, the Liver and the Spleen; for the cases of Deficiency of both the Heart and the Spleen, the Heart and the Spleen; for the cases with impaired the Kidney due to fear and terror, the Heart and the Kidney. Next, what should be differentiated clearly is whether the disease is Cold, Heat, Deficiency or Excess. Stagnation of Liver Qi, Damp Heat in the Gallbladder belong to Excess Syndrome and Heat Syndromes; decline of Fire from the Gate of Life, Deficiency of both the Heart and the Spleen belong to Deficiency Syndrome and Cold Syndromes. Then, according to individual symptoms and signs and their tongue conditions, the syndromes are differentiated and categorized. In addition, when diagnosing this disease, try to distinguish it with premature ejaculation which refers to that before or at the beginning of sexual intercourse, the penis can erect, but because of too-early ejaculation, penis becomes relaxed and further sexual intercourse fails. Impotence disease here refers to astysia or not-hard-enough erection which leads to the failure of sexual intercourse while the male wants to.

Treatment Based on Syndrome Differentiation

To treat impotence, principles of treatment should be set up according to different etiopathogenesis and main points of Syndrome Differentiation. For the cases with stagnation of Liver Qi, soothing the Liver and regulating the flow of Qi are considered to be the main thing; for the cases with decline of Fire from the Gate of Life, warming and replenishing Kidney Yang; for the cases with Damp Heat in the Gallbladder, clearing Heat and promoting diuresis; for the cases with Deficiency of both the Heart and the Spleen, tonifying and benefiting the Heart and the Spleen; for the cases with impaired the Kidney due to fear and terror, tranquilizing and reliving mental stress.

• *Stagnation of Liver Qi*

Main Symptoms and Signs: No male sexuality, mental depression, fullness in the chest and hypochondrium, restlessness and irritability, susceptible to sigh, pale and red tongue, thin white tongue coating, and stringy pulse.

Analysis of the Symptoms and Signs: The Liver stores Blood and governs tendons, and the Liver Channel links to sexual genitals. The stagnation of Liver Qi leads to flaccidity of the external genitals. The stagnation of Liver Qi results in disorder of Liver Qi, and in turn results in disturbance of visceral function. This is the reason of depressed mental state, fullness in the chest and hypochondrium; Fire-transmission due to stagnation of Liver Qi causes restlessness and irritability; unsmoothness of the flow of Liver Qi results in susceptibility to sigh. Tongue and pulse conditions indicate stagnation of Liver Qi.

Treatment Principles: Soothing the Liver and promoting the flow of Liver Qi; removing obstruction in the channels to boost the flaccid genitals.

Prescription: Sini San Jia Wugong Xiangfu (Powder for

56

Treating Cold Limbs supplemented with Centipede and Cyperus Tuber)

Bupleurum root (Radix Bupleuri) 9g, bitter orange (Fructus Aurantii) 9g, white peony root (Radix Paeoniae) 9g, prepared licorice (Radix Glycyrrhizae Praeparata) 3g, centipedefern (Scolopendra) 2g and cyperus tuber (Rhizoma Cuperi) 9g. All the above drugs are decocted in water for oral administration, one dose per day.

Analysis of the Prescription: Bupleurum root (Radix Bupleuri) soothes the Liver and promotes the flow of Liver Qi. White peony root (Radix Paeoniae) softens the Liver and replenishes Yin. Bitter orange (Fructus Aurantii) relieves the depressed Liver, dispels the stagnation of Spleen Qi, regulates functional activities of the Middle Jiao. If used together with bupleurum root (Radix Bupleuri), bitter orange (Fructus Aurantii) can strengthen its function of soothing the Liver and promoting the flow of Liver Qi. Licorice (Radix Glycyrrhizae) coordinates the effects of all the drugs. If used along with white peony root (Radix Paeoniae), licorice (Radix Glycyrrhizae) can reduce acute pain. If Used together with cyperus tuber (Rhizoma Cuperi), licorice (Radix Glycyrrhizae) can strengthen the function of relieving the depressed Liver. Centipede exerts its effects in the Liver and removes obstruction in the Liver Channel. The whole prescription soothes the Liver and promotes Liver Qi circulation, removes obstruction in the channel, and braces up the flaccid genitals.

Modifications of the Prescription: For the cases of Fire-transmission due to stagnation of Liver Qi, moutan bark (Cortex Moutan Radicis) 9g and capejasmine (Fructus Gardeniae) 9g are added for clearing Heat from the Liver Channel; for the cases of Cold in the Liver Channel, evodia fruit (Fructus Evodiae) 6g, common fennel fruit (Fructus Foeniculi) 6g, cinnamon bark (Cortex Cinnamomi) 6g and lindera root (Radix Linderae) 9g are added.

• *Decline of Fire from the Gate of Life*

Main Symptoms and Signs: Inability to make penis erect, cold body and limbs, cold lower abdomen, cold genital area and glens penis, hyposexuality, thin and cold sperma, mental depression, soreness and weakness of waist and knees, dizziness and tinnitus, pale tongue with white coating, deep, thready, and feeble pulse.

Analysis of the Symptoms and Signs: Congenital defect, or excessive intercourse results in Deficiency of Kidney Essence. Yin can not supplement Yang and Yang aspect is not prosperous; therefore, flaccidity of external genitals is caused. Cold is Yin pathogen, and it easily impairs Yang Qi. Vegetarian dietary and Yang Deficiency, or the attack of pathogenic pathogenic Cold, or overeating cold and raw food will result in Yang Deficiency and Qi and breakdown of Qi activities. Therefore, it results in general cold, and cold limbs, lower abdomen, genital area, and glens penis. Deficiency of Kidney Qi results in excessive consumption of Kidney Essence. Therefore, sexuality is low and sperma is thin and cold. Excessive consumption of Kidney Essence leads to poor nourishment of the brain. Therefore, mental depression, dizziness, and tinnitus occur. Waist is the place where the Kidney is located, and knees are the collaterals of the Kidney. Deficiency of vital energy of waist and knees, pale tongue with white coating, deep thready and feeble pulse indicate decline of Fire from the Gate of Life.

Treatment Principles: Warming the Kidney to replenish Essence; invigorating Yang to cure flaccidity.

Prescription: Yougui Wan (Bolus for Reinforcing the Kidney Yang)

Aconite root (Radix Aconiti Praeparata) 6g, cinnamon bark (Cortex Cinnamomi) 6g, prepared rehmannia root (Radix Rehmanniae Praeparata) 15g, dogwood fruit (Fructus Corni) 9g, Chinese yam (Ehizoma Dioscoreae) 15g, wolfberry fruit (Fructus Lycii) 9g, dodder seed (Semen Cuscutae) 9g, antler glue (Colla Cornus Cervi) 9g (parched), Chinese angelica root (Radix Angelicae Sinensis) 9g and eucommia bark (Cortex Eucommiae) 9g. All the above drugs are decocted in water for oral administration, one dose per day.

Analysis of the Prescription: Aconite root (Radix Aconiti Praeparata), cinnamon bark (Cortex Cinnamomi) warm and reinforce Kidney Yang and relieve Cold. Prepared rehman-

58

nia root (Radix Rehmanniae Praeparata) sweet in taste warms and nourishes the Kidney to replenish Essence. Dogwood fruit (Fructus Corni) nourishes the Liver and the Kidney. Chinese yam (Ehizoma Dioscoreae) tonifies the Middle Jiao and invigorates the Spleen. Wolfberry fruit (Fructus Lycii) nourishes Liver Blood. Dodder seed (Semen Cuscutae) reinforces the Kidney and benefits Essence. Antler glue (Colla Cornus Cervi) warms the Kidney and replenishes Essence. Chinese angelica root (Radix Angelicae Sinensis) nourishes Blood and promotes the circulation of Blood. Eucommia bark (Cortex Eucommiae) tonifies the Liver and the Kidney and strengthens muscles and joints. The whole prescription warms and reinforces Kidney Yang, replenishes Essence and cures impotence.

• Damp Heat in the Gallbladder and the Liver

Main Symptoms and Signs: Penis unable to erect, or not hard enough, though it can erect; damp scrotum, distention and pain with dragging feeling, vexation, bitter taste, heavy body and limbs, scanty dark urine, red tongue with yellowish greasy coating, slippery rapid pulse.

Analysis of the Symptoms and Signs: Damp Heat in the Liver and Gallbladder gets stagnated and steams urogenital region, therefore, penis is unable to erect, or not hard enough though it can erect. Damp Heat going downward makes scrotum damp and causes dragging and distending pain. Hepatic Fire flames up, therefore, the mouth feels bitter and the patient feels vexed. Damp Heat troubles the whole body; therefore, heavy body and limbs are resulted in. Damp Heat going downward to the Bladder causes scanty dark urine. Tongue and pulse conditions indicate Damp Heat in the Liver and Gallbladder.

Treatment Principles: Purging the Liver of pathogenic Fire to normalize the functioning of the Gallbladder.

Prescription: Longdan Xiegan Tang (Decoction of Gentian for Purging Liver Fire)

Gentian root (Radix Gentianae) 9g, capejasmine fruit (Fructus Gardeniae) 9g, scutellarium root (Radix Scutellariae) 9g, bupleurum root (Radix Bupleuri) 9g, fiveleaf akebia stem (Caulis Akebiae) 6g, plantain seed (Semen Plantagi-

59

nis) (Wrapped) 9g, oriental water plantain (Rhizoma Alismatis) 9g, Chinese angelica root (Radix Angelicae Sinensis) 9g, dried rehmannia root (Radix Rehmanniae) 12g and licorice (Radix Glycyrrhizae) 6g. All the above drugs are decocted for oral administration, one dose per day.

Analysis of the Prescription: Scutellarium root (Radix Scutellariae), gentian root (Radix Gentianae), capejasmine fruit (Fructus Gardeniae) purge the Liver of the pathogenic Fire. Bupleurum root (Radix Bupleuri) soothes the Liver and promotes the flow of Liver Qi. Fiveleaf akebia stem (Caulis Akebiae), plantain seed (Semen Plantaginis), oriental water plantain (Rhizoma Alismatis) remove Damp Heat. Dried rehmannia root (Radix Rehmanniae), Chinese angelica root (Radix Angelicae Sinensis) nourishes Yin and Blood. Licorice (Radix Glycyrrhizae) coordinates the effects of various drugs. All the drugs used together not only purge and remove but also replenish and nourish—purging the Liver of the Excess Fire, removing Damp Heat from the Middle Jiao. If Liver Fire is purged, and Damp Heat are relieved, impotence is cured.

• *Deficiency of Both the Heart and the Spleen*

Main Symptoms and Signs: Feeble erection of the penis, tiredness and poor appetite, sallow complexion, wakeful sleep, amnesia, severe palpitation, loose stool, pale tongue with thin white coating, thready and weak pulse.

Analysis of the Symptoms and Signs: Depression impairs the Heart and the Spleen, and this affects the Yangming Channel and the Chong Channel. That surely results in Deficiency of the Sea of Qi and Blood from foodstuff. The impairment of Deficiency of Qi and Blood causes the urogenital region to lack moistening. So erection of penis is feeble. Deficiency of the Spleen causes Qi to decline and Blood to reduce. Therefore, the Heart has nothing for nourishment and sallow complexion, tiredness, poor appetite, loose stool all occur. Pale tongue with thin white tongue coating, and thready and feeble pulse are signs of Deficiency of Heart Qi and Spleen Qi.

Treatment Principles: Benefiting Qi and Replenishing Blood; invigorating the Spleen and nourishing the Heart.

60

Prescription: Guipi Tang (Decoction for Invigorating the Spleen)

Astragalus root (Radix Astragali Seu Hedysari) 30g, dangshen (Radix Codonopsis Pilosulae) 18g, Chinese angelica root (Radix Angelicae Sinensis) 9g, longan aril (Arillus Longan) 9g, bighead atractylodes rhizome (Rhizoma Atractylodis Macrocephalae) 9g, auklandia root (Radix Aucklandiae) 6g, poria (Poria) 9g, licorice (Radix Glycyrrhizae) 6g, fresh ginger (Rhizoma Zingiberis Recens) 3 pieces and 5 Chinese dates (Fructus Ziziphi Jujubae). All the above drugs are decocted in water for oral administration, one dose per day.

Analysis of the Prescription: Astragalus root (Radix Astragali Seu Hedysari), dangshen (Radix Codonopsis Pilosulae) replenish Qi and reinforce the Spleen. Chinese angelica root (Radix Angelicae Sinensis), longan aril (Arillus Longan) nourish Blood and regulate the nutrient metabolism. Bighead atractylodes rhizome (Rhizoma Atractylodis Macrocephalae), auklandia root (Radix Aucklandiae) invigorate the Spleen and regulate the flow of Qi. Poria (Poria), polygala root, and Chinese dates (Fructus Ziziphi Jujubae) tonify the Spleen and the Stomach to enrich digestion and transportation. Prosperous Qi leads to profuse Blood. The whole prescription reinforces the Spleen and nourishes the Heart, benefits Qi and cures flaccidity.

• *Impaired the Kidney due to Fear and Terror*

Main Symptoms and Signs: Penis unable to erect, or not hard enough though it erects; palpitations due to fright, dream-disturbed sleep, timidness and doubting mania, pale tongue with thin white coating, stringy and thready pulse.

Analysis of the Symptoms and Signs: Terror impairs the Heart and the Kidney, and also makes Qi go downward. As a result, urogenital region lacks nourishment. This is the reason of impotence or not-hard-enough erection. The the Gallbladder governs decision-making. Terror impairs motions, and so decision-making runs loose from control. This leads to doubting mania. The impaired Heart causes mental derangement. This is the reason of palpitations and susceptibility to fright, dream-disturbed sleep.

61

Treatment Principles: Reliving mental stress; reinforcing the Kidney to brace up flaccidity.

Prescription: Xuan Zhi Tang Jia Longgu, Muli, Wukong (Decoction for Dispelling Mental Stress supplemented with Dragon's Bone, Oyster Shell and Centipede)

Prepared rehmannia root (Radix Rehmanniae Praeparata) 12g, morinda root (Radix Morindae Officinalis) 9g, ginseng (Radix Ginseng) 6g, bighead atractylodes rhizome (Rhizoma Atractylodis Macrocephalae) 9g, Chinese angelica root (Radix Angelicae Sinensis) 9g, Chinese yam (Ehizoma Dioscoreae) 15g, poria (Poria) 9g, stir-fried Chinese date (Fructus Ziziphi Jujubae) seed 15g, polygala root (Radix Polygalae) 6g, bupleurum root (Radix Bupleuri) 9g, cimicifuga rhizome (Rhizoma Cimicifugae) 9g, dragon's bone (Os Draconis) 30g, oyster shell (Concha Ostreae) 30g and centipedes (Scolopendra) 2 pieces. All the above drugs are decocted in water for oral administration, one dose per day.

Analysis of the Prescription: Prepared rehmannia root (Radix Rehmanniae Praeparata) and morinda root (Radix Morindae Officinalis) nourish the Kidney and replenish Yang. Ginseng (Radix Ginseng), bighead atractylodes root, Chinese angelica root (Radix Angelicae Sinensis), Chinese yam (Ehizoma Dioscoreae) and poria (Poria) regulate the flow of Qi, and invigorate the Spleen and nourish Blood. Wild date seed, polygala root (Radix Polygalae), dragon's bone (Os Draconis) and oyster shell (Concha Ostreae) relieve mental stress. Bupleurum root (Radix Bupleuri) and cimicifuga rhizome (Rhizoma Cimicifugae) strengthen Yang to regulate the flow of Liver Qi. Centipede exerts its effects on the Liver, removing obstruction in the Liver Collaterals to cure impotence. The whole prescription invigorates the Kidney, nourishes the Heart, relieves mental stress and elevates the Spleen Yang and cures impotence.

Current Research
1. Research Institute of TCM Drugs of Shandong Province and Qilu Pharmaceutics Plant, Jinan, Shandong, have jointly worked out a Yang-invigorating drug: Xiongbao (Yang-Strengthening Capsules) Which was used clinically to 103

62

cases with erection disorder. The total effective rate was 83.
3%, among which the recent curative rate was 41.3%. 77
cases with sexual disorder were also treated whose total effective rate was 90.9%. The control group took Nan Bao
(Impotence-Curing Capsule). 30 Cases with erection disorder were treated in this group. The total effective rate was
46.7%, which was lower than that of the group taking Yang-Strengthening Capsule. Statistical processing showed $P < 0.01$. There were marked differences between the two groups.

Yang-Strengthening Capsule was worked out on the basis
of TCM theory, relating to TCM clinical prescriptions and
modern research achievements. The prescription includes
mainly epimedium (Herba Epimedii), dog's calculus (Calculus Canis), ram testes (Testis Caprae seu Ovis), Chinese
chives seed (Semen Allii Tuberosi), fresh water shrimp,
whose effective parts, processed into capsules, are extracted
by means of modern scientific methods. The drug is taken orally, 3 times per day, and 3-4 capsules each time (36 capsules/box). The drug is taken successively for one month
which accounted for one course of treatment.

Yang-Strengthening Capsule showed best effects on Syndrome of Deficiency of Kidney Yang and decline of Fire from
the Gate of Life. It is also effective for Syndrome of stagnation of Liver Qi, but not effective for Syndrome of Damp
Heat in the Liver and the Gallbladder. The drug also had
certain effect on the patients without symptoms.

Thin layer scanning was used to determine icariine content, the main effective element, and it was also found at the
same time that Yang-Strengthening Capsule contains 22
kinds of amino acids and 12 kinds of trace elements such as
iron, copper, zinc, manganese. This shows that Yang-Strengthening Capsule contains rich amino acids and many
kinds of inorganic elements necessary to human body. These
amino acids have the function of reinforcing and benefiting
body's physiological functions. That Yang-Strengthening
Capsule invigorates the Kidney, strengthens Yang, and
counteracts against aging is closely related to the many
kinds of trace elements in it. The acute and subacute toxic
experiments on young rats and matured rats showed that the

63

drug has no any toxic response to animal's hemogram, the Liver functions and the internal organs. It was also found that the drug can noticeably reduce SGPT activity. Pharmacodynamics study also showed that Yang-Strengthening Capsule can promote and maintain the growth and development of the matured rat's scrotum, prostate, and testicles, increase the power of the testicles to produce sperma, increase the number of spermatogonia whose activity is also increased. It was found, too, that this drug can decrease the formation amount of malonic aldehyde in brain tissue fluid in rat, and increase the matured rats' power of macrophagocytes to phagocytize red cells, and have anti-senility and body's immunostrengthening functions.

There have been no side effects found since the drug was used clinically. The Liver and the Kidney examinations of 30 patients showed normal after they took the drug. Basal study also showed that there are no toxic effects. This indicates that Yang-Strengthening Capsule is really a safe, effective, new drug in treating sexual disorder (Jin Weixin, 1990).

2. Yanling Changchun Dan (Pills for Prolonging Life Span and Keeping Youthful) was worked out by Professor Ren Jixue of Changchun TCM College according to the effective prescriptions over many years. The herbs included in this prescription are pilose antler (Cornu Cervi Pantotrichum), sea horse (Hippocampus), gecko (Gecko), tortoise Plastron (Plastrum Testudinis), sun-dried ginseng (Radix Ginseng), dried shrimp, epimedium leaf (Herba Epimedii), cnidium fruit (Fructus Cnidii), etc. The drug invigorates the Kidney and strengthens Yang, makes the body robust and healthy, prolongs life span and slows the process of aging, and is specialized at curing impotence, premature ejaculation, male's sterility, etc. The drug was used to 165 cases with impotence. After the treatment, 40 (24.24%) were recovered. Effects were shown on 26 (15.75%). 80 (48.48%) were improved. 19 (11.5%) failed to response to the drug. The total effective rate was 88.5%. This drug is produced by Dongfeng Pharmaceutics Plant of Jilin Province, in capsule form, weighting 0.3g each, 4-6 pills each time, 3 times a day. One month is one course of treatment.

Laboratory research shows that this drug can increase the damp weight of cutaneous glands of young white rats, and increase young rat's plasma testosterone level. This suggests that this drug has gonadotropic hormonal effect. What's more, this drug also promotes the formation of DNA and protein, increases younger rat's circulatory antibody IgG level and increases the times of seeking for drinking of male fruit flies. It can be seen that this drug has anti-senility and protein metabolism regulating functions (Nan Zheng, 1989).

3. A clinical observation of 117 cases with impotence treated with Xianzi Dihuang Tang Jiawei (Modified Decoction of Epimedium (Herba Epimedii), Curculigo, Cnidium, Wolfberry, Rehmannia, and Astragalus) showed that 83 (71%) were cured and 19 (16%) gained effects. 15 (13%) failed to be cured. The total effective rate was 87%. The prescription includes wolfberry fruit (Fructus Lycii) 15g, prepared rehmannia root (Radix Rehmanniae Praeparata) 15g, astragalus root (Radix Astragali Seu Hedysari) 15g. According to complicated syndromes, impotence is divided into the following types: Simple impotence, impotence due to decline of Fire from the Gate of Life, impotence due to Kidney Deficiency and impairment of the Heart and the Spleen, impotence due to Kidney Deficiency and stagnation of Liver Qi, impotence due to Kidney Deficiency and downward flow of Damp Heat. The drugs are modified according to different types, among which the first, second, and the third showed better effects, and the remaining two types showed poor effects. The longest course of treatment was 90 days, and the shortest, 21 days, averaged 54 days (Tang Qingming, etc., 1990).

4. Huichun Zhuangyang Ling Yihao (Pill No. I for Youth Recovery and Replenishing Yang) was used to treat 102 cases with impotence. The patients were diagnosed by using Deficiency of Kidney Essence and decline of Fire from the Gate of Life as the standards. The prescription includes epimedium (Herba Epimedii), pilose antler (Cornu Cervi Pantotrichum), ginseng (Radix Ginseng), glossy privet fruit (Fructus Ligustri), red peony root (Radix Paeoniae Rubra), achyranthes root (Radix Achyranthis Bidentatae), polygala

65

root (Radix Polygalae), etc. The drug was taken 2-3 times a day, 4 pills each time, and 14 days made up a course of treatment. The drug was taken successively over 2-5 courses of treatment. The result of treatment showed that 65 (63. 5%) got obvious curative effect; 26 (26%) got effect; and 11 (10.5%) failed to be cured. The total effective rate was 89.5%. After follow-up studies, there were no cases of reoccurrence.

5. Under the guidance of rheological modern medicine, method of promoting the circulation of Blood to remove Blood Stasis, used to treat impotence, has gained good results, too. To treat the Kidney, the Liver, the Spleen, or Damp Heat, drugs that promote the circulation of Blood should be appropriately added though there are no obvious symptoms and signs of Blood Stasis Syndrome. For the cases with Blood Stasis or no recovery though treated for a long period of time, promoting the circulation of Blood to remove Blood Stasis is regarded as the main thing, to improve microcirculation inside the penis and therefore to boost its function (Jiao Yanbo, 1987).

Seminal emission

Seminal emission refers to emission without sexual intercourse. It includes spermatorrhea and oneirogmus. It is stated in *Complete Works of Zhang Jingyue* (*Jing Yue Quan Shu*) that "oneirogmus and spermatorrhea both are seminal emission. Though the manifestations are different in clinic, the causes are the same." This shows that these two kinds of emission manifest differently in the degree of seriousness. The etiology and pathogenesis are on the whole the same. Generally, spermatorrhea is more severe than oneirogmus.

The earliest record of this disease is seen in the *Yellow Emperor's Internal Classic* (*Huang Di Nei Jing*). In *Benshen*, a chapter of *Miraculous Pivot* (*Ling Shu·Ben Shen*), it says, "Palpitations due to fright and overanxiety impair Vitality, furtherly causing fear and terror, thus seminal emission occurs. Fear and terror which are not relieved will

66

impair Essence, causing soreness of bones and flaccidity and cold sensation of limbs, also, seminal emission occurs." The Chinese term "Yi Jing" (emission) comes from *Emission*, a chapter of *Standards of Diagnosis and Treatment (Zheng Zhi Zhun Sheng · Yi Jing)* written by Wang Kentang (Ming Dynasty), which states, "Emission because of dreaming to do sexual intercourse with ghost is called oneirogmus, and nocturnal emission with no effect of dreaming is called spermatorrhea. However, they all belong to emission." The diseases are mostly caused by unconsolidation of gate for ejaculation due to Kidney Deficiency, breakdown of the normal physiological coordination between the Heart and the Kidney, impairment of the Heart and the Spleen caused by overstrain, and downward flow of Damp Heat.

Etiology and Pathogenesis
• *Breakdown of Normal Physiological Coordination between the Heart and the Kidney*

Overstrain, mental disorder, vain hopes cause excessive consumption of Heart Yin and due to hyperactivity of Heart Fire. The flaring Heart Fire does not go down to the Kidney and Kidney Yin does not go up to relieve Heart Fire. Therefore, the Ministerial Fire interferes with the upper area and the Ministerial Fire of the Liver and the Kidney responses down; as a result, the semen-storing organs are disturbed, and sperma can not be stored, and runs out induced by dreaming. *Oneirogmus and Spermatorrhea*, a chapter of *Additional Works of Synopsis of Prescriptions of the Golden Chamber (Jin Yi Yi · Meng Yi Hua Jing)*, says, "Palpitation is because of vitality impairment, and sperma is emitted down."

• *Unconsolidation of Gate for Ejaculation due to Kidney Deficiency*

Congenital defect, excessive sexual intercourse, frequent masturbation, excessive consumption of Kidney Essence, breakdown of storing and secretion, unconsolidation of Essence Gate for ejaculation—all of this leads to emission. Also, lasting emission is caused by other syndromes, which leads to excessive consumption of Kidney Essence and in turn

67

impairs Yang. So, Essence Gate will be not consolidated for Deficiency of Kidney Yang, and at last, spermatorrhea occurs.

• *Deficiency of Heat Qi and Spleen Qi*

Overstrain impairs and consumes excessively Yin and Blood, so hyperactivity of Fire is caused. Deficiency Fire interferes the semen-storing organs, leading to seminal emission. Also, anxiety impairs the Spleen. This leads to sinking of Qi of the Middle Jiao and it will fail to control seminal fluid; and as a result, emission occurs. In *Emission*, a chapter of *Complete Works of Zhang Jingyue (Jing Yue Quan Shu)*, written by Zhang Jiebin (Ming Dynasty), it states, "This is because of insufficiency of Qi in the Middle Jiao, or due to Deficiency and impairment of the Heart and the Spleen."

• *Downward Flow of Damp Heat*

Because of pathogenic Damp or overdrinking or overeating rich food, dysfunctions of the Middle Jiao, the Spleen, and the Stomach are caused, because of which Damp Heat are produced in the Interior, and they disturb the semen-storing organs. As a result, Essence Gate for ejaculation is not consolidated and emission occurs.

Main Points of Diagnosis

The main characteristic of this disease is seminal emission without sexual intercourse. Cases of emission are different in degree of seriousness, illness course, or staleness and Excess or Deficiency. For the cases in a short illness course and bodily Excess, they often suffer from oneirogmus which is mild. For the cases with lingering course and weak body, they often suffer from spermatorrhea which is comparatively serious. Spermatorrhea develops from oneirogmus. Emission will take place 3-4 times every month at least, or one time every 2-3 days, or every night or several times in the same night, or during wake time if it is severe. In the process of onset, development of this disease, it often transforms each other. For instance, the flaring Heart Fire will surely consume and burn Kidney Yin. If this continues for a long time, it will lead to Kidney Deficiency which will lose its function to store Essence, and it will change to other syndromes. Attention should be paid in the diagnosis.

In the diagnosis of emission, it should be distinguished with physiological emission. Unmarried grown-ups or those living separately after marriage go through 1-2 times of emission but there are no uncomfortable feelings after it, this is physiological phenomenon. Sometimes, when men get sexually excited, there may be urethral secretion, or secretory fluid from prostate without sexual stimulation. This is not regarded as pathologic change. Only does pathological emission take place complicated with corresponding symptoms, emission can be determined with confirmation.

Treatment Based on Syndrome Differentiation

To treat emission, invigorating the Kidney to control nocturnal emission is regarded as a main thing. The general principles for treatment are to the upper, clearing Heart Fire and tranquilizing and easing mental stress; to the middle, regulating the Spleen and the Stomach; to the lower, invigorating the Kidney to control nocturnal emission. For instance, at early stage, what is often seen is Heart Fire and the Ministerial Fire disturbance, breakdown of normal physiological coordination of the Heart and the Kidney. Therefore, needed are clearing Heart Fire and tranquilizing and easing mental stress, nourishing Yin and relieving Fire, normalizing the physiological coordination between the Heart and the Kidney. If the disease is prolonged which excessively consumes Kidney Essence, the Kidney will fail to store Essence due to Kidney Deficiency, and Essence Gate for ejaculation will not be consolidated, either. So, reinforcing the Kidney to arrest seminal emission is needed. Just as ancient people said, "Dream-disturbed sleep indicates Excess Syndrome, and no dreaming suggests Deficiency Syndrome." "The Heart should be treated if dreaming, and the Kidney should be treated if no dreaming." This is for reference during the treatment.

• *Breakdown of Normal Physiological Coordination between the Heart and the Kidney*

Main Symptoms and Signs: Nocturnal emission while

dreaming, mental depression, tiredness, weakness, dream-disturbed sleep, dizziness, palpitation, scanty dark urine, red tongue with slight coating, thready and rapid pulse.

Analysis of the Symptoms and Signs: Flaring Heart Fire consumes the Heart Yin, and Heart Fire can not go down to the Kidney, and Kidney Water can not go up to help the Heart. Deficiency of Kidney Water producing hyperactivity of Heart Fire disturbs the uterus, and nocturnal emission while dreaming takes place. Dream-disturbed sleep and mental tiredness cause mental depression, bodily tiredness and weakness. Heart Fire moving about inside and mental derangement causes dream-disturbed sleep. The excessive consumption of Heart Blood causes poor nourishment of the brain. This is the reason of dizziness and palpitation. Heart Fire moves down to the Small Intestines. This leads to scanty dark urine. The conditions of the tongue and pulse indicates Heart Fire.

Treatment Principles: Nourishing Yin and clearing Fire; normalizing the physiological coordination of the Heart and the Kidney.

Prescription: Huanglian Qingxin Yin He Sancai Fengsui Dan (Decoction of Coptis Root for Relieving Heart Fire Together with Pills of Three Marvelous Drugs for Strengthening Mallow)

Coptis root (Rhizoma Coptidis) 3g, dried rehmannia root (Radix Rehmanniae) 12g, Chinese angelica root (Radix Angelicae Sinensis) 9g, wild jujube seed (Semen Ziziphi Spinosae) 15g, poria with hostwood (Poria Cum Ligno Hospite) 9g, dangshen (Radix Codonopsis Pilosulae) 18g, polygala root (Radix Polygalae) 6g, lotus seed (Semen Nelumbinis) 6g, asparagus root (Radix Asparagi) 9g, prepared rehmannia root (Radix Rehmanniae Praeparata) 12g, phellodendron bark (Cortex Phellodendri) 6g, amomum fruit (Fructus Amomi) 6g and prepared licorice (Radix Glycyrrhizae Praeparata) 3g. All the above drugs are decocted in water for oral administration, one dose per day.

Analysis of the Prescription: Coptis root (Rhizoma Coptidis) can clear away Fire from the Heart and the Stomach. Dried rehmannia root (Radix Rehmanniae) nourishes Yin and removes Heat. Chinese angelica root (Radix Angelicae Sinensis) replenishes Blood and promotes the circulation of Blood. Wild jujube seed (Semen Ziziphi Spinosae), poria (Poria) with hostwood, polygala root (Radix Polygalae) relieve mental stress. Dangshen (Radix Codonopsis Pilosulae) rhizome, licorice (Radix Glycyrrhizae) ease the Mind and replenish Qi. Lotus seed (Semen Nelumbinis) nourishes the Heart to calm the Mind, reinforces the Kidney to arrest seminal emission. Asparagus root (Radix Asparagi), prepared rehmannia root nourish water and replenish Yin. Phellodendron bark (Cortex Phellodendri) strengthens Yin and reduces Fire. Amomum fruit (Fructus Amomi) removes obstruction and invigorates the Spleen.

• *Unconsolidation of Gate for Ejaculation due to Kidney Deficiency*

Main Symptoms and Signs: Spermatorrhea while dreaming, pale complexion, listlessness and weakness, dizziness and tinnitus, insomnia and amnesia, frequent urination at night, pale tongue, deep and thready pulse.

Analysis of the Symptoms and Signs: The Kidney fails to store Essence due to Deficiency. This causes spermatorrhea while dreaming. Deficiency of Yang Qi causes pale complexion for there is no Yang Qi to go up to the face. Kidney Deficiency leads to listlessness and physical weakness. Deficiency of Kidney Yin causes excessive consumption of Kidney Essence, and the Sea of Marrow has nothing to fill up. Therefore, dizziness and tinnitus, insomnia and amnesia are caused. Deficiency of Kidney Yang makes the Bladder fail to control closure and opening; therefore, problem of frequent night urination occurs. Tongue and pulse conditions indicate Kidney Deficiency.

Treatment Principles: Replenishing Kidney Essence and controlling nocturnal emission.

Prescription: Jinsuo Gujing Wan He Shuilu Erxian Dan (Golden Lock Bolus for Keeping the Kidney Essence Supplemented with Pill of Euryales and Rosa Laevigatae)

Gordon eurales seed (Semen Euryales) 12g, lotus stamen (Stamen Nelumbinis) 9g, flatstem milkvetch seed (Semen Astragali Complanati) 9g, calcined dragon's bone (Os Dra-

71

conis Fossilia Ossis Mastodi, calcined) 30g, calcined oyster shell (Concha Ostreae) 30g, lotus seed (Semen Nelumbinis) 9g and cherokee rose-hip (Fructus Rosae Laevigatae) 12g. The above drugs are decocted in water for oral administration, one dose daily.

Analysis of the Prescription: Euryales seed (Semen Euryales) and lotus stamen (Stamen Nelumbinis) invigorate the Kidney and arrest nocturnal emission. Flatstem milkvetch seed (Semen Astragali Complanati) and lotus seed (Semen Nelumbinis) benefit the Kidney to control emission. Cacined dragon's bone (Os Draconis) and calcined oyster shell (Concha Ostreae) arrest discharge by astringing. Cherokee rose-hip (Fructus Rosae Laevigatae) invigorates the Kidney and controls nocturnal emission.

• *Deficiency of Heart Blood and Spleen Qi*

Main Symptoms and Signs: Spermatorrhea, severe palpitation, insomnia and amnesia, shallow complexion, tired limbs, poor appetite and loose stool, pale tongue with thin coating, weak and feeble pulse.

Analysis of the Symptoms and Signs: Overstrain consumes Heart Blood and impairs Yin leading to Deficiency Fire. Deficiency Fire disturbs the semen-storing organs; or anxiety impairs the Spleen, which leads to Deficiency of Spleen Qi and the failure of the Kidney to govern the sperma. Therefore, spermatorrhea is caused. Overanxiety will cause restlessness which causes severe palpitation, insomnia and amnesia. Deficiency of Spleen Qi will cause insufficiency of digestion source. This is the reason of sallow complexion, poor appetite and loose stool. The Spleen does not spread to the limbs and so they are tired and weak. The signs of the tongue and the pulse suggest Deficiency of Heart Qi and Spleen Qi.

Treatment Principles: Replenishing Blood and tonifying Qi; invigorating the Spleen and nourishing the Heart.

Prescription: Guipi Tang Jiajian (Modified Decoction for Invigorating the Spleen)

Astragalus root (Radix Astragali Seu Hedysari) 30g, dangshen (Radix Codonopsis Pilosulae) 30g, Chinese angelica root (Radix Angelicae Sinensis) 9g, longan aril (Arillus

Longan) 9g, bighead atractylodes rhizome (Rhizoma A-tractylodis Macrocephalae 9g, aucklandia root (Radix Aucklandiae) 6g, poria with hostwood (Poria cum Ligno Hospite) 9g, polygala root (Radix Polygalae) 6g, wild jujube seed (Semen Ziziphi Spinosae) 15g, prepared licorice (Radix Glycyrrhizae Praeparata) 6g, Chinese yam (Ehizoma Dioscoreae) 15g and platycodon root (Radix Platycodi) 9g. The above drugs are decocted in water for oral administration, one dose per day.

Analysis of the Prescription: Astragalus root (Radix Astragali Seu Hedysari), dangshen (Radix Codonopsis Pilosulae) tonify Qi and reinforce the Spleen. Chinese angelica root (Radix Angelicae Sinensis), longan aril (Arillus Longan) nourish Blood and regulate the nutrient. Bighead atractylodes rhizome (Rhizoma Atractylodis Macrocephalae), aucklandia root (Radix Aucklandiae) invigorate the Spleen and regulate Qi flow, tonic but not obstructive. Poria with hostwood (Poria cum Ligno Hospite), polygala root (Radix Polygalae), wild jujube seed (Semen Ziziphi Spinosae) ease and tranquilize anxiety. Chinese yam (Ehizoma Dioscoreae) tonifies the Spleen and benefits the Kidney. Platycodon root (Radix Platycodi) ascending up Lucid Yang. The whole prescription enriches Blood and tonifies Qi and relieves mental stress and arrests spermatorrhea.

• *Downward Flow of Damp Heat*

Main Symptoms and Signs: Spermatorrhea, bitter and greasy feeling in the mouth, dark urine with burning sensation, turbid and foul stools, yellow and greasy coating of the tongue, soft rapid pulse.

Analysis of the Symptoms and Signs: Downward flow of Damp Heat disturbs the semen-storing organs. This causes spermatorrhea. Retention of Damp Heat in the Interior causes bitter and sticky feeling in the mouth. Damp Heat flows down to the small intestines. This causes dark urine with burning sensation, turbid and dripping. Damp Heat flows down to the large intestines. This causes loose foul stool. Yellow and greasy tongue coating, soft and rapid pulse are signs of Damp Heat.

Treatment Principles: Clearing Heat and promoting di-

73

uresis; invigorating the Spleen to promote the flow of clear Qi.

Prescription: Bixie Fenging Yin (Yam Decoction for Clearing Turbid Urine)

Seven-lobed yam (Rhizoma Dioscoreae Septemlobae) 9g, phellodendron bark (Cortex Phellodendri) 6g, poria (Poria) 9g, plantain seed (Semen Plantaginis) (wrapped) 9g, lotus seed (Semen Nelumbinis) 9g, red sage root (Radix Salviae Militiorrhizae) 15g, grassleaved sweetflag rhizome (Rhizoma Acori Graminei) 9g and bighead atractylodes rhizome (Rhizoma Atractylodis Macrocephalae) 9g. The above drugs are decocted in water for oral administration, one dose daily.

Analysis of the Prescription: Seven-lobed yam (Rhizoma Dioscoreae Septemlobae), phellodendron bark (Cortex Phellodendri), poria (Poria) and plantain seed (Semen Plantaginis) clear away Heat and promote diuresis. Lotus seed (Semen Nelumbinis), red sage root (Radix Salviae Militiorrhizae), grassleaved sweetflag rhizome (Rhizoma Acori Graminei) remove Fire from the Heart and ease mental stress, reduce turbid urine and cause resuscitation. Bighead atractylodes rhizome (Rhizoma Atractylodis Macrocephalae) invigorates the Spleen and promotes diuresis.

Current Research

1. 145 cases with nocturnal emission were treated by Ji Ji Tang (Decoction for Strengthening the Heart and the Kidney) worked out by the author himself. According to therapy that oneirogmus concerning with the Heart and spermatorrhea is related to the Kidney. The Kidney and the Heart are mainly be treated in combination based on Syndrome Differentiation on Qi and Blood, Yin and Yang. In this way, the total effective rate was 100%, among which curative rate was 88.2%. Prescription includes prepared rehmannia root (Radix Rehmanniae Praeparata), mashed with amomum fruit (Fructus Amomi) 30g, dogwood fruit (Fructus Corni) 12g and dried Chinese yam (Ehizoma Dioscoreae) 12g, poria (Poria) 9g, bighead atractylodes rhizome (Rhizoma Atractylodis Macrocephalae) 15g, Chinese angelica root (Radix An-

74

gelicae Sinensis) 10g, schisandra fruit (Fructus Schisandrae) 4g, white peony root (Radix Paeoniae) 9g, ophiopogon root (Radix Ophiopogonis) 9g, Chinese date seed (Fructus Ziziphi Jujubae) 30g, polygala root (Radix Polygalae) 9g, morinda root (Radix Morindae Officinalis) 9g, desertliving cistanche (Herba Dendrobii) 9g, ginseng (Radix Ginseng) 9g, lotus seed (Semen Nelumbinis) 12g and dried human placenta (Placenta Hominis) 15g (Chen Runwen, 1990).

2. An observation of 36 cases with nocturnal emission treated through acupuncture according to Syndrome Differentiation: According to the patients' etiological factors and Syndromes, they were divided into seven types: ① Breakdown of normal physiological coordinations between the Heart and the Kidney; ② Deficiency and impairment of Kidney Yin; ③ Unconsolidation of Kidney Qi; ④ Hyperactivity of Live Fire; ⑤ Downward flow of Damp Heat; ⑥ The impairment of the Heart and the Spleen due to overstrain; ⑦ Blood Stasis and Qi stagnation. Principles of Treatment: Invigorating the Kidney to arrest nocturnal emission was taken as the main factor. The main points are Guanyuan (REN 4), Dahe (KID 12) and Zhishi (BL 52). For the cases of Type 1, added were points that nourish Yin and remove Fire. The supplementary points were Shenshu (BL 23) and Sanyinjiao (SP 6). Filiform needles were used by means of uniform reinforcing-reducing method. For the cases of Type 2, added were points that nourish and replenish Kidney Yin, and the supplementary points used were Shenshu (BL 23), Sanyinjiao (SP 6) and Taixi (KID 3). Filiform needles were used with reinforcing method. For the cases of Type 3, added were points that invigorate and benefit Kidney Essence and strengthen the control of nocturnal emission. The supplementary points used were Shenshu (BL 23) and Mingmen (DU 4). Filiform needles were used by means of reinforcing method (Shenshu BL 23 and Mingmen DU 4 can be moxibusted). For the cases of Type 4, added were points that purge the Liver of pathogenic Fire, and the supplementary points were Ganshu (BL 18), Jianshi (PC 5) and Taichang (LIV 3). Filiform needles were used by means of reducing method. For the cases of Type 5, added were points that clear Heat

and promote diuresis, and the supplementary points were Ciliao (BL 32), Fenglong (ST 40), Xingjian (LIV 2) and Yinlingquan (SP 9). Filiform needles were used by means of reducing method. For the cases of Type 6, added were points that regulate and tonify the Heart and the Spleen, replenish Qi and Essence. The supplementary points were Xinshu (BL 15), Pishu (BL 20), Jueyinshu (BL 14). Filiform needles were used by means of reinforcing method. For the cases of Type 7, added were the points that regulate the flow of Qi and promote Blood circulation. The supplementary points were Geshu (BL 17), Qihai (REN 6) and Xuehai (SP 1). Filiform needles were used by means of reducing method. The treatment was carried out one time every other day, and 20 minutes each time, 10 times account for one course of treatment. The results showed that 20 cases (51. 5%) were cured. The treatment was effectual on 4 cases (11. 1%). 9 cases (25%) gained effects. 3 cases (8. 3%) failed to respond to the treatment. The total effective rate was 91.6%. This shows that acupuncture points are specific. Guanyuan is the crossing area of Three Yin Channels of Foot and Ren Channel, the essential source of Qi in human body. The acupoint is selected and used, Kidney Qi will be strengthened. The supplementary points Zhishi (BL 52), Dahe (KID 12) can consolidate Essence Gate for ejaculation. Clinically, different points and different prickling and needling methods should be selected and used according to different syndromes so that curative effects can be improved (Wang Shijing, 1990).

3. Nocturnal emission treated with acupuncture by Syndrome Differentiation.

Spermatorrhea without differences of daytime and nighttime, and emission while thinking, bodily thin and weak, thready and feeble pulse, accompanied by palpitations and impotence, etc. Prickled are Guanyuan (REN 4), Zusanli (ST 36), Shenshu (BL 23), Sanyinjiao (SP 6), Tinggong (SI 19) and Taichong (LIV 3), which were divided into two groups. The two groups were needled alternately every day.

Spermatorrhea without dreaming, and soreness and weakness of the lumbar area, palpitations, insomnia, distending pain in the lower abdomen, cold glens penis, mostly weak pulse. Qihai (REN 6), Guanyuan (REN 4), Zhongji (REN 3), Ciliao (BL 32), Neiguan (PC6), Sanyinjiao (SP 6) were divided into two groups which were needled alternately every day. Dreaminess, oneirogmus, and with the lingering of it, listlessness, dizziness and tinnitus. Punctured were Neiguan (PC 6), Sanyinjiao (SP 6), moxibusted Xinshu (BL 15) and Zhishi (BL 52) (Zhu Guangyao, 1990).

Prospermia

Prospermia means too early ejaculation during sexual intercourse or ejaculation before sexual life. As what is stated in Shen's Works on the Impotence of Life Preservation (Shen Shi Zun Sheng Shu), "Ejaculation before sexual activities, or emission too early during sexual intercourse." This disorder is caused by poor storage and consolidation of Essence due to Kidney Deficiency, or flaring of the Ministerial Fire due to impairment and Deficiency of Kidney Essence. This results in hyperactivity of Fire and Deficiency of Yin, and breakdown of storing and releasing of the Kidney.

Etiology and Pathogenesis
• *Unconsolidation of Kidney Qi*
Marrying too early or habit of masturbation impairs the Kidney. This causes Deficiency and Decline of Kidney Qi and dysfunction of Essence storing. As a result, premature ejaculation takes place.
• *Hyperactivity of Yang due to Yin Deficiency*
Congenital Yin Deficiency, or excessive sexual activities leads to impairment and Deficiency of Kidney Yin which in turn causes hyperactivity of Fire. The flaring of the Ministerial Fire burns the Uterus and forces spermia to flow out.
• *Damp Heat of the Liver Channel*
Lingering stagnation of Liver Qi forms Heat. Heat and Damp accumulate in the Interior, and it leads to dysfunction of releasing and transporting. Premature ejaculation occurs.

77

Main Points of Diagnosis

During sexual intercourse, or before touching of the penis, or when inserting just happens, ejaculation takes places. This is the main point in the diagnosis. It has not been agreed in confirmation as to the standard length of sexual intercourse before prospermia happens. Generally, the time length of sexual intercourse of the male with normal health condition before ejaculation is 2-6 minutes, the normal range. Some doctors hold, time length can not be solely taken as a standard. If the both experience sexual satisfaction, it is the most suitable time length.

When diagnosis of this disease is done, it should be distinguished with impotence, nocturnal emission. Impotence refers to astysia of penis, or not hard enough erection, which makes sexual intercourse fail. Nocturnal emission refers to seminal emission without doing sexual intercourse. Premature ejaculation refers to too early ejaculation in the process of sexual intercourse.

Treatment Based on Syndrome Differentiation

Prospermia has the difference in Deficiency and Excess. According to the rules "Tonifying is needed for the cases with Deficiency Syndrome, and releasing is needed for the cases with Excess Syndrome," for the cases of Deficiency Syndrome, reinforcing the Kidney to arrest spontaneous emission is considered to be the main therapeutic principle, and for the cases of Excess Syndrome, clearing Heat and removing Fire are regarded as therapeutic principle.

• *Unconsolidation of Kidney Qi*

Main Symptoms and Signs: Premature ejaculation, hyposexuality, soreness and weakness of the waist and the knees, pale complexion, thin profuse urine, and dropping urine, pale tongue with white coating, deep and weak pulse.

Analysis of the Symptoms and Signs: Dysfunction of Essence storing due to unconsolidation of the Kidney causes prospermia. Deficiency of Kidney Qi causes weakness of Fire from the Gate of Life. This is the reason of hyposexuality, soreness and weakness of the waist and the knees. Deficiency of Kidney Yang results in the fact that Yang Qi can not reach

78

the face; therefore, the complexion is pale. Tongue and pulse conditions indicate Deficiency of Kidney Qi.

Treatment Principles: Reinforcing the Kidney to arrest spontaneous emission.

Prescription: Jingui Shenqi Wan Jiawei (Modified Pill for Restoring Kidney Qi)

Aconite root (Radix Aconiti Praeparata) 3g, cinnamon bark (Cortex Cinnamomi) 3g, prepared rehmannia root (Radix Rehmanniae Praeparata) 12g, dogwood fruit (Fructus Corni) 9g, Chinese yam (Ehizoma Dioscoreae) 15g, moutan bark (Cortex Moutan Radicis) 9g, poria (Poria) 9g, alismaceae (Rhizoma Alismatis) 9g, mantise egg-case (Ootheca Mantidis) 9g and schisandra fruit (Fructus Schisandrae) 9g. The above drugs are decocted in water for oral administration, one dose daily.

Analysis of the Prescription: Aconite root (Radix Aconiti Praeparata) and cinnamon bark (Cortex Cinnamomi) warm Yang and the Kidney to promote Yang and encourage Kidney Qi. Prepared rehmannia root (Radix Rehmanniae Praeparata) nourishes the Kidney and replenishes Essence. Dogwood fruit (Fructus Corni) and Chinese yam (Ehizoma Dioscoreae) restore and enrich Essence and Blood of the Kidney, the Liver and the Spleen to arrest seminal emission. Moutan bark (Cortex Moutan Radicis) purges pathogenic Fire from the Liver and produces Heat such as dogwood fruit (Fructus Corni). Poria (Poria) removes Damp from the Spleen to help Chinese yam (Ehizoma Dioscoreae) in invigorating the Spleen. Alisaceae removes Kidney Fire, and avoids being affected by wettness and greasiness of prepared rehmannia root (Radix Rehmanniae Praeparata). Mantise egg-case (Ootheca Mantidis) restores the Kidney and stops spontaneous emission. Schisandra fruit (Fructus Schisandrae) reinforces the Kidney and strengthens the function of Essence storing, benefits Qi and nourishes the Heart. The whole prescription benefits the Kidney and arrests emission and treats prospermia.

• *Hyperactivity of Yang due to Deficiency of Yin*

Main Symptoms and Signs: Premature ejaculation, easy erection, dizziness and giddiness, dysphoria with feverish sensation in chest, palms and soles, soreness and weakness of the waist and the knees, insomnia and night sweating, red tongue with slight coating, thready and rapid pulse.

Analysis of the Symptoms and Signs: Hyperactivity of Fire due to Deficiency of Yin disturbs the semen-storing organs, and causes dysfunction of sperm storing. This is the reason of prospermia. Because of hyperactivity of Yang caused by Yin Deficiency, erection of penis is easy. Heat due to Deficiency of Yin causes dysphoria with feverish sensation in chest, palms and soles. There is no Essence to nourish Vitality and the brain, then, dizziness and giddiness, insomnia and night sweating are induced. Kidney Deficiency also causes poor nourishment to the organs; therefore, soreness and weakness of the waist and knees are caused. Tongue and pulse conditions indicate Interior Heat which is brought about by Yin Deficiency.

Treatment Principles: Nourishing Yin and removing Fire.

Prescription: Zhibo Dihuang Tang Jiawei (Modified Decoction of Anemarrhena, Phellodendron, and Rehmannia)

Rhizome of wind-weed (Rhizoma Anemarrhenae) 9g, phellodendron bark (Cortex Phellodendri) 9g, dried rehmannia root (Radix Rehmanniae) 12g, dogwood fruit (Fructus Corni) 9g, Chinese yam (Ehizoma Dioscoreae) 15g, moutan bark (Cortex Moutan Radicis) 9g, poria (Poria) 9g, Alismaceae (Rhizoma Alismatis) 9g, dried dragon's bone (Os Draconis) 30g, parched oyster shell (Concha Ostreae) 30g and flatstem milkvetch seed (Semen Astragali Complanati) 9g. The above drugs are decocted in water for oral administration.

Analysis of the Prescription: The same as the above corresponding content.

• *Damp Heat of the Liver Channel*

Main Symptoms and Signs: Premature ejaculation, sexual hyperesthesia, dizziness and restlessness, bitter taste and dry pharynx, dark urine, pain during urination and tingling penis, red tongue with yellow and greasy coating, stringy rapid pulse.

Analysis of the Symptoms and Signs: Damp Heat of the Liver Channel burns gate for ejaculation, so sperma is forced

80

to flow out. Liver Fire moves about in the Interior, so hyperesthesia is caused. The Fire disturbs the clear Yang above. So dizziness is caused. Fire also interferes with the Heart and the Vitality, it naturally leads to dysphoria with feverish sensation in chest, palms and soles. Damp Heat steams up, so the mouth feels bitter and pharynx feels dry. Damp Heat flows down, and it causes dark urine, pain during urination and tingling penis. Tongue and pulse conditions show Damp Heat Syndrome.

Treatment Principles: Clearing Heat to promote diuresis.

Prescription: Longdan Xiegan Tang (Decoction of Gentiana For Purging Liver Fire)

Gentian root (Radix Gentianae) 9g, scutellaria root (Radix Scutellariae) 9g and capejasmine (Fructus Gardeniae) 9g, bupleurum root (Radix Bupleuri) 9g, Alismaceae (Rhizoma Alismatis) 9g, Caulis clematidis armandii (Caulis Akebiae) 6g and plantain seed (Semen Plantaginis) (wrapped) 9g, Chinese angelica root (Radix Angelicae Sinensis) 9g, dried rehmannia root (Radix Rehmanniae) 12g and dried licorice (Radix Glycyrrhizae) 6g. The above drugs are decocted in water for oral administration, one dose daily.

Analysis of the Prescription: Gentian root (Radix Gentianae) purges the Liver of the pathogenic Fire, and removes Damp Heat in the Lower Jiao. Scutellaria root (Radix Scutellariae), capejasmine (Fructus Gardeniae) bitter in taste and cold in nature remove Fire. Bupleurum root (Radix Bupleuri) removes obstruction in the Liver and the Gallbladder. Alismaceae (Rhizoma Alismatis), Caulis clematidis armandii (Caulis Akebiae), plantain seed (Semen Plantaginis) relieve Damp Heat and remove Fire through urination. Chinese angelica root (Radix Angelicae Sinensis) nourishes Blood and promotes the circulation of Blood. Dried rehmannia root (Radix Rehmanniae) nourishes Yin and clears Heat. Dried licorice (Radix Glycyrrhizae) coordinates the effects of all the drugs. The whole prescription purges Liver Fire, and removes Damp Heat.

81

Non-ejaculation

Non-ejaculation is also termed "inability to ejaculate," both referring to the failure of sending out seminal fluid during coitus. General Treatise on Etiology and Symptology (Zhu Bing Yuan Hou Lun) states, "The seminal fluid is congested in the glens penis but not ejaculated, thus causing no pregnancy." This disease is predominantly caused by hyperactivity of Fire due to Yin Deficiency, accumulation of Blood Stasis, and decline of Fire from the Gate of Life.

Etiology and Pathogenesis

• *Hyperactivity of Fire due to Yin Deficiency*

Excessive sexual intercourse or masturbation causes excessive consumption of Kidney Yin. Yin Deficiency, in turn, leads to hyperactivity of the Ministerial Fire. The Ministerial Fire thus fails to nourish the Heart. With the breakdown of coordination between the Kidney and the Heart, Essence Gate for ejaculation loses its normal level of discharge and retention. In this case, a coitus can take place but without ejaculation.

• *Blood Stasis*

Constant intemperance of sexual intercourse causes stagnancy of Qi and Blood Stasis in the ejaculatory duct, thus making ejaculation impossible.

• *Decline of Fire from the Gate of Life*

Congenital defect, lasting Yang Deficiency, with internal injury caused by overstrain, exhaust Fire from the Gate of Life to such an extent that Kidney Yang declines. Deficiency of Kidney Yang leads to an imbalance of functional activity of Qi and inability to ejaculate.

Main Points of Diagnosis

No emission of the seminal fluid during coitus is the main symptom of non-ejaculation. In clinical practice, the diagnosis should be based on the analysis of the overall condition of the body, tongue, and pulse.

82

For non-ejaculation, there are no orgasm and ejaculatory action. In case with ejaculatory feeling accompanied by a climax but no actual sperm sent out, this may be because the sperm has gone back to the Bladder, thus resulting in retrograde ejaculation. This can also be identified by taking an examination of urine after coitus to find out if there is any sperm in the urine.

In diagnosing this disease, the doctor should at first inquire about the patient's ejaculatory action. There are cases in which after the insertion of the penis, no up-and-down movement follows, or the movement is not full enough, so that no ejaculation is achieved.

Treatment Based on Syndrome Differentiation

The differentiation and treatment of non-ejaculation should also be based on its chief manifestations, combined with the overall symptoms and signs, especially those of the tongue and the pulse in order to recognize the location of the disease and its condition of Deficiency or Excess. Then a therapy can be worked out and given.

• *Hyperactivity of Fire due to Deficiency of Yin*

Main Symptoms and Signs: Inability to ejaculate, sexual hyperesthesia, ever-hardened penis, irritability, dream-disturbed sleep, yellow urine and dry stool, red and uncoated tongue, and thready pulse.

Analysis of the Symptoms and Signs: Yin Deficiency causes hyperactivity of the Ministerial Fire, which, in turn, fails to nourish the Heart. The breakdown of coordination between the Kidney and Heart makes it impossible for Essence Gate for ejaculation to display the functions of discharge and retention normally; coitus, then, does not end in ejaculation. Yin Deficiency and Yang Excess lead to hyperesthesia and ever-stiff penis. The troubled internal heat causes irritability, therefore, reduces sleep. Yellow urine and dry stool, red tongue with the coating peeled, and thready pulse are also symptoms and signs of Deficiency of Yin and hyperactivity of Fire.

Treatment Principles: Nourishing Yin to reduce pathogenic Fire.

83

Prescription: Zhibo Dihuang Wan Jiajian (Modified Pill of Anemarrhena, Phellodendron, Rehmannia)

Anemarrhena rhizome (Rhizoma Anemarrhenae) 9g, phellodendron bark (Cortex Phellodendri) 9g, prepared rehmannia root (Radix Rehmanniae Praeparata) 12g, dogwood fruit (Fructus Corni) 9g, Chinese yam (Ehizoma Dioscoreae) 15g, moutan bark (Cortex Moutan Radicis) 9g, poria (Poria) 9g and oriental water plantain rhizome (Rhizoma Alismatis) 9g. The above drugs are decocted in water for oral administration, one dose daily.

Modifications of the Prescription: In case with irritability, bupleurum (Radix Bupleuri) 9g, scutellaria root (Radix Scutellariae) 9g are added. In case with insomnia and frequent dreams during sleep, parched date kernel (Semen Ziziphi Spinosae) 30g is added. In case with stagnation of Liver Qi causing Fire transmission, gentian root (Radix Gentianae) 9g, capejasmine fruit (Fructus Gardeniae) 9g, dried rehmannia root (Radix Rehmanniae) 12g, Caulis clematidis armandii (Caulis Akebiae) 6g and bamboo leaf 9g are added.

Analysis of the Prescription: The functions of Modified Pill of Anemarrhena, Phellodendron, Rehmannia are the same as what has already been explained in the previous chapters. Bupleurum (Radix Bupleuri) and scutellaria (Radix Scutellariae) can soothe the Liver and reduce Heart Fire. Parched date kernel (Semen Ziziphi Spinosae) can nourish the Heart and calm the Mind. Gentian and capejasmine fruit (Fructus Gardeniae) can reduce Liver Heat and purge the Ministerial Fire. Dried rehmannia rhizome (Radix Rehmanniae), caulis clematidis armandii (Caulis Akebiae) and bamboo leaf (Herba Lophatheri) can nourish Yin and reduce Heat through relaxing the bowels and conducting Heat out along the urine.

• *Blood Stasis*

Main Symptoms and Signs: Inability to ejaculate, distending pain of the penis, oppression of chest and discomfort, irritability, dark-purple tongue or ecchymosis on the tongue proper with thin coating, deep and choppy pulse.

Analysis of Symptoms and Signs: The stasis due to linger-

84

ing sickness, and the Qi Stagnation, and Blood Stasis blocks the ejaculatory duct, thus causing an inability to ejaculate and distending pain of the penis. The hepatic congestion and Qi stagnation give rise to oppression of chest and discomfort and irritability. All the conditions of the tongue and pulse have the symptoms and signs of stagnation of Qi and Blood Stasis.

Treatment Principles: Promoting Blood circulation to eliminate Blood Stasis.

Prescription: Xuefu Zhuyu Tang Jiajian (Modified Decoction for Removing Blood Stasis in Chest), including:

Dried rhizome of rehmannia (Radix Rehmanniae) 12g, Chinese angelica root (Radix Angelicae Sinensis) 9g, red peony root (Radix Paeoniae Rubra) 9g, Chuanxiong rhizome (Rhizoma Ligustici Chuanxiong) 9g, peach kernel (Semen Persicae) 9g, safflower (Flos Carthami) 9g, achyranthes and achyranthes root (Radix Achyranthis Bidentatae) 9g, bupleurum root (Radix Bupleuri) 9g, bitter orange (Fructus Aurantii) 9g, platycodon root (Radix Platycodi) 9g and licorice root (Radix Glycyrrhizae) 6g. The above drugs are decocted in water for oral administration, one dose per day.

Modifications of the Prescription: In case with inability to ejaculate due to hepatic congestion, cyperus tuber (Rhizoma Cuperi) 9g, curcuma root (Radix Curcumae) 9g, pangolin scales (Squama Manitis) 12g and cudrania root (Radix Cudraniae) 9g are added. In case with inability to ejaculate due to Damp Heat retardation, gentian root (Radix Gentianae) 9g, scutellaria root (Radix Scutellariae) 9g, capejasmine fruit (Fructus Gardeniae) 9g, plantain seed (Semen Plantaginis) (wrapped) 15g, moutan bark (Cortex Moutan Radicis) 18g and vaccaria seed (Semen Vaccariae) 18g are added.

Analysis of the Prescription: Chinese angelica root (Radix Angelicae Sinensis), chuanxiong rhizome, red peony root (Radix Paeoniae Rubra), peach kernel (Semen Persicae) and safflower (Flos Carthami) in the prescription promote the circulation of Blood and remove Blood Stasis. Achyranthes and achyranthes root (Radix Achyranthis Bidentatae)

85

not only promotes Blood circulation, but also guides the extravasated Blood to go downwards. Bupleurum root (Radix Bupleuri) relieves the depressed Liver, soothes the Liver and regulates the flow of Qi, thus sending up the Lucid Yang. Platycodon root (Radix Platycodi) and fruit of citron or trifoliate orange promote the functional activities of Qi. Qi in motion facilitates Blood circulation, and Blood in motion ensures normal seminal flow. Dried rhizome of rehmannia eliminates pathogenic Heat from Blood. Licorice root (Radix Glycyrrhizae) coordinates the actions of various ingredients in the prescription. Cyperus tuber (Rhizoma Cuperi) and curcuma root (Radix Curcumae) not only relieve the depressed Liver, soothe the Liver and regulate the flow of Qi, but also relieve stuffiness of the chest and reduce stagnation. Pangolin scales (Squama Manitis) and cudrania root (Radix Cudraniae) remove lumps and soften hardness, as well as improve the condition of Essence Gate for ejaculation. Gentian root (Radix Gentianae), scutellaria root (Radix Scutellariae) and capejasmine fruit (Fructus Gardeniae) remove Fire from the Liver and Gallbladder, and relieve the Lower Jiao syndrome and Damp Heat. Moutan bark (Cortex Moutan Radicis) and plantain seed (Semen Plantaginis) remove pathogenic Heat from Blood. Vaccaria seed (Semen Vaccariae) dredges the channels, ensures Qi and Blood to flow through the channels, removes obstruction in the ejaculatory duct and guides the sperm to ejaculate.

• *Decline of Fire from the Gate of life*

Main Symptoms and Signs: Inability to ejaculate, hyposexuality, normal erection of the penis or inability to maintain an erection, sublumbar Cold, lassitude in the loins and knees, languidness, tender tongue with white coating, deep and thready pulse.

Analysis of the Symptoms and Signs: Insufficiency of Kidney Yang causes the decline of Fire from the Gate of Life and disturbance in Qi transformation, and makes it difficult to open Essence Gate for ejaculation, which ultimately leads to an inability to ejaculate, hyposexuality, and inability to maintain an erection. The decline of Fire from the Gate of Life, the loin losing its nourishment, and warmth and asthe-

86

nia all contribute to the sublumbar Cold and lassitude. Light texture of tongue with white coating and deep and thready pulse are also the symptoms and signs of the decline of Fire from the Gate of Life.

Treatment Principles: Warming and recuperating the Gate of Life.

Prescription: Jingui Shenqi Wan Jiawei (Modified Kidney Qi-Tonifying Pill)

Prepared lateral root of aconite (Radix Aconiti Lateralis Praeparata) 3g, cinnamon bark (Cortex Cinnamomi) 3g, prepared rehmannia root (Radix Rehmanniae Praeparata) 12g, dogwood fruit (Fructus Corni) 9g, Chinese yam (Ehizoma Dioscoreae) 15g, moutan bark (Cortex Moutan Radicis) 9g, poria (Poria) 9g, oriental water plantain (Rhizoma Alismatis) rhizome 9g, epimedium (Herba Epimedii) 18g and vaccaria seed (Semen Vaccariae) 18g. The above drugs are decocted in water for oral administration, one dose per day.

Analysis of the Prescription: The effects of the drugs in the prescription listed above are the same as what has been described previously. Morinda root (Radix Morindae Officinalis) and epimedium (Herba Epimedii) warm and invigorate Kidney Yang. Vaccaria seed (Semen Vaccariae) removes obstruction in the ejaculatory duct and facilitates ejaculating sperm.

Current Research

1. Liu Minghan (1987) advanced that non-ejaculation during sexual intercourse is due to "the malfunction of Essence Gate for ejaculation." This is quite consistent with the idea of modern medicine that "non-ejaculation may be related either to the intensified inhibition of the cerebral cortex on the ejaculatory center, or to the functional exhaustion of the spinal center." In order to treat functional non-ejaculation, Liu established the main therapy which is to restore the function of Essence Gate for ejaculation to arrest spermatorrhea. On the basis of removing obstruction for invigoration, and of including invigoration in removing obstruction, according asinvigoration is applied if it is needed, or removing ob-

87

struction is carried out if it is needed, or the two sides are combined, and also according to the specific cases, he has established some subprinciples: Warming the Kidney to restore the function of Essence Gate for ejaculation, nourishing the Kidney to restore the function of Essence Gate for ejaculation, reducing Blood Stasis to restore the function of ejaculation, relieving depression to restore the function of Essence Gate for ejaculation and clear Damp Heat to restore the function of Essence Gate for ejaculation. Accordingly, he has processed Tongjing Ling Yihao, Erhao, Sanhao, Sihao, Wuhao (Effective Prescriptions No. I, No. II, No. III, No. IV, No. V for Restoring the Function of the Gate for Ejaculation). Besides TCM herbal drugs, according to the exposition that "The Liver governs the normal flow of Qi," "The Liver controls channels and vessels of the external genitals," "The Kidney stores the reproductive Essence and foodstuff," "The Heart dominates mental activities," and "Treating the brain means treating the Heart," he succeeded in carrying out a treatment with neuropathology, acupuncture, massage, pricking therapy, and electromassage combined in light of theory of the channels and collaterals of TCM, thus achieving the effect of invigorating the Liver and the Kidney; nourishing the Heart and replenishing Blood; removing the stagnation and soothing the Liver; adjusting the emotional state; and regulating the reproductive center to restore its normal functions of storing Essence and eliminating wastes.

In 1990, with Tongjing Ling as the medication, Liu Minghan and others treated 130 cases with functional non-ejaculation, and carried out a clinical control test. The curative rate of the medicine group was 98. 46% ; whereas, that of the control group was 84. 62%. The tablet prescription for Tongjing Ling includes earthworm 10. 2kg, whole worm 10. 2kg, fasciolopsis 10. 2kg, Chinese angelica root (Radix Angelicae Sinensis) 15. 3kg, white peony root (Radix Paeoniae) 15. 3kg, centipedefern (Scolopendra) 1. 6kg, desertliving cistanche (Herba Dendrobii) 30. 6kg, achyranthes root (Radix Achyranthis Bidentatae) 30. 6kg, ephedra root 10. 2kg, grassleaved sweetflag rhizome 10. 2kg, prepared licorice (Radix Glycyrrhizae Praeparata) (Radix Glycyrrhizae) 10. 2kg, sweetgum fruit 15. 3kg, red sage root (Radix Salviae Militiorrhizae) 30. 6kg, and epimedium (Herba Epimedii) 20. 4kg. All the above drugs are put together and processed into 100,000 tablets, each weighing 0. 5mg, and sealed and stored in cool place.

2. In 1990, Shui Houdi reported a controlled observation of 100 cases of non-ejaculation treated respectively with TCM drugs and western medicines. The 100 patients were divided into three groups: ① The Acupunctured Group: The patients in this group were treated with acupuncture and digital acupoint pressure, and it was further divided into two subgroups according to acupoints: the master point of the first subgroup was Dahe (KID 12) or Zhongji (REN 3), the supplementary points were Ligou (LIV 5) and Taichong (SP 3). The main acupoint of the second subgroup was Yongquan (KID 1). The supplementary points were Qugu (REN 2) and Sanyinjiao (SP 6). If erection was difficult, or if erection was possible but not hard enough, another acupoint was then added: Ciliao (BL 32). If there were symptoms of anxiety and restlessness, dream-disturbed sleep, constant dreaming, and mental stress, then the acupoints Fengchi (GB 20) and Neiguan (PC 6) should be applied. The acupoints of the two sub-groups were used alternately. Acupuncture therapy was carried out once a day with No. 30, 2 *cun* (2/3 decimeter) filiform needle inserted down 1. 2-1. 8 *cun* (0. 4-0. 6 decimeters). The needling is applied to Yongquan until the whole body becomes hot and sweats a little; then the patient is told to press and move his testicles, as well as the hairy areas of both sides of the external genitals, and to use digital pressing massage on Huiyin (REN 1) twice a day, 30 minutes each time. ② The Group Medicated With TCM: With relieving spasm and removing obstruction in the channels as therapeutic principle, the doctor processed a special medicine—Paijing Wuyou San (No-Worry-Powder for Ejaculation)—whose prescription includes the same portions of pangolin scales (Squama Manitis), earthworm (Lumbricus), Chinese angelica root (Radix Angelicae Sinensis), white peony root (Radix Paeoniae), licorice

(Radix Glycyrrhizae), and 1/2 portion of centipedefern (Scolopendra). All the above drugs were ground into powder, and taking twice a day, 5g a time, after being mixed with 100ml of boiled water; or with wine first, then with boiled water. ③ The Group Treated with Western Medicine: The group was treated with urological routine treatment, including inculcation of sexual knowledge, taking sexual hormones, electromassage treatment, and intramuscular injection of strychnine or galanthamine. The patients also took ephedrine or levodopa orally, and received other specific treatments. One course of treatment of each of the above three groups was one month. The cases with no effects in one month were considered to be the failure cases. The results of the experiment, are as follows: In the acupunctured group, 25 of 30 cases were cured, causing the best curative rate of 83.3%. As for the TCM group, 17 of 30 cases were cured, leading to a curative rate of 56.7%. The result of the 40 cases in the group treated with western medicine was not good, with no effect on 35 cases, and with effect on 5 cases, causing a curative rate of 12.5%. The average curative period needed from the beginning of the treatment to the first ejaculation was 7.28 ± 4.57 days for the acupunctured group, 10.3 ± 7.01 days for the TCM group. It is one advantage of acupuncture treatment that the curative period was shorter than that of the TCM group.

3. In 1990, Wu Jinceng and others reported a clinical research on functional non-ejaculation treated with Maqian Tong Guan San (Nux-vomica Seed Powder) in 172 cases. In the medicated group with 141 cases, 130 were cured, leading to a curative rate of 92.19%. 4 cases (2.83%) were improved. 7 cases (4.96%) gained no effect. The total effective rate was 95.03%. In the control group, treated with western medicine, 10 of 31 cases were cured, causing a curative rate of 32.26%. 1 patient (3.22%) was improved. 20 patients (64.52%) had no improvement. The total effective rate was 35.48%. Nux-vomica Seed Powder includes nux-vomica seed (Semen Strychni) 0.3g, centipedefern (Scolopendra) 0.5g and borneol (Borneolum) 0.1g. The ingredients were ground into powder, and taking one and a

90

half hours before the patients went to bed. The prescription for the potions includes giant knotweed rhizome (Rhizoma Polygoni Cuspidati) 15kg, grassleaved sweetflag rhizome (Rhizoma Acori Graminei) 9kg, dried ephedra (Herba Ephedrae) 9kg, dried licorice (Radix Glycyrrhizae) 6kg and refined white sugar 15kg. The herbs were decocted to 50 cubic liters. The patients drank 50ml of the drug one hour and a half before sexual intercourse. One course of treatment was 20 days. The longest period of treatment among the cases of the treated group was 200 days. Among them, the longest continuous treatment period was 90 days. There were no side effects, but more than half of the cases of the control group had side reactions with different symptoms.

4. In 1988, Qi Guangchong and others applied electromassage to treat 50 non-ejaculation cases. The cured cases after the treatment were 34 (68%). 16 cases (32%) failed to respond to the treatment. The therapy is as follows: Stimulate strongly the sexy areas, such as the laterals above the glens penis, the meatus urinarius periphery, the frenum area of the glens penis, the middle part (near the urethra) of the penis. Patients can massage and stimulate those areas continuously, intermittently, or slidingly etc. in the most comfortable, hedonia-irritating way. Through observation, to treat nonejaculation by means of electromassage has no obvious side effects. Very few patients had glens penis hyperemia or edema due to excessively heavy pressing application of the electromassager, and these symptoms disappeared automatically in one or two days.

Oligospermia

Oligospermia refers to sperm count (density) lower than 20 millions/ml. In the past, it was believed that sperm count should not be lower than 60 milliosn/ml. In recent years, experts, both national and international, regard the sperm count 20-200 millions/ml as the normal range. If sperm count is lower than this standard, it shows that spermatogenic function of the testicles decreases remarkably, and fer-

91

tility chances are markedly reduced. TCM calls it "syndrome of less number of of spermatozoa", or "syndrome of thinness of seminal fluid", or "syndrome of cold sperm".

Sperm density influences fertility greatly, but sperm count is not constant, for under the influences of various objective factors, the same individual can show different results at a different time and in a different environment. These factors include ascetic period of time, physical condition, mental factors, good or bad rest, determination technology, etc. So generally, a final judgment can be made after 3 times of successive examination. When judging the fertility of a patient, comprehensive consideration of the indices of rate of sperm motility, sperm activity, sperm abnormality rate, so that correct conclusion can be made.

Etiology and Pathogenesis

Oligospermia belongs to the realm of Deficiency Syndrome. This disease is caused by Kidney Deficiency, and Deficiency of Qi and Blood.

• *Decline of the Kidney Yang*

Congenital defect or excessive sexual activities impairs or excessively consumes Kidney Essence. Ordinary Yang Deficiency cause decline of Fire from the Gate of Life. Or five kinds of lingering consumptive diseases and seven kinds of impairment affect the Kidney, or Kidney Yang fails to warm Spleen Yang because of insufficiency of it, and this finally leads to decline of Fire from the Gate of Life, insufficiency of Kidney Yang, the formation of Interior Cold. As a result, cold spermia, thin spermia and oligospermia are induced.

• *Excessive Consumption of the Kidney Essence*

The lingering internal impairment due to excessive sexual activity affects the Kidney, or during the latter stage of febrile diseases, the extreme Heat impairs Yin and causes excessive consumption of Kidney Essence, and this finally leads to oligospermia.

• *Deficiency of both Qi and Blood*

Insufficiency of the congenital Essence, lack of acquired Essence, or and ordinary Deficiency of both Qi and Blood or the lingering diseases cause weak body, and Deficiency of

92

both the Heart and the Spleen, thus Deficiency of Qi and Blood is caused. Therefore, Qi fails to keep normal circulation of Blood, and Blood does not form spermia, so oligospermia is induced.

Main Points of Diagnosis
1. Those who suffer from sterility after marriage and sperm count is lower than 20 millions/ml after sperm determination.
2. Those whose rate of sperm motility, sperm activity, etc. are normal or abnormal.
3. Those having symptoms of various syndromes of this and typical signs of the tongue and pulse of this disease.

Treatment Based on Syndrome Differentiation
• *Insufficiency of the Kidney Yang*
Main Symptoms and Signs: No pregnancy long after marriage, thin and cold spermia, reduced sperm number, overall physical tiredness, susceptibility to catch cold, cold limbs, soreness and weakness of lumbar area and knees, or hyposexuality, impotence, spermatorrhea, clear profuse urine, pale tongue with white coating, deep thready or deep slow pulse.
Analysis of the Symptoms and Signs: Insufficiency of Kidney Yang leads to the decline of Fire from the Gate of Life, which can't produce spermia. This is the reason of cold, reduced spermia, and sterility is caused. Because of insufficiency of Kidney Yang, astysia is caused and sexual intercourse is impossible. Therefore, hyposexuality, impotence and spermatorrhea are caused. Kidney Deficiency leads to overall physical tiredness. Yang Qi doesn't spread to the whole body; therefore, the cold limbs are caused. The waist is the place where the Kidneys are located, and the knees are linked with the Kidney, so if Deficiency of Kidney Yang happens, soreness and weakness of the waist and the knees are caused. Kidney Deficiency causes the Bladder to lose warming; as a result, clear and profuse urine is caused. Tongue and pulse conditions show the symptoms and signs of Deficiency of Kidney Yang.

93

Treatment Principles: Warming the Kidney to replenish Yang.

Prescription: Da Lao'er Wan He Yougui Wan Jiajian (Modified Bolus for Prolonging Life supplemented with Bolus for Reinforcing the Kidney Yang)

Antler glue (Colla Cornus Cervi) 9g (melted by heat), morinda root (Radix Morindae Officinalis) 9g, papermulberry fruit (Fructus Broussonetiae) 9g, aconite root (Radix Aconiti Praeparata) 6g, cinnamon bark (Cortex Cinnamomi) 6g, dodder seed (Semen Cuscutae) 9g, prepared rehmannia root (Radix Rehmanniae Praeparata) 12g, wolfberry fruit (Fructus Lycii) 15g, Chinese yam (Ehizoma Dioscoreae) 15g, eucommia bark (Cortex Eucommiae) 12g, Chinese angelica root (Radix Angelicae Sinensis) 9g, polygala root (Radix Polygalae) 6g, grassleaved sweetflag rhizome (Rhizoma Açori Graminei) 9g and common fennel (Fructus Foenicuii) 6g. The above drugs are decocted in water for oral administration, one dose per day, and successively 24-30 doses account for one course of treatment.

Analysis of the Prescription: Antler glue (Colla Cornus Cervi), morinda root (Radix Morindae Officinalis), papermulberry fruit (Fructus Broussonetiae), aconite root (Radix Aconiti Praeparata), cinnamon bark (Cortex Cinnamomi) and dodder seed (Semen Cuscutae) reinforce Kidney Yang. This is called "benefiting the source of Fire to remove Yin Cold." Prepared rehmannia root (Radix Rehmanniae Praeparata), wolfberry fruit (Fructus Lycii), Chinese yam (Ehizoma Dioscoreae), eucommia bark (Cortex Eucommiae) and Chinese angelica root (Radix Angelicae Sinensis) nourish Yin and Blood. This is called, "a best way to treat Yang is to treat Yin, then when Yang is supported by Yin, metabolism will be endless." Polygala root (Radix Polygalae), grassleaved sweetflag rhizome, common fennel (Fructus Foenicuii) induce the above drugs to reach the Kidney Channel, go through the sperm-storing organs, regulate Qi flow and remove Phlegm, remove obstruction from the orifice for discharging seminal fluid, and enhance the function of restoring the Kidney, strengthening Yang and replenishing Essence will be achieved.

94

• *Excessive Consumption of Kidney Essence*

Main Symptoms and Signs: No pregnancy long after marriage, reduced sperm number, sperma non-liquefaction, or more dead spermia, soreness and weakness of the waist and the knees, hot feeling on the palms of hands and feet, dizziness and tinnitus, dry throat and night sweating, red tongue with little or no coating, thready and rapid pulse.

Analysis of the Symptoms and Signs: The Kidney stores Essence, governs reproduction. The excessive consumption of Kidney Essence causes spermia to be reduced, and at last sterility. Flaring Fire due to Deficiency of Yin burns and impairs Kidney Essence, so seminal fluid is not liquefied and dead spermia increase. The waist holds the Kidney and the knees and is linked with the Kidney Channels. So excessive consumption of Kidney Yin causes soreness and weakness of the waist and the knees. Hyperactivity of Fire due to Deficiency of Yin causes hot feeling on palms of hands and feet. The Kidney has its specific orifice in the ears. The insufficiency of Kidney Essence causes dizziness and tinnitus. The Kidney channel links up to throat. Hyperactivity of Fire due to Yin Deficiency, causes the body fluids unable to go up; as a result, throat is dry, and the fluid is forced out. This is the reason of night sweating. Red tongue with little or no coating, thready pulse indicate Yin Deficiency, and rapid pulse suggests hyperactivity of Fire.

Treatment Principles: Nourishing the Kidney to replenish Kidney Essence.

Prescription: Jinshi Yiehua Shengjing Tang (Jin's Decoction for Replenishing Essence and Sperma Liquefaction)

Moutan bark (Cortex Moutan Radicis) 9g, wolfberry bark (Cortex Lycii Radicis) 9g, white peony root (Radix Paeoniae) 9g, dried rehmannia root (Radix Rehmanniae) 12g, ophiopogon root (Radix Ophiopogonis) 9g, scrophularia root (Radix Scrophulariae) 9g, fleece flower root (Radix Polygoni Multiflori) 15g, mulberry fruit (Fructus Mori) 15g, wolfberry fruit (Fructus Lycii) 15g, dogwood fruit (Fructus Corni) 9g, epimedium (Herba Epimedii) 15g, poria (Poria) 9g, lophatherum (Herba Lophatheri) 9g, dried oyster shell (Concha Ostreae) 30g, red sage root (Radix

95

Salviae Militiorrhizae) 30g, honeysuckle flower (Flos Lonicerae) 18g and forsythia fruit (Fructus Forsythiae) 12g. The above drugs are decocted in water for oral use, one dose per day. One course of treatment requires taking 24-30 doses successively.

Analysis of the Prescription : Moutan bark (Cortex Moutan Radicis), wolfberry bark (Cortex Lycii Radicis), white peony root (Radix Paeoniae), dried rehmannia root (Radix Rehmanniae), ophiopogon root (Radix Ophiopogonis) and scrophularia root (Radix Scrophulariae) clear Heat and cool Blood, nourish Yin and produce fluid. Fleece-flower root (Radix Polygoni Multiflori) and mulberry fruit (Fructus Mori) tonify Liver and Kidney Yin. Wolfberry fruit (Fructus Lycii) sweet in taste and neutral in nature nourishes and reinforces Kidney Essence, nourishes Yin and benefit Blood. Dogwood fruit (Fructus Corni) not only invigorates the Liver and the Kidney, but also astringes and arrests discharge, but also replenishes Yang. Epimedium (Herba Epimedii), pungent and sweet in taste and warm in nature, warms and replenishes Kidney Yang. Red sage root (Radix Salviae Militiorrhizae) promotes the circulation of Blood and removes Blood Stasis. Dried oyster shell (Concha Ostreae) soothes the Liver and checks exuberance of Yang, softens hardness and resolves lumps, astringes and arrests discharge. Poria (Poria), tasteless, reinforces the Spleen and induces diuresis. Honeysuckle flower (Flos Lonicerae) and forsythia fruit (Fructus Forsythiae) clear Heat and remove Toxins. Lophatherum removes Heat and promotes diuresis and relieves anxiety so that it offers a passage for Heat to escape. The above drugs nourish Yin and clear Heat, reinforce the Kidney and replenish Essence.

• *Deficiency of both Qi and Blood*

Main Symptoms and Signs : No pregnancy long after marriage, reduced spermia number, sallow complexion, pale nail, listlessness, palpitations and shortness of breath, pale thick tender tongue, thready and weak pulse.

Analysis of the Symptoms and Signs : The ancient doctors said, "Congenital Essence provides for acquired Essence, and acquired Essence reinforces congenital Essence." The formation of the acquired Essence depends on the congenital Essence, and the enriching of the acquired Essence relies on the congenital Essence. Because of Deficiency of Qi and Blood, the acquired Essence can not replenish the congenital Essence, so the number of spermia is reduced and sterility is caused. Deficiency of both Qi and Blood causes the body to lack nourishment of refined nutrients; as a result, the complexion is sallow, the nails are pale, listlessness and physical tiredness are caused. Deficiency of Qi and Blood also causes the Heart not to be nourished by Blood. This is the reason of palpitations and shortness of breath. Deficiency of both Qi and Blood causes pale, thick, tender tongue. Blood and Qi can not substantiate the channel passages, so the pulse is thready and weak.

Treatment Principles: Replenishing Qi and Blood.

Prescription: Heche Zhongzi Wan (Pill of Dried human placenta (Placenta Hominis) for pregnancy)

Dried human's placenta (Placenta Hominis) 15g, Chinese angelica root (Radix Angelicae Sinensis) 9g, dogwood fruit (Fructus Corni) 9g, psoralea fruit (Fructus Psoraleae) 9g, asparagus root (Radix Asparagi) 9g, dried rehmannia root (Radix Rehmanniae) 12g, ginseng (Radix Ginseng) 6g, wolfberry fruit (Fructus Lycii) 15g, dodder seed (Semen Cuscutae) 9g, prepared rehmannia root (Radix Rehmanniae Praeparata) 12g, Chinese yam (Ehizoma Dioscoreae) 15g, raspberry (Fructus Rubi) 9g, schisandrae fruit 9g, morinda root (Radix Morindae Officinalis) 9g, achyranthes root 12g, phellodendron bark (Cortex Phellodendri) 9g, poria (Poria) 9g, cynomorium 9g, bighead atractylodes rhizome (Rhizoma Atractylodis Macrocephalae) 9g, tangerine peel (Pericarpium Citri Reticulatae) 9g, eucommia bark (Cortex Eucommiae) 9g and cinnamon bark (Cortex Cinnamomi) 3g. The above drugs are decocted in water for oral administration, one dose daily. One course of treatment requires taking 24-30 doses successively.

Analysis of the Prescription: Dried human's placenta (Placenta Hominis) reinforces the Kidney and benefits Essence, replenishes Qi and nourishes Blood. Ginseng (Radix Ginseng), Bighead atractylodes rhizome (Rhizoma

Atractylodis Macrocephalae), poria (Poria), prepared rehmannia root (Radix Rehmanniae Praeparata) and Chinese angelica root (Radix Angelicae Sinensis) tonify Qi and nourish Blood. Cinnamon bark (Cortex Cinnamomi), morinda bark, psoralea fruit (Fructus Psoraleae), eucommia bark (Cortex Eucommiae), cynomorium, wolfberry fruit (Fructus Lycii), dodder seed (Semen Cuscutae) and dogwood fruit (Fructus Corni) warm the Kidney and replenish Yang, invigorate the Liver and the Kidney. Raspberry (Fructus Rubi), schisandrae fruit reinforce the Kidney to arrest spontaneous emission, benefit Qi and promote the production of the body fluids. Dried rehmannia root (Radix Rehmanniae), asparagus root (Radix Asparagi), psoralea fruit (Fructus Psoraleae) nourish Yin and promote the production of the body fluids. Chinese yam (Ehizoma Dioscoreae) invigorates the Spleen and the Kidney. Tangerine peel (Pericarpium Citri Reticulatae) promotes Qi flow, reinforces the Spleen, and removes Phlegm. Achyranthes root promotes the circulation of Blood, removes Blood Stasis, and reinforces the Liver and the Kidney. Phellodendron bark (Cortex Phellodendri) clears Heat and removes Fire. This is called the method that the congenital Essence provides for the acquired Essence and the acquired Essence nourishes the congenital Essence.

Besides the above three types, clinically, there are also Syndrome of Damp Heat in the Lower Jiao, and Syndrome of Qi Stagnation and Blood Stasis, each having its own clinical symptoms and signs. For the treatment of Damp Heat in the Lower Jiao, on the basis of using prescription of restoring the Kidney to arrest spontaneous emission or prescription of replenishing Qi and nourishing Blood, added are drugs that clear Heat, remove Toxins, cool Blood, and promote diuresis, such as rhizome of wind-weed, phellodendron bark (Cortex Phellodendri), moutan bark (Cortex Moutan Radicis), red sage root (Radix Salviae Militiorrhizae), red peony root (Radix Paeoniae Rubra), honeysuckle flower (Flos Lonicerae), forsythia fruit (Fructus Forsythiae), patrinia, dandelion herb, seven-lobed yam, coix seed, etc. For the case with accumulation of Qi and Blood Stasis, on the basis of using the prescriptions of restoring the Kidney to arrest spontaneous emission, and of replenishing Qi and Blood, added are such drugs that promote the circulation of Blood and remove Blood Stasis, benefit Yin and promote the production of spermia as moutan bark (Cortex Moutan Radicis), red sage root (Radix Salviae Militiorrhizae), red peony root (Radix Paeoniae Rubra), achyranthes root (Radix Achyranthis Bidentatae), motherwort, siberian solomonseal rhizome, dendronbium, etc. Some of the patients have no symptoms for differentiation. Sperma determination examination can be an indicator. If simple sperm count is reduced, or accompanied by lowered rate of sperm motility, and low sperm activity, it is treated by using the prescriptions for Syndrome of Deficiency of Kidney Yang and Syndrome of Deficiency of both Qi and Blood. For the case with pyocytes, red cells or accompanied by seminal fluid not liquefied, and high sperm abnormality rate, generally, they are treated according to the prescription for Damp Heat or prescription for accumulation of Qi and Blood Stasis in accordance with clinical symptoms.

Current Research

1. The article titled Use Sheng Jing Tang (Decoction for Promoting Spermiogenesis) and Yie Hua Tang (Decoction for Sperma Liquefaction) to Treat Sterility in Male reported that 151 cases with oligospermia were treated through spermatogenic decoction. The average period of treatment was 60 days. The total effective rate was 95.4%. The female pregnancy rate was 31.1%. Prescription: Wolfberry fruit (Fructus Lycii) 15g, dodder seed (Semen Cuscutae) 9g, Chinese raspberry (Fructus Rubi) 9g, schisandra fruit (Fructus Schisandrae) 9g, mulberry Fruit (Fructus Mori) 9g, Chinese angelica root (Radix Angelicae Sinensis) 12g, prepared rehmannia root (Radix Rehmanniae Praeparata) 12g, fleeceflower root (Radix Polygoni Multiflori) 15g, dangshen (Radix Codonopsis Pilosulae) 15g, astragalus root (Radix Astragali Seu Hedysari) 18g, epimedium (Herba Epimedii) 12g and tangerine peel (Pericarpium Citri Reticulatae) 9g. All the above herbal drugs were decocted in water for oral administration, one dose per day. One course of treatment

requires taking 24-30 doses of it. The whole prescription invigorates the Kidney and replenishes Essence, benefits Yin and promotes the production of body fluids and replenishes Qi and Blood as well. Besides improving sperm density, this prescription can also enhance sperm survival rate, sperm activity to the varying degree, increase sperm penetrating power, quicken sperm velocity, but on the whole, does not influence sperm abnormality rate and sperma liquefying time. Sheng Jing Tang (Decoction for Promoting Spermiogenesis) can markedly increase the testicle's weight in animal, and makes hemoglobin content increase, and prolong weight carrying fatigue swimming time of the young rats, and also it shows no effect to the weight of testicular tissues of the grown-up rat, and causes the weight of the epididymis tissues increase obviously Radioimmunoassay shows Sheng Jing Tang (Decoction for Promoting Spermiogenesis) can noticeably increase the animal's plasma testosterone content, which shows that it has the function similar to that of androgen hormone. The prescription mentioned above exerts the above functions just through the kinetogenesis toward the epididymides (Jin Weixin, etc., 1988).

2. To search for the rules of Syndrome Differentiation and treatment about sterility in male, Hunan TCM College reviewed all the related documents and data, totaled 163 pieces, of the last 10 years', selected 8, 500 sterile cases with complete data among 10, 000 cases, then generalized and analyzed systematically about them by etiological factors, Syndrome Differentiation, prescriptions which are commonly used, and administration for drugs. The analysis showed that among the cases, the proportion with sperma abnormality was the highest, up to 58.27%. This suggests that abnormal change of spermia is the main cause of sterility. The statistical result also showed that among the syndromes of sterility, Deficiency Syndrome amounted up to over half of them, in which, Kidney Deficiency was the main side, up to 40% or so. In the case with Kidney Deficiency, cases of Deficiency of Kidney Yang dominated. Especially in the syndrome of sperma quality abnormality, this inclination displayed dominantly. Of course, there were also many cas-

100

es of Excess Syndrome together with Deficiency Syndrome, with Blood Stasis and Damp Heat on two extremes. Blood Stasis was related to the Liver, and the latter is linked to the Spleen. This indicates that the affected area of male's sterility is located at the Kidney and involves the Liver and the Spleen. Kidney Deficiency is the source, and Blood Stasis, Damp Heat are the signs. The analysis of the prescriptions, the drug administration showed that no matter what prescription or drug was used, both showed a centralized inclination. Among the set prescriptions used, the total frequency of Pill of Six Ingredients Including Rehmannia (Including Kidney Qi-tonifying Pill, Pill of Anemarrhena, Phellodendron, and Rehmannia, etc.) was up to 84 times, among which, the frequency of Wuzi Yanzong Wan (Bolus of Five Seed Drugs for Pregnancy) was 42 times. As far as the inclination of the drugs used is concerned, if the frequency of 10 times is regarded as the basis, the numbers of commonly used drugs are fewer than 55 kinds. Arranged by the frequencies of the prescriptions appearing, the drugs tonifying Yang include epimedium (Herba Epimedii), dodder seed (Semen Cuscutae), antler glue (Colla Cornus Cervi), desertliving cistanche (Herba Dendrobii), curculigo rhizome (Rhizoma Curculiginis), cinnamon bark (Cortex Cinnamomi), morinda root (Radix Morindae Officinalis), aconite root (Radix Aconiti Praeparata), cynomorium (Herba cynomorii), etc. The drugs invigorating Yin are prepared rehmannia root (Radix Rehmanniae Praeparata), wolfberry fruit (Fructus Lycii), dogwood fruit (Fructus Corni), schisandra fruit (Fructus Schisandrae), raspberry (Fructus Rubi), dried rehmannia root (Radix Rehmanniae), glossy privet fruit (Fructus Ligustri), etc. Drugs invigorating the Spleen, benefiting Qi, nourishing Blood are poria (Poria), Chinese yam (Ehizoma Dioscoreae), Chinese angelica root (Radix Angelicae Sinensis), astragalus root (Radix Astragali Seu Hedysari), bighead atractylodes rhizome (Rhizoma Atractylodis Macrocephalae), white peony root (Radix Paeoniae), etc. Drugs removing Blood Stasis are moutan bark (Cortex Moutan Radicis), safflower (Flos Carthami), sweetgum fruit (Fructus Liquidambaris), red sage root

(Radix Salviae Militiorrhizae), red peony root (Radix Paeoniae Rubra), peach kernel (Semen Persicae), etc. Tasteless diuretics are Alismaceae (Rhizoma Alismatis), coix-seed and Caulis clematidis armandii (Caulis Akebiae). Drugs removing Damp Heat in the Lower Jiao are phellodendron bark (Cortex Phellodendri), rhizome of wind-weed (Rhizoma Anemarrhenae), gentian root (Radix Gentianae), capejasmine (Fructus Gardeniae), etc. (Li Biao, etc., 1988).

3. Hebei Provincial Hospital researched the mechanism of the drugs invigorating the Kidney and replenishing Yang in the treatment of sterility. It collected 110 papers about Chinese herbs treating sterility, in which 78% of them used the method of invigorating the Kidney, and 22% used other methods. Among 500 cases of sterility treated, 80% of them suffered from Kidney Deficiency. 72% of them were given the drugs that reinforce the Kidney and replenish Yang. The curative effects were fine. The determination of zinc level in seminal serum provides the needed basis for the diagnosis of sterility. The seminal serum zinc level of the sterile patients was lower than that of the normal group. After using drugs restoring the Kidney and invigorating Yang, zinc level increased compared with that before treatment. Sperm density, sperm survival rate, and sperm activity improved remarkably. The determination of zinc, manganese contents showed that the content of zinc in dodder seed (Semen Cuscutae), morinda root (Radix Morindae Officinalis), curculigo rhizome (Rhizoma Curculiginis), flatstem milkvetch seed (Semen Astragali Complanati), etc. is high and epimedium (Herba Epimedii), morinda root (Radix Morindae Officinalis), flatstem milkvetch seed (Semen Astragali Complanatus), desertliving cistanche (Herba Dendrobii) contain much manganese. The experiments of the effects of the drugs restoring the Kidney and invigorating Yang on hypophysis sexual gland axis proved that morinda root (Radix Morindae Officinalis), curculigo rhizome (Rhizoma Curculiginis), desertliving cistanche (Herba Dendrobii), wolfberry fruit (Fructus Lycii), Chinese angelica root (Radix Angelicae Sinensis), obviously influence the weight of hypophysis, with that of Chinese angelica root (Radix Angelicae Sinen-

sis) being the greatest. Dodder seed (Semen Cuscutae), epimedium (Herba Epimedii), morinda root (Radix Morindae Officinalis), curculigo rhizome (Rhizoma Curculiginis), flatstem milkvetch seed Semen Astragali Complanati), desertliving cistanche (Herba Dendrobii), wolfberry fruit (Fructus Lycii), Chinese angelica root (Radix Angelicae Sinensis) show effects on prostate, with that of dodder seed (Semen Cuscutae), wolfberry fruit (Fructus Lycii), curculigo rhizome (Rhizoma Curculiginis) being the greatest. Dodder seed (Semen Cuscutae), epimedium (Herba Epimedii), flatstem milkvetch seed (Semen Astragali Complanati), desertliving cistanche (Herba Dendrobii), wolfberry fruit (Fructus Lycii), Chinese angelica root (Radix Angelicae Sinensis) also show effects upon seminal vesicle. These eight drugs show less obvious influence on rat's testicles (Guo Lianshu, 1988).

4. Jiangsu Provincial TCM Hospital treated the sterile cases with sperma abnormality with Jujing Tang (Decoction for Collecting Essence) that reinforces both the Spleen and the Kidney according to theory, "The congenital Essence nourishes the acquired Essence, and the acquired Essence provides for the congenital Essence." The cure effect was quite good. The essential drugs in the prescription are rehmannia root, wolfberry fruit (Fructus Lycii), fleece-flower root (Radix Polygoni Multiflori), dried human's placenta (Placenta Hominis), epimedium (Herba Epimedii), flatstem milvetch seed (Semen Astragali Complanati), poria (Poria), siberian solomonseal rhizome (Rhizoma Polygonati), coix seed (Semen Coicis), etc. The prescription is modified according to different Syndrome types. For the case with Yin Deficiency, tortoise Plastron (Plastrum Testudinis), rhizome of wind-weed (Rhizoma Anemarrhenae) are added; Yang Deficiency, antler glue (Colla Cornus Cervi) and cynomorium (Herba Cynomorii); Spleen Deficiency, poria (Poria) and Chinese yam (Ehizoma Dioscoreae); Qi Deficiency, dangshen (Radix Codonopsis Pilosulae) and astragalus rhizome (Radix Astragali Seu Hedysari); Blood Deficiency, white peony root (Radix Paeoniae), and donkeyhide gelatin (Colla Corii Asini); blood loss, glossy privet

fruit (Fructus Ligustri) and eclipta (Herba Ecliptae); hyperactivity of Liver Yang, abalone shell (Concha Haliotidis) and gastrodia tuber (Rhizoma Gastrodiae); the stagnation of Liver Qi, cyperus tuber (Rhizoma Cuperi) and curcuma root (Radix Curcumae). The prescription is also modified according to symptoms: For the case with thin seminal fluid and reduced sperma and sperm number, air bladder glue of fish is added, to invigorate the Kidney and replenish Essence; low rate of sperm motility and weak sperm activity, Wuzi Bushen Wan (Bolus of Five Seed Drugs for Restoring the Kidney) to reinforce both Yang and Yin; the increase of seminal fluid volume, high adhesion of seminal fluid, and non-liquefaction of sperma, myrobalan, black plum, licorice (Radix Glycyrrhizae) sweet and sour in taste to promote Yin-transmission; high sperm abnormality rate and with pyoctes, ailanthus bark, Bi Yu San (Green Jade Powder) to remove Damp Heat. The author systematically treated and observed 82 cases of sterility with sperma abnormality. The total effective rate was 85.4% and the recovery rate was 58.6% (Xu Fusong, 1989).

Azoospermia

If several times of sperma examination (usually more than 3 times) find no spermia, this is called azoospermia, which is clinically divided into true azoospermia and pseudo azoospermia. The former refers to that the testicles can not produce spermia, and the latter to that the testis can produce spermia, but they can not flow out because of obstruction in spermatic duct. If fructose can be determined in seminal serum, it means that ejaculatory duct is patent or seminal vesicle still can function, but the possibility of obstruction in other areas of the spermia passage, and scrotum examination and vasography should be done. After contrast examination, if the lumen is unobstructive, spermia can be seen under microscope after puncturing the material in the Interior of epididymides, it suggests that obstruction occurs at the epididymides, then, epididymides-spermatic duct anastomosis is carried out. If there is no obstruction in the epididymides, then, pathologic change occurs at testicles. Determination of plasma FSH shows it is obviously higher than the normal value, which indirectly suggests severe impairment of testicular convoluted seminiferous tubule. Only after FSH increases does it need to determine plasma LH and testosterone. If sperma pH is lower than 7.5, and fructose negative, it suggests seminal vesicle defect or hypodevelopment of ejaculatory duct.

Patients with azoospermia should undergo testicular pathological examination, spermatic duct contrast, immunoassay of endocrine hormone, sperma biochemical examination, etc. For those whose testicles do lose their spermatogenic function and genital duct is congenitally abnormal, drug treatment is not given. If testicles do have certain spermatogenic function, then, Syndrome Differentiation and treatment are conducted in accordance with the treatment of azoospermia. For those patients with no syndromes for differentiation, the method of azoospermia treatment is applied.

Drum-Tower Hospital of Beijing divided azoospermia into Deficiency of Vital Essence and Energy, Deficiency of Yin and Essence and Damp Heat according to theory of Syndrome Differentiation. 66 cases were treated with Sheng Jing Zan Yu Wan (Pill for Spermatogeny and Supporting Fertility). 4 cases were cured, 6 gained effects, and 37 gained obvious effects, and 19 failed to be cured. The total effective rate was 71.2%. The prescription includes essentially the following drugs: Epimedium (Herba Epimedii), desertliving cistanche (Herba Dendrobii), curculigo rhizome (Rhizoma Curculiginis) and wolfberry fruit (Fructus Lycii). For the case with insufficiency of Vital Qi, aconite root (Radix Aconiti Praeparata), cinnamon bark (Cortex Cinnamomi), morinda root (Radix Morindae Officinalis) and dodder seed (Semen Cuscutae) are added. For the case with Yin and Essence insufficiency, prepared fleece-flower root (Radix Polygoni Multiflori Praeparata), prepared rehmannia root (Radix Rehmanniae Praeparata), glossy privet fruit (Fructus Ligustri) and rhizome of wind-weed (Rhizoma Anemar-

105

rhenae) are added. For the case with Damp Heat in the semem-storing organs, phellodendron bark (Cortex Phellodendri), rhizome of wind-weed (Rhizoma Anemarrhenae), gentian root (Radix Gentianae) and wild chrysanthemum flower (Flos Chrysan-themi Indici) are added. For the case with obstruction in the channels, peach kernel (Semen Persicae), safflower (Flos Carthami), red sage root (Radix Salviae Militiorrhizae) and tail of Chinese angelica root (Radix Angelicae Sinensis) are added (Chen Wenbo, 1987).

Syndrome of Too Many Dead Spermia

If sperma assay shows that the number of dead spermia is over 40%, it is regarded as "syndrome of too many dead spermia". Sperm activity is closely related to seminal serum quality. Seminal serum is made of the combined secretion from seminal vesicles, epididymides, prostate, bulbourethral gland, and paraurethral duct. It is not only the transmitter to transport spermia but also contains the essential substances that maintain spermia survival and stimulate spermia activity. It is believed that fructose content in seminal serum is even closely related to sperm activity. TCM holds that this disease is caused by congenital defect or weak body after disease or excessive sexual intercourse or overeating.

Etiology and Pathogenesis
1. Insufficiency of congenital Essence or weak body after illness results in insufficiency of Kidney Qi. Therefore, Essence has nothing for nourishment, which leads to weak Vital Essence and Energy, and finally to syndrome of too many dead spermia.
2. Excessive sexual intercourse, frequent masturbation result in impairment and excessive consumption of Kidney Essence, hyperactivity of Fire which burns and impairs spermia. Finally, it leads to this disease.
3. Overeating, or addiction to food hot, pungent in taste results in production of Damp Heat in the Interior. The

106

Damp Heat steams the semen-storing organs, and this impairs the spermia, and syndrome of too many dead spermia is caused.

Main Points of Diagnosis
The number of dead spermia being over 40% after seminal assay is the main basis in the diagnosis of this disease. At the same time, the disease is complicated with low sperm activity, high sperm abnormality rate. The results of other assay items can be normal or abnormal. There may be white cells, pyocytes or red cells. Clinical manifestations are not the same. Part of patients also have testitis, epididymitis, prostatitis or seminal vesiculitis. Some patients have no clinical symptoms at all.

Treatment Based on Syndrome Differentiation
• *Insufficiency of Kidney Qi*
Main Symptoms and Signs: Seminal assay shows the number of dead spermia is over 40%. Many are accompanied by low sperm activity, high sperm abnormality rate, or by hyposexuality, impotence, prospermia, cold limbs, aversion to cold, sallow complexion, pale tongue with white coating and deep thready pulse.

Analysis of the Symptoms and Signs: Deficiency of Kidney Qi causes Essence to fail to be nourished, so there is little and feeble Vital Essence and Energy, and the number of dead spermia increases. Insufficiency of Kidney Yang causes hyposexuality, impotence, premature ejaculation, cold limbs and aversion to cold and sallow complexion. Tongue and pulse conditions reflect the signs of insufficiency of Kidney Qi.

Treatment Principles: Warming the Kideny and replenishing Kidney Qi.

Prescription: Wuzi Yanzong Wan Jiawei (Modified Bolus of Five Seed Drugs for Pregnancy)

Wolfberry fruit (Fructus Lycii) 9g, dodder seed (Semen Cuscutae) 9g, raspberry (Fructus Rubi) 9g, plantain seed (Semen Plantaginis) (wrapped) 9g, schisandra fruit (Fructus Schisandrae) 9g, epimedium (Herba Epimedii) 15g,

107

morinda root (Radix Morindae Officinalis) 9g, prepared a-conite root (Radix Aconiti Praeparata) 3-6g, cinnamon bark (Cortex Cinnamomi) 3-6g, tangerine peel (Pericarpium Citri Reticulatae) 9g, dangshen (Radix Codonopsis Pilosulae) 18g and astragalus rhizome (Radix Astragali Seu Hedysari) 30g. The above drugs are decocted in water for oral administration, one dose daily. One course of treatment needs 24-30 doses.

Analysis of the Prescription: This prescription warms and restores Kidney Qi. Epimedium (Herba Epimedii), morinda root (Radix Morindae Officinalis), prepared aconite root (Radix Aconiti Praeparata) and cinnamon bark (Cortex Cinnamomi) warm and invigorate Kidney Yang, activate the flow of Kidney Qi and spermia finally. Dangshen (Radix Codonopsis Pilosulae) and astragalus rhizome (Radix Astragali Seu Hedysari) replenish Qi and reinforce the Spleen to strengthen sperm activity. Tangerine peel (Pericarpium Citri Reticulatae) regulates Qi flow and stomach function, and remove Phlegm. The whole prescription warms and restores Kidney Qi, activates the spermia and increases spermia activity, and reduces the number of the dead spermia.

• *Hyperactivity of Fire due to Deficiency of Yin*

Main Symptoms and Signs: Seminal assay shows that the number of dead spermia is over 40%, or the number of abnormal spermia increases, or accompanied by hypersexuality, or nocturnal emission, blood spermia, frequent micturation, urgent micturation, pain from urination, dragging pain in perineum area, dizziness and tinnitus, soreness and weakness in the waist and the knees, dysphoria with feverish sensation in chest, palms and soles, dry mouth and sore throat, red tongue with little or no coating, thready and rapid pulse.

Analysis of the Symptoms and Signs: Impairment and excessive consumption of Kidney Essence causes hyperactivity of Fire due to Deficiency of Yin. The Fire burns spermia and causes the dead spermia or abnormal spermia to increase. Hyperactivity of the Ministerial Fire causes hypersexuality. The Heat burns seminal fluid, which is forced to flow out and causes nocturnal emission. The Fire burns the sperm-storing organs, and it impairs Blood Vessels and it causes blood spermia. The Fire disturbs perineum, so it causes pain with dragging feeling in that area. The Heat moves to the small intestines; that causes frequent micturation, urgent micturation, pain from urination. Dizziness, tinnitus, soreness and weakness of the waist and the knees suggest Kidney Deficiency. Dysphoria with feverish sensation in chest, palms and soles, dry mouth, and sore throat suggest Yin Deficiency. Tongue and pulse conditions display the signs of hyperactivity of Fire coming from Yin Deficiency.

Treatment Principles: Nourishing Yin to reduce Fire.

Prescription: Zhibo Dihuang Tang Jiajian (Modified Decoction of Anemarrhena, Phellodendron and Rehmannia)

Rhizome of wind-weed (Rhizoma Anemarrhenae) 9g, phellodendron bark (Cortex Phellodendri) 9g, dried rehmannia root (Radix Rehmanniae) 12g, moutan bark (Cortex Moutan Radicis) 9g, Alismaceae (Rhizoma Alismatis) 9g, dandelion herb (Herba Taraxaci) 15g, honeysuckle flower (Flos Lonicerae) 24g, poria (Poria) 15g, Herba Paris Polyphyllae 9g and dried licorice (Radix Glycyrrhizae) 6g. The above drugs are decocted in water for oral administration, one dose daily. One course of treatment requires 24-30 doses.

Analysis of the Prescription: Rhizome of wind-weed (Rhizoma Anemarrhenae), phellodendron bark (Cortex Phellodendri) remove Deficiency Fire from the Kidney. Alismaceae (Rhizoma Alismatis) promotes diuresis and clear Heat. Dandelion herb, honeysuckle flower (Flos Lonicerae), poria (Poria), Herba Paris Polyphyllae clear Heat and remove Toxins. Licorice (Radix Glycyrrhizae) clears Heat and removes Toxins, coordinates the effects of all the drugs. The whole prescription nourishes Yin, reduces Fire and removes Toxins, and reduces the number of dead spermia, and enhances spermia activity.

• *Accumulation of Heat in the Interior*

Main Symptoms and Signs: Seminal assay shows that the number of dead spermia is over 40%, or it is accompanied by the increase of abnormal spermia, or impotence and prospermia, fullness of chest, poor appetite and poor digestion, greasy feeling in the mouth, difficult stool, red tongue with yellowish and greasy coating, slippery and rapid pulse.

Analysis of the Symptoms and Signs: Damp Heat steams the sperm-storing organs. This impairs the spermia; as a result, the numbers of dead spermia and abnormal spermia increase. The downward flow of Damp Heat makes urogenital region relax. This causes impotence. Damp Heat force the spermia flow outwards, or premature ejaculation is caused. Restlessness and fullness in chest and stomach, poor appetite and poor digestion, sticky greasy mouth, retention of feces are symptoms of Damp Heat in the Spleen and the Stomach. Red tongue with yellow and greasy tongue coating, slippery and rapid pulse are signs of accumulation of Damp Heat in the Interior.

Treatment Principles: Removing Heat and eliminating Damp.

Prescription: Zini Qingre Huashi Tang (Self-made Decoction for Removing Heat and Eliminating Damp)

Poria (Poria) 15g, Herba Paris Polyphyllae 9g, scutellaria root (Radix Scutellariae) 9g, coptis root (Rhizoma Coptidis) 3g, phellodendron bark (Cortex Phellodendri) 6g, plantain seed (Semen Plantaginis) (wrapped) 15g, dried rehmannia root (Radix Rehmanniae) 12g, moutan bark (Cortex Moutan Radicis) 9g, epimedium (Herba Epimedii) 12g, morinda root (Radix Morindae Officinalis) 9g, dodder seed (Semen Cuscutae) 9g, tangerine peel (Pericarpium Citri Reticulatae) 9g and dried licorice (Radix Glycyrrhizae) 6g. The above drugs are decocted in water for oral administration, one dose daily, and one course of treatment requires taking 24-30 doses successively.

Analysis of the Prescription: Poria (Poria), Herba Paris Polyphyllae, scutellaria root (Radix Scutellariae), coptis root (Rhizoma Coptidis), phellodendron bark (Cortex Phellodendri), plantain seed (Semen Plantaginis) clear Heat and remove Toxins, promote diuresis and purge Fire. Dried rehmannia root (Radix Rehmanniae), moutan bark (Cortex Moutan Radicis) nourish Yin, clear Heat and cool Blood. Epimedium (Herba Epimedii), morinda and dodder seed (Semen Cuscutae) invigorate the Kidney and replenish

110

Essence to prosper spermia. Dried licorice (Radix Glycyrrhizae) clears Heat, removes Toxins, coordinates the effects of all the drugs. The prescription as a whole clears Heat, eliminates Damp, invigorates the Kidney, replenishes Essence, removes dead spermia and produces survival spermia.

Current Research

1. According to clinical observation of 182 cases of the with syndrome of too many dead spermia treated with Yishen Zhuangjing Tang (Self-made Decoction for Benefiting the Kidney and Replenishing Essence), taken one dose per day, and 30 days making up a course of treatment. After clinical treatment for 3 course of treatment, 67 cases were cured, and 57 gained effects, and 36 responded markedly to the treatment, and 22 failed to be cured. The total effective rate was 87.9%. Prescription: Epimedium (Herba Epimedii) 15g, dodder seed (Semen Cuscutae) 12g, atractylodes rhizome (Rhizoma Atractylodis) 15g, prepared rehmannia root (Radix Rehmanniae Praeparata) 30g, Chinese angelica root (Radix Angelicae Sinensis) 12g, peach kernel (Semen Persicae) 9g, safflower (Flos Carthami) 6g and chuanxiong rhizome (Rhizoma Ligustici Chuangxiong) 6g. For the case with Kidney Deficiency, prepared fleece-flower root (Radix Polygoni Multiflori) and cynomorium (Herba Cynomorii) are added. For the case with Qi Deficiency, dangshen (Radix Codonopsis Pilosulae) and Chinese yam (Ehizoma Dioscoreae) are added. For the case with severe Blood Stasis, zedoary (Rhizoma Zedoariae) and burreed tuber (Rhizoma Sparganii) are added (Ou Chun, 1990).

2. According to observation of 300 cases with syndrome of too many dead spermia treated with Zini Yinyanghuo Tang (Self-made Epimedium (Herba Epimedii) Decoction), after the treatment, 120 patients (40%) became pregnant, 140 (46.6%) responded effectively to the treatment, and 40 (13.3%) failed to be cured. The total effective rate was 86.7%. Prescription: Epimedium (Herba Epimedii) 30g, desertliving cistanche (Herba Dendrobii) 15g, dodder seed (Semen Cuscutae) 30g, glossy privet fruit (Fructus Ligustri) 15g,

wolfberry fruit (Fructus Lycii) 15g, prepared fleece-flower root (Radix Polygoni Multiflori) 20g, white peony root (Radix Paeoniae) 15g, astragalus rhizome 15g, Chinese angelica root (Radix Angelicae Sinensis) 20g, dogwood fruit (Fructus Corni) 15g, dipsacus root (Radix Dipsaci) 20g, eclipta (Herba Ecliptae) 15g, plantain seed (Semen Plantaginis) (wrapped) 30g and licorice (Radix Glycyrrhizae) 6g. The above drugs were decocted in water for 2 times, and 500ml decoction should be obtained each time. The two decoctions were mixed together. The liquid was divided into two parts, and drunk in the morning and at night respectively. One dose was for each day. One course of treatment needed 30 doses. Modification: For the case accompanied by unconsolidation of the gate ejaculation, nocturnal emission, spermatorrhea, premature ejaculation, added were desertliving cistanche (Herba Dendrobii) plus cynomorrium (Herba Cynomorii), gordon euryale seed (Semen Euryales), Cherokee rose-hip (Fructus Rosae Laevigatae); for the case with impotence, psoralea fruit (Fructus Psoraleae), morinda root (Radix Morindae Officinalis), walnut kernel (Semen Juglandis), pilose antler (Cornu Cervi Pantotrichum); for the case with azoospermia, poor sperm activity, dried human's placenta (Placenta Hominis), antler glue (Colla Cornus Cervi), tortoise-plastron glue (Colla Plastri Testudinis), etc.; for the case of Qi Deficiency, astragalus rhizome (Radis Astragali Seu Hedysari), stir-fried bighead atractylodes rhizome (Rhizoma Atractylodis Macrocephalae), poria (Poria); for the case accompanied by prostatitis, seminal vesiculitis, honeysuckle flower (Flos Lonicerae), rhizome of wind-weed (Rhizoma Anemarrhenae), phellodendron bark (Cortex Phellodendri), dandelion herb (Herba Taraxaci) (Zhou Hong, 1990).

3. 31 cases with low spermia activity were treated with Zini Zujing Tang (Self-Made Spermia-Strengthening Decoction). Prescription: Dodder seed (Semen Cuscutae) 12g, wolfberry fruit (Fructus Lycii) 10g, mulberry (Fructus Mori) 12g, raspberry (Fructus Rubi) 12g, plantain seed (Semen Plantaginis) (wrapped) 12g, schisandra fruit (Fructus Schisandrae) 12g, curculigo rhizome (Rhizoma Curculigi-

112

nis) 15g, epimedium (Herba Epimedii) 15g, astragalus rhizome (Radix Astragali Seu Hedysari) 30g, prepared rehmannia root (Radix Rehmanniae Praeparata) 30g, glossy privet fruit (Fructus Ligustri) 12g, dipsacus root (Radix Dipsaci) 18g, Chinese angelica root (Radix Angelicae Sinensis) 15g, dangshen (Radix Codonopsis Pilosulae) 30g and two goat's testicles. Modifications: For the case with few spermia, siberian solomonseal rhizome (Rhizoma Polygonati) and fleece-flower root (Radix Polygoni Multiflori) are added; for the case with high sperm abnormality rate, honeysuckle flower (Flos Lonicerae) and forsythia fruit (Fructus Forsythiae) are added; for the case with spermia non-liquefaction, or poor liquefaction, red sage root (Radix Salviae Militiorrhizae) and achyranthes root (Radix Achyranthis Bidentatae) are added; for the case with Deficiency of Kidney Yang, aconite root (Radix Aconiti Praeparata) and cinnamon bark (Cortex Cinnamomi) are added; for the case with Deficiency of Kidney Yin, dogwood fruit (Fructus Corni) is added. For the case of Blood Deficiency, donkeyhide gelatin is added; for the case of Qi Deficiency, Chinese yam (Ehizoma Dioscoreae) and bighead atractylodes rhizome (Rhizoma Atractylodis Macrocephalae) are added. The above drugs are decocted in water for oral administration, one dose per day. One month accounted for one course of treatment. 19 were cured, and seven gained effects, and five failed to be treated. The shortest period of time was one course of treatment, and the longest was four courses of treatment, averaged 2.6 courses of treatment (Yang Jiping, 1990).

Non-liquefaction of Seminal Fluid

When freshly ejaculated, the seminal fluid does not liquefy within 60 minutes or still contains non-liquefying coagula after 60 minutes at room temperature, it is called the syndrome of non-liquefaction of seminal fluid. Non-liquefaction of seminal fluid is one of the common causes that lead to sterility and accounts for approximately 2.1-42.56% of the

113

causes of sterility on the ground of statistics. This abnormal delay of liquefying process results in sterility because it causes the spermatozoa to agglutinate or immobilize, thus decelarating or restraining the normal flow of spermatozoa through the uterus neck, which finally leads to sterility. At present, a great difference exists between different regions in diagnosing non-liquefaction of seminal fluid because of having no objective standards in observing and judging the seminal viscosity and the time concerning liquefaction of seminal fluid.

Modern medicine holds that the liquefying substances of ejaculation originate from the secretory juice of prostate and bulbourethral glands. If these accessory glands get infected, it may lead to partial or complete non-liquefaction of seminal fluid. The statistics taken by some people shows 90% of the patients with non-liquefaction of semen suffer from from prostatitis while about 12% of patients with prostatitis have syndrome of non-liquefaction of semen. TCM does not have similar account of non-liquefaction of seminal fluid, but it is more or less related to stranguria with turbid urine, cold semen and warm semen.

Etiology and Pathogenesis
1. Excessive sexual intercourse may give rise to Yin Deficiency and Excess Fire which heats the semen, thus making it thicker and difficult to liquefy.
2. Constitutional insufficiency of Kidney Yang leads to Deficiency Coldof the uterus. So, Yang is unable to resolve Yin, thus causing non-liquefaction of semen.
3. The downward flow of Damp Heat blocks the Yang channel, which causes seminal fluid and turbid discharges to mix up, thus producing non-liquefaction of semen.

Main Points of Diagnosis
Normal semen is an even mobile liquid in which there are no fibers when pushed up or there are a few fibers which break up as soon as they are pushed up. If the semen does not liquefy, it must be thick and viscous, containing gel-like structures, or occasionally appearing as flakes and lumps,

114

and does not liquefy after being ejaculated for over an hour. The observation concerning the time of liquefaction must be done by fixed personnel at regular times and under fixed temperature and the correctness of the diagnosis should also be emphasized.

Treatment Based on Syndrome Differentiation
  • *Impairment of Kidney Yin*
  Main Symptoms and Signs: No pregnancy long after marriage, viscous semen that does not liquefy, the number of spermatozoa and their survival rate and mobility being normal or abnormal, dizziness, tinnitus, flaccidity of lumbar area and legs, dysphoria with feverish sensation in chest, palms and soles, dry mouth, night sweating, insomnia, forgetfulness, hypersexuality, red tongue with slight or no coating on it, thready and rapid pulse.

  Analysis of the Symptoms and Signs: Since the Kidney stores reproductive Essence and, dominates reproduction, insufficiency of Kidney Essence may cause abnormal and eventually lead to sterility. Yin Deficiency producing deficient Fire, burning Kidney Essence to be thicker with difficulty to liquefy. Kidney Deficiency leads to insufficiency of the Sea of Marrow, causing poor nourishment of the brain, thus dizziness and tinnitus occur. Since the lumbar area is the place where the Kidney is located, and the knees are linked with the Kidney, impairment of Kidney Yin will cause the lumbar area to have nothing for nourishment, and the lassitude results. Yin Deficiency producing deficient Heat may give rise to dysphoria with feverish sensation in chest, palms and soles, insomnia, amnesia and hypersexuality. As the Kidney Channel goes up as far as the throat, pharynx and larynx, Yin Deficiency producing excessive Heat will cause the body fluids to fail to be carriedup, thus dry mouth occurs. If the body fluids is discharged by force, night sweating results. Red tongue with slight coating on it and thready pulse are the signs of Deficiency of Yin, and rapid pulse is the sign of excessive Interior Heat.

  Treatment Principles: Nourishing Yin by purging the pathogenic Fire.

115

Prescription: Yiehua Tang (Decoction for Semen Liquefaction)

Anemarrhena rhizome (Rhizoma Anemarrhenae) 9g, phellodendron bark (Cortex Phellodendri) 9g, dried rehmannia
root (Radix Rehmanniae) 12g, red sage root (Radix Salviae
Militiorrhizae) 30g, red peony root (Radix Paeoniae Rubra)
9g, ophiopogon root (Radix Ophiopogonis) 9g, trichosanthes root (Radix Trichosanthis) 9g, white peony root (Radix
Paeoniae) 9g, plantain herb (Herba Plantaginis) 15g, scrophularia root (Radix Scrophulariae) 9g, prepared rehmannia
root (Radix Rehmanniae Praeparata) 12g, wolfberry fruit
(Fructus Lycii) 15g, epimedium (Herba Epimedii) 15g and
lophatherum (Herba Lophatheri) 9g. All the above drugs are
decocted in water for oral administration, taken one dose
per day and continuously for 24-30 days accounting for one
course of treatment.

Analysis of the Prescription: In the prescription, anemar-
rhena rhizome (Rhizoma Anemarrhenae), phellodendron
bark (Cortex Phellodendri) and dried rehmannia root (Radix
Rehmanniae) nourish Yin and clear Heat. Red sage root
(Radix Salviae Militiorrhizae) and red peony root (Radix
Paeoniae Rubra) promote Blood circulation to remove Blood
Stasis. Ophiopogon root (Radix Ophiopogonis), trichosanthes root (Radix Trichosanthis) and white peony root (Radix
Paeoniae) increase the body fluids. Plantain herb (Herba
Plantaginis) and scrophularia root (Radix Scrophulariae)
clear Heat and Toxins, replenish Yin to increase the formation of body fluids. Prepared rehmannia root (Radix
Rehmanniae Praeparata) and wolfberry fruit (Fructus Lycii)
restore the Kidney and strengthen Essence, nourish Yin and
benefit Blood. Epimedium (Herba Epimedii) restores Yang
for warming and resolving and has gonadotropic function.
Lophatherum (Herba Lophatheri) clears Heat and relieves
restlessness, thus purging Interior Heat. As a whole, the
prescription has the effects of nourishing Yin, purging
pathogenic Heat, clearing Heat, and promoting the production of body fluids as well as replenishing Essence and Blood
to promote liquefaction of semen.

• *Insufficiency of Kidney Yang*

116

Main Symptoms and Signs: Cold semen and sterility, viscous semen that does not liquefy, the number of spermatozoa, the survival rate and mobility being normal or abnormal, impotence and premature ejaculation, flaccidity of lumbar area and legs, aversion to cold, polyuria at night, profuse urination not scanty in amount, pale tongue with thin white coating, thready and weak pulse.

Analysis of the Symptoms and Signs: Insufficiency of Kidney Yang gives rise to cold sperma and sterility. Yang Deficiency can not revolve Yin, so semen becomes viscous and does not liquefy. Yin Deficiency makes penis fail to erect, thus impotence, and the failure of reinforcement and astringency of the Kidney results in premature ejaculation. Deficiency of Yang cannot warm the body, so aversion to cold arises. It cannot warm the reproductive organs, so scrotum and testicles feel cold. Kidney Deficiency causes the Bladder to lose its control function, thus polyuria at night and micturation with clear urine not scanty in amount result. Light tongue with thin white coating on it, and thready weak pulse are all the signs of insufficiency of Kidney Yang.

Treatment Principles: Replenishing Essence and Qi; warming the Kidney and dispelling Cold.

Prescription: Shengjing Tang Jiawei (Modified Decoction for Promoting Generation of Vital Essence)

Epimedium (Herba Epimedii) 15g, dipsacus root (Radix Dipsaci) 15g, prepared rehmannia root (Radix Rehmanniae Praeparata) 12g, fleece-flower root 15g, mulberry (Fructus Mori) 15g, pilose asiabell root (Radix Codonopsis Pilosulae) 15g, astragalus root (Radix Astragali Seu Hedysari) 18g, Chinese angelica root (Radix Angelicae Sinensis) 9g, raspberry (Fructus Rubi) 9g, schisandra fruit (Fructus Schisandrae) 9g, wolfberry fruit (Fructus Lycii) 15g, dodder seed (Semen Cuscutae) 9g, tangerine peel (Pericarpium Citri Reticulatae) 9g, plantain seed (Semen Plantaginis) (wrapped) 9g, morinda root (Radix Morindae Officinalis) 9g, prepared aconite root (Radix Aconiti Praeparata) 3-6g, lindera root (Radix Linderae) 6g, common fennel fruit (Fructus Foeniculi) 6g and evodia fruit (Fructus Evodiae) 9g. All the above drugs are decocted in water for oral ad-

117

ministration, one dose daily, and one course of treatment requiring taking it successively for 24-30 doses.

Analysis of the Prescription: In the prescription, epimedium (Herba Epimedii) and dipsacus root (Radix Dipsaci) warm the Kidney to invigorate Yang, promote the formation of Kidney Yang. Prepared rehmannia root (Radix Rehmanniae Praeparata), fleece-flower root, mulberry (Fructus Mori) tonify and nourish Kidney Yin and the Liver Yin. Pilose asiabell root (Radix Codonopsis Pilosulae) and astragalus root (Radix Astragali Seu Hedysari) invigorate Qi and enrich Blood. Chinese angelica root (Radix Angelicae Sinensis) nourishes Blood and promotes the circulation of Blood. The combination of Chinese angelica root (Radix Angelicae Sinensis) and astragalus root (Radix Astragali Seu Hedysari) makes a decoction for nourishing Blood. Since Essence and Blood have a common source, Vital Essence is replenished while Blood is being enriched. Raspberry (Fructus Rubi) and schisandra fruit (Fructus Schisandrae) reinforce the Kidney, control nocturnal emission, supplement Qi and promote the production of body fluids. Wolfberry fruit (Fructus Lycii) replenishes Kidney Essence, nourishes Yin and Blood. Dodder seed (Semen Cuscutae) not only replenishes Yin but also strengthens Yang Qi. It warms but not causes Dryness, nourishes but not causes stagnation. Together with tangerine peel (Pericarpium Citri Reticulatae), it promotes the flow of Qi, strengthens the Spleen and reduces Phlegm; and with plantain seed (Semen Plantaginis) (wrapped), it clears Deficiency Fire in the Kidney. As a whole, the prescription replenishes Essence and restores the Kidney, tonifies and nourishes Yin, promotes the production of body fluids, as well as invigorates Qi and enriches Blood. In addition, with morinda root (Radix Morindae Officinalis), prepared aconite root (Radix Aconiti Praeparata) and lindera root (Radix Linderae), it warms the Kidney to strengthen Yang, with common fennel fruit (Fructus Foeniculi) and evodia fruit (Fructus Evodiae), it promotes the flow of Qi, warms the Middle Jiao and Kidney Yang to warm up the semen.

• *Downward Flow of Damp Heat*

118

Main Symptoms and Signs: No pregnancy long after marriage, viscous semen that does not liquefy, the number of spermatozoa, their survival rate and motility being normal or abnormal, ejaculate with pyocytes, white blood cells, burning sensation, difficulty and pain in micturation, frequent and dribbling urination, yellow-red turbid urine, even hematuria or contracture of lower abdomen, physical fatigue and somnolence, yellow or curdy tongue coating, soft or slippery rapid pulse.

Analysis of the Symptoms and Signs: The downward flow of Damp Heat disturbs the sperm-storing organs, and Damp Heat accumulate in it, causing seminal fluid and turbid urine to get mixed up with the result that the ejaculate does not liquefy, and has pus cells and white blood cells. Burning sensation during urination, difficulty and pain in urination, frequent and dribbling urination, yellowish and red turbid urine are all caused by downward flow of Damp Heat in bladder. The downward flow of Damp Heat impairs Blood Vessels, causing blood to overflow internally, thus hematuria, Damp Heat fumes and steams, so yellow or curdy tongue coating and soft or slippery pulse occurs.

Treatment Principles: Clearing Heat and eliminating Damp to promote diuresis; nourishing Yin to reduce Fire.

Prescription: Longdan Xiegan Tang He Zhibo Dihuang Tang (Decoction for Purging Liver Fire supplemented with Decoction of Anemarrhena, Phellodendron and Rehmannia) (See the above corresponding contents)

Analysis of the Prescription: See the analysis of Longdan Xiegan Tang (Decoction for Purging Liver Fire) in impotence.

Current Research

1. Modern medicine believes that high viscosity or non-liquefaction of human semen may restrain the mobility of spermatozoa. Spermatozoa seem to be trapped in such high-viscosity semen and move about sluggishly or vibrate in the same place without forward progression, thus greatly affecting the fertilization of spermatozoa. Non-liquefaction of semen mostly develops in the patients with prostatitis and sem-

119

inal vesiculitis. After these patients are treated with the effective antibiotics for 6-12 weeks, the number of pus cells or white blood cells in succus prostaticus of approximately half the patients decreases remarkably or they disappear, thus their semen viscosity is lower, the time period of semen liquefaction is shortened or reaches the normal level. It is reported that the patients, whose freshly ejaculated semen has high viscosity and does not liquefy after one hour, can be treated with mucolytic detergent alevaive which is unharmful to live cells and whose pH is consistent with the persistence of sperm mobility and has strong effect on lowering semen viscosity. Before sexual intercourse, dropping a little alevaive in vagina with a ringer will effectively lower the viscosity of ejaculate. Bunge once reported an effective treatment of non-liquefaction of semen. They found human saliva has the ability to liquefy semen sample, so rinsing vagina with α-amylase before coitus would make ejaculate liquefy. It was also reported recently that infusing α-amylase vagina suppositorium 50mg, or α-amylase solution 1ml into vagina after coital connection during ovulatory period had an effect in creating non-liquefaction of semen because α-amylase may increase glycogen in the section of vagina or cervix uteri thus increasing the source of power for spermatozoa mobility. It was also reported that infusing 3-5ml of diluted chymotrypsin or cacao butter suppositorium into vagina before coital encounter will make semen liquefy, thus achieving fertilization. It was reported abroad that placing semen sample pressure in syringe, injecting it into a glass container with syringe needle No. 18 or No. 19, pouring the sample into the syringe again to repeat the process several times until the semen looked like a liquid which does not impair spermatozoa, then using the semen to do artificial insemination will achieve pregnancy. The author used a smooth glass stitch to slowly stirred the semen sample in the same direction for several minutes with the result that most semen liquefied; meanwhile, spermatozoa mobility was enhanced. The author also added different kinds of enzyme preparation (hyaluronidase, chymotrypsin and amylase) to observe their effects on semen viscosity, and the time period of liquefaction with the result that different patients had different cure effects to different enzymes, and there was no regular pattern in them, but every enzyme preparation has cure effect on this syndrome. Recently, it was reported at home and abroad that taking large doses of vitamin C has achieved good cure effect on treating non-liquefaction of semen, but the dose is comparatively too large, 0.3g each time and the time period is too long, 3 times a day and continuously for 1-2 months. There have been reports to use acidum pipemidicum, belladoma tablets, belladonna mixture to treat non-liquefaction of semen effectively or in combination with ultrashort wave physiotherapy and acupuncture therapy. In a small number of patients, non-liquefaction results from seminal immunological factors. The antisperm antibodies in these patients are positive or abnormal when examined after coital connection in addition to semen non-liquefaction. With the treatment of antiinflammatory therapy and antiimmune therapy with the drugs of both TCM and the western medicines, not only did the antisperm area become normal on immunological examination, but also the time of liquefaction of semen turned to be normal as well (Jin Weixin's experience of treatment).

2. 30 sterile cases were treated with Yiehua Shengjing Tang (Decoction for Liquefaction of Seminal Fluid and Ascending of Spermatozoa) with the result that conception took place in the spouses of 18 patients, and spouses of 6 patients whose seminal test was all normal did not get pregnant, and 6 failed to be cured, with a total effective rate of 80% (The pregnancy rate was 60%), and the ineffective rate being 20%. Drugs are moutan bark (Cortex Moutan Radicis) 9g, wolfberry bark (Cortex Lycii Radicis) 9g, red peony root (Radix Paeoniae Rubra) 9g, white peony root (Radix Paeoniae) 9g, dried rehmannia root (Radix Rehmanniae) 12g, ophiopogon root (Radix Ophiopogonis) 12g, scrophularia root (Radix Scrophulariae) 12g, oyster shell (Concha Ostreae) 30g, wolfberry fruit (Fructus Lycii) 15g, red sage root (Radix Salviae Militiorrhizae) 30g, dodder seed (Semen Cuscutae) 9g, honeysuckle flower (Flos Lonicerae) 30g, forsythia fruit (Fructus Forsythiae) 12g, selfheal spike

121

(Spica Prunellae) 9g, bupleurum root (Radix Bupleuri) 9g, lophatherum (Herba Lophatheri) 9g, poria (Poria) 9g and epimedium (Herba Epimedii) 12g. The above drugs were decocted in water for oral use, one dose per day, to be taken continuously over 24-30 doses as one treatment course. This prescription is made of Qingjing Tang (Decoction for Removing Obstruction from the Channel), Qing Luo San (Powder for Removing Scrofula), Zengyie Tang (Decoction for Ascending Semen) and Liuwei Dihuang Wan (Bolus of Six Ingredients Including Rehmannia), which pays attention not only to the tonification of the Kidney, the Liver and the Spleen, but also to the reinforcement of Kidney Yang and replenishing Kidney Essence so that tonification contains purgation, which is included in the reinforcement. Therefore, this prescription has the effect of not only promoting liquefaction but also promoting the formation of spermatozoa and increasing the survival rate of the spermatozoa (Jin Weixin, 1984).

3. Beijing Gu Lou TCM Hospital diagnosed and treated 100 cases of non-liquefaction of semen by overall Syndrome Differentiation. They treated the patients of Yin Deficiency with dried rehmannia root (Radix Rehmanniae), wolfberry fruit (Fructus Lycii), glossy privet fruit (Fructus Ligustri), anemarrhena rhizome (Rhizoma Anemarrhenae) and phellodendron bark (Cortex Phellodendri); treated patients of Damp Heat type with modifications of atractylodes rhizome, phellodendron bark (Cortex Phellodendri), coix seed (Semen Coicis), poria (Poria), oriental water plantain (Rhizoma Alismatis), dandelion herb (Herba Taraxaci), wild chrysanthemum flower (Flos Chrysanthemi Indici); treating the patients of Yin Deficiency with epimedium (Herba Epimedii), curculigo rhizome (Rhizoma Curculiginis), prepared aconite root (Radix Aconiti Praeparata), cinnamon bark (Cortex Cinnamomi), pilose antler (Cornu Cervi Pantotrichum), prepared rehmannia root (Radix Rehmanniae Praeparata) and wolfberry fruit (Fructus Lycii). The effective rate was 88%, of which 74 cases of Yin Deficiency had an effective rate of 86.5%, 23 cases of Damp Heat had an effective rate of 91.3%, and 3 cases of Yang Deficiency had an

122

effective rate of 100% (Chen Wenbo, 1989).

4. 20 cases of non-liquefaction of semen (Four of them had pustales " + —||| "shown through routine examination) were treated with Shaofu Zhouyu Tang Jia Huangbo (Decoction for Removing Blood Stagnation in Lower Abdomen Supplemented with Phellodendron Bark) with 20 days being one course of treatment. The result of the treatment showed that 17 cases (85%) had their semen became normal in routine examination. Prescription drugs include common fennel fruit (Fructus Foeniculi) 6g, dried ginger (Rhizoma Zingiberis) 3g, corydalis tuber (Rhizoma Corydalis) 6g, myrrh (Myrrha) 5g, chuanxiong rhizome (Rhizoma Ligustici Chuangxiong) 6g, Cinnamon Twig (Ramulus Cinnamomi) 3g, red peony root (Radix Paeoniae Rubra) 10g, cat-tail pollen (Pollen Typhae) 9g, trogopterus dung (Faeces Trogopterori) 6g, Chinese angelica root (Radix Angelicae Sinensis) 12g, siberian solomonseal rhizome (Rhizoma Polygonati) 30g. Modifications: For the case with pustales in routine semen test due to Yang Deficiency and pathogenic Damp causing non-liquefac tion, seven-lobed yam (Rhizoma Dioscoreae Hypoglaucae) 15g, grassleaved sweetflag rhizome (Rhizoma Acori Graminei) 10g, pyrrosia leaf (Folium Pyrrosiae) 20g and plantain seed (Semen Plantaginis) (wrapped) 20g. After the treatment, when liquefaction could take place, but the mobility rate of spermatozoa was low, astragalus root (Radix Astragali Seu Hedysari) 30g, epimedium (Herba Epimedii) 30g, were added to supplement Qi and strengthen Yang to restore the functional activity of Qi. If the number of spermatozoa was too small, together with Wu Zi Bushen Wan (Bolus of Five Seed Drugs for Restoring the Kidney) was taken to replenish Vital Essence to restore the Kidney (Sun Huanming, 1985).

5. A clinical observation of the effects of 43 cases of non-liquefaction of semen treated with TCM drugs was carried according to the description below. The patients were divided into three Syndromes according to theory of Syndrome Differentiation and treatment: ① For the cases of Deficiency of Liver and Kidney Yin, the prescription Yujing Tang (Decoction for Nourishing Vital Essence) was applied, and the

123

drugs include eclipta (Herba Ecliptae), glossy privet fruit (Fructus Ligustri), mulberry (Fructus Mori), Chinese angelica root (Radix Angelicae Sinensis), fleece-flower root (Radix Polygoni Multiflori), white peony root (Radix Paeoniae), cnidium fruit (Fructus Cnidii), anemarrhena rhizome (Rhizoma Anemarrhenae), epimedium (Herba Epimedii), poria (Poria), flatstem milvetch seed (Semen Astragali Complanati) and licorice (Radix Glycyrrhizae). ② For the case of Spleen and Kidney Yang, the prescription Shengjing Yie Hua Tang (Decoction for Promoting the Generation of Vital Essence and Liquefaction of Semen) was applied. The drugs include astragalus root (Radix Astragali Seu Hedysari), pilose asiabell root (Radix Codonopsis Pilosulae), poria (Poria), bighead atractylodes rhizome (Rhizoma Atractylodis Macrocephalae), cimicifuga rhizome (Rhizoma Cimicifugae), Chinese angelica root (Radix Angelicae Sinensis), siberian solomonseal rhizome (Rhizoma Polygonati), psoralea fruit (Fructus Psoraleae), dodder seed (Semen Cuscutae), wolfberry fruit (Fructus Lycii), common fennel fruit (Fructus Foeniculi) and licorice (Radix Glycyrrhizae). ③ For the case with stagnation of Damp Heat, the prescription Bixie Fenqing Yin Jiajian (Modified Decoction of Seven-lobed Yam for Clearing Away Turbid Urine) was applied, and the drugs include seven-lobed yam (Rhizoma Dioscoriae Hypoglaucae), grassleaved sweetflag rhizome (Rhizoma Acori Graminei), lindera root (Radix Linderae), oriental wormwood (Herba Artemisiae Scopariae), giant knotweed rhizome (Rhizoma Polygoni Cuspidati), curcuma root (Radix Curcumae), dandelion herb (Herba Taraxaci), tribulus fruit (Fructus Tribuli), anemarrhena rhizome (Rhizoma Anemarrhenae), vaccaria seed (Semen Vaccariae), plantain seed (Semen Plantaginis), Japanese raspberry root (Radix Rubi Parvifolii), poria (Poria), licorice (Radix Glycyrrhizae) top. The drugs were taken orally one dose per day and 2 times a day, and 20 days accounting for one course of treatment. The total effective rate was 86.3%. After the treatment, 13 had their wives pregnant, with a pregnancy rate of 30.23% (Wang Mingxiang, 1990).

Diminution of Seminal Fluid

Generally speaking, the normal amount of semen (ejaculation of one time) is 2-6ml. If the amount is less than 1. 5ml, it is called diminution of seminal fluid. The amount of semen ejaculated each time by a normal male is not always the same, and it is closely related to the frequency of coitus, the degree of sexual excitement, mental factors and physical conditions.

TCM does not have special exposition of this disease. It is often found in oligospermatism, cold sperm, and thinness of seminal fluid.

Etiology and Pathogenesis
• *Deficiency and Impairment of the Kidney Essence*

It occurs because of the insufficiency of the congenital Essence, or excessive coitus which excessively consumes Kidney Essence, thus causing this disease.

• *Deficiency of both Qi and Blood*

Insufficiency of the congenital Essence together with poor nourishment after birth, or constitutional Deficiency of Qi and Blood, or weak physical constitution due to lingering disease, or overanxiety which impairs and exhausts the Heart and the Spleen leading to Deficiency of both the Heart and the Spleen and Deficiency of both Qi and Blood,—all of this causes diminution of seminal fluid.

• *The Blockage of the Sperma Duct due to Blood Stasis*

Addiction to fat-rich diet gives rise to either Interior Heat which flows down to the uterus, or to the affection of external pathogenic Damp Heat which steams or fumigates the sperm-storing organs, causing sticky and turbid sperma which stagnates and blocks the sperma duct, and thus causing diminution of seminal fluid.

Main Points of Diagnosis
All the cases whose amount of seminal fluid is less than 1. 5ml after being examined for 3 times can be diagnosed as

125

diminution of seminal fluid. However, it should be distinguished with diminution of seminal fluid caused by such factors as excessive coitus, spermatorrhea, seminal emission, incomplete ejaculation, ways to obtain seminal fluid.

Treatment Based on Syndrome Differentiation
• *Deficiency and Impairment of Kidney Essence*

Main Symptoms and Signs: Sterility after marriage, the amount of semen being less than 1.5ml, flaccidity of lumbar area and legs, fatigue and acratia, dizziness and tinnitus, reddish tongue with thin white coating on it, deep and thready pulse.

Analysis of the Symptoms and Signs: Since the Kidney stores reproductive Essence and foodstuff, and dominates reproduction, Deficiency of Kidney Essence may cause little amount of semen to be ejaculated and sterility occurs. As the loin is the place where the Kidney is located, insufficiency of Kidney Essence may produce flaccidity of lumbar area and legs. Fatigue and acratia occur because of Deficiency of Kidney Essence. Now that Kidney Qi flows to the ears, Kidney Deficiency may give rise to dizziness and tinnitus. Tongue and pulse conditions suggest Deficiency of Kidney Essence.

Treatment Principles: Restoring the Kidney and replenishing the Vital Essence.

Prescription: Zengjing Tang (Decoction for Increasing Seminal Fluid) (Prescription based on clinical experience of the author)

Fish air bladder glue (parched) 9g, tortoise plastron glue (Colla Plastri Testudinis) (parched) 9g, human placenta (Placenta Hominis) powder (to be taken with water) 6g, dogwood fruit (Fructus Corni) 9g, eucommia bark (Cortex Eucommiae) 9g, wolfberry fruit (Fructus Lycii) 15g, dodder seed (Semen Cuscutae) 12g, prepared rehmannia root (Radix Rehmanniae Praeparata) 12g, Chinese angelica root (Radix Angelicae Sinensis) 9g, siberian solomonseal rhizome (Rhizoma Polygonati) 15g, mulberry (Fructus Mori) 15g, ophiopogon root (Radix Ophiopogonis) 12g, ginseng (Radix Ginseng) 6g and Chinese yam (Rhizoma Dioscoreae) 15g. The above drugs are decocted in water for oral adminis-

126

tration, one dose daily, to be taken successively over 1-3 months.

Analysis of the Prescription: Fish air bladder glue, tortoise plastron glue (Colla Plastri Testudinis) and human placenta (Placenta Hominis) nourish the Kidney and replenish its Essence. Dogwood fruit (Fructus Corni), wolfberry fruit (Fructus Lycii), dodder seed (Semen Cuscutae) and eucommia bark (Cortex Eucommiae) nourish the Liver and restore the Kidney. Prepared rehmannia root (Radix Rehmanniae Praeparata), Chinese angelica root (Radix Angelicae Sinensis), siberian solomonseal rhizome (Rhizoma Polygonati), mulberry (Fructus Mori) and ophiopogon root (Radix Ophiopogonis) nourish Yin and replenish Blood. Ginseng (Radix Ginseng), Chinese yam (Rhizoma Dioscoreae) replenish Qi and reinforce the Spleen. The whole prescription restores the Kidney and replenishes Kidney Essence, and increases and benefits the seminal fluid.

• *Deficiency of both Qi and Blood*

Main Symptoms and Signs: No pregnancy long after marriage, the seminal fluid ejaculated each time being less than 1.5ml, pale complexion, fatigue and acratia, dizziness and palpitation, pale tongue with thin and white coating, deep and thready pulse.

Analysis of the Symptoms and Signs: Since sperma and Blood have the same source, Deficiency of both Qi and Blood causes the break-down of sperma transformation from its source, so the amount of sperma is less and fertility is impossible. Because Deficiency of Qi and Blood occurs, they can not reach the head and the face, pale complexion results. Blood can not nourish the Heart, and it fails to nourish the brain; therefore, dizziness and tinnitus occur. Because of Deficiency of Qi and Blood, the functions of the viscera decline, and fatigue occurs. Tongue and pulse conditions suggest insufficiency of Qi and Blood.

Treatment Principles: Replenishing Qi and nourishing Blood.

Prescription: Ba Zhen Tang Jiawei (Modified Decoction of Eight Valuable Ingredients)

Prepared rehmannia root (Radix Rehmanniae Praeparata)

12g, Chinese angelica root (Radix Angelicae Sinensis) 9g, white peony root (Radix Paeoniae Alba) 9g, Chuanxiong rhezome (Rhizoma Ligustici Chuanxiong) 9g, ginseng (Radix Ginseng) 6g, bighead atractylodes rhizome (Rhizoma Atractylodis Macrocephalae) 9g, poria (Poria) 9g, licorice (Radix Glycyrrhizae) 6g, dried human placenta (Placenta Hominis) 6g (to be taken with water), siberian solomonseal rhizome (Rhizoma Polygonati) 30g, astragalus root (Radix Astragali Seu Hedysari) 30g, antler glue (Colla Cornus Cervi) (parched) 9g and ophiopogon root (Radix Ophiopogonis) 12g. The above drugs are decocted in water, one dose daily, to be taken successively over 1-3 months.

Analysis of the Prescription: Dried rehmannia root, Chinese angelica root (Radix Angelicae Sinensis), white peony root (Radix Paeoniae Alba) and chuanxiong rhezome (Rhizoma Ligustici Chuanxiong) comprise of Siwu Tang (Decoction of Four Ingredients) to replenish and nourish Blood. Ginseng (Radix Ginseng), bighead atractylodes rhizome, poria (Poria), licorice (Radix Glycyrrhizae) consist of Si Junzi Tang (Decoction of Four Marble Ingredients) to replenish Qi and reinforce the Spleen. Human's placenta, antler glue (Colla Cornus Cervi) reinforce the Kidney and replenish Kidney Essence. Siberian solomonseal rhizome (Rhizoma Polygonati) and ophiopogon root (Radix Ophiopogonis) nourish Yin and nourish Blood. Astragalus root (Radix Astragali Seu Hedysari) replenishes Qi and increases Yang. The whole prescription replenishes Qi, nourishes Blood, restores the Kidney and replenishes Kidney Essence and increases the seminal fluid.

• *The Blockage of the Sperma Duct due to Blood Stasis*

Main Symptoms and Signs: No pregnancy long after marriage, the seminal fluid ejaculated each time being less than 1.5ml, straining pain or distending pain of the lower abdomen, scrotum and testicles, chest tightness and poor appetite, dry mouth and throat, dim tongue with petechia or ecchymosis, white or greasy coating, deep and tense pulse, or deep and choppy pulse.

Analysis of the Symptoms and Signs: Blood Stasis blocking in the ejaculatory tract causes abnormal emission of se-

128

men, which leads to oligospermia and sterility. Since ejaculatory tract is blocked, straining pain or distending pain in lower abdomen, scrotum, and testicles occurs. Stagnant Heat gives rise to oppression in chest, poor appetite, dry mouth and throat. Tongue and pulse conditions suggest the blockage of ejaculatory tract due to Blood Stasis.

Treatment Principles: Removing obstruction and activating the channels.

Prescription: Shu Jing Tang (Decoction for Removing Obstruction in Ejaculatory Tract, the prescription from the author's clinical experience)

Parched pangolin scales (Squama Manitis) 12g, sweetgum fruit (Fructus Liquidambaris) 15g, Chinese angelica root (Radix Angelicae Sinensis) 9g, spatholobus stem (Caulis Spatholobi) 15g, cyathula root (Radix Cyathulae) 15g, red peony root (Radix Paeoniae Rubra) 9g, red sage root (Radix Salviae Militorrhizae) 30g, peach kernel (Semen Persicae) 9g, safflower (Flros Carthami) 9g, chuanxiong rhezome (Rhizoma Ligustici Chuanxiong) 9g, prepared cyperus tuber (Rhizoma Cyperi Praeparata) 9g, prepared frankincense (Resina Olibani Praeparata) 9g, prepared myrrh (Myrrha Praeparata) 9g and centipede (Scolopendra) 2 pieces. The above drugs are decocted in water for oral administration, one dose per day, and taking continuously over 1-3 months.

Analysis of the Prescription: Parched pangolin scales (Squama Manitis), sweetgum fruit (Fructus Liquidambaris) remove obstruction in ejaculatory tract. Chinese angelica root (Radix Angelicae Sinensis), spatholobus stem (Caulis Spatholobi), cyathula root (Radix Cyathulae) nourish Blood and activate the circulation of Blood, and guide Blood to flow downward. Red peony root (Radix Paeoniae Rubra), red sage root (Radix Salviae Militor rhizae), peach kernel (Semen Persicae), safflower (Flos Carthami), chuanxiong rhezome (Rhizoma Ligustici Chuanxiong) activate Blood circulation and remove Blood Stasis and promote Qi flow. Prepared cyperus tuber (Rhizoma Cyperi Praeparata) soothes the Liver, regulates Qi flow, and alleviates pain. Prepared frankincense (Resina Olibani Praeparata), prepared myrrh

129

(Myrrha Praeparata) remove Blood Stasis and pain. Centipede (Scolopendra) removes obstruction in collaterals and resolves lumps and alleviates pains. The whole prescription activates the circulation of Blood and removes Blood Stasis, removes obstruction in ejaculatory tract, and finally the increase of seminal fluid is achieved.

Immunosterility

Autoimmune response caused by antisperm antibody has been widely stressed at present, and has been confirmed to be one of the causes leading to sterility. It was reported that 4-7% of sterile men has agglutination of spermatozoa. The Central Laboratory of Affiliated Hospital of Shandong University of TCM detected the antisperm antibodies in 204 couples of reproductive age who have normal sexual life and no organic lesion after marriage, only to find that the positive rate of male serum and seminal antisperm antibodies is 2.94% and that of female serum and seminal antisperm antibodies is 20.10%. According to the result of seminal immunoglobulin detection of 666 cases, the IgG is above the normal level in most patients' seminal serum which contains varying degrees of white cells and pyocytes, and approaches the normal level in the seminal serum which dose not contain them. In the semen of a small number of azoospermia and spermacrasia cases, IgG increases remarkably, some are 5-8 times of that of normal seminal serum, and complement C_3 can also be detected, but IgG is close to the normal level. Azim and others have discovered that sera and seminal plasma IgG of infertile men whose antisperm antibodies in sperm agglutination and circulation were positive was remarkably higher than those of control group, and IgA was also found in seminal serum; therefore, they advanced that the presence of IgA and Complement C_3 was to a certain degree related to spermagglutination and the presence of antisperm antibodies was related to the increased level of IgG, IgA and Complement C_3. During detection, they found that IgA level in seminal plasma of the patients of azoospermia and spermacrasia increased remarkably; therefore, they put forward that there may be a little part of IgA forming in genital duct while most IgA is exudated from blood. Consequently, the quantitative determination of im-munoglobulin and Complement C_3 in seminal plasma is contradictory to the diagnos is of male immunological sterility. It has been confirmed through a lot of laboratory studies and clinical observations that the exclusive routine seminal examination is not comprehensive in diagnosing sterility, because sera and genital duct antisperm antibodies also affect significantly male's fertility. Thus, it can be seen that the detection of antisperm antibodies in seminal plasma and sera, determination of immunoglobulin, complement C_3 in seminal plasma as well as spermagglutination and immobilization test should be performed together with routine seminal examination to achieve a routine conclusion through comprehensive analysis of multiple indices.

Laboratory studies have shown that sperm density, sperm mobility, the number of white cells and pyocytes are closely related to the positive rate of antisperm antibodies, i.e. the lower the sperm density and sperm motility are the more white cells and pyocytes there are, the higher the positive rate of antisperm antibodies is. The amount of semen and the time of liquefaction have nothing to do with the positive rate of antisperm antibodies. The male gonadal inflammation and urethra infection are the most common causes that lead to the positive rate of antisperm antibodies.

Modern medicine has had no satisfactory treatment for immunological sterility yet. Immunosuppressive therapy, treatment of infection of reproductive system, the use of contraceptives, intrauterine artificial insemination are the common therapeutic measures. The immunosuppressive therapy mostly has no specificity. It suppresses abnormal immune responses as well as normal ones. It not only causes the whole immunological system to be suppressed to a certain degree, but also has greater toxicity and more side effects. If it is used over a long period of time, serious complication may result. On the contrary, using TCM drugs has

131

some advantages. Through overall regulation, it can not only increase the weakened immunologic homeostasis, but also eliminate the harmful autoimmunity, and avoid side effects. It is confirmed through a lot of clinical observations and laboratory studies that drugs for promoting Blood circulation and removing Blood Stasis have some suppressive effects on substances that cause humoral immunity and cellular immunity, and better curative effect on immunologic diseases. The effect of removing Blood Stasis of therapy is quite similar to the homeostasis of immunity, so it has common curative significance in treating immunological diseases, particularly the autoimmunological diseases. Drugs for nourishing Yin and removing Heat from Blood can suppress immunologic hyperfunction, and counteract against allergic lesion. Drugs for clearing Heat and Toxins can suppress immunoreaction, some can also strengthen the phagocytic function of the white cells, and remarkably increase the phagocytic function of reticuloendothelial system, and a few can increase lymphocyte transformation rate. Drugs for expelling Wind, removing Damp and clearing Cold have the effect of counteracting against allergies, diminishing inflammation, suppressing the releasing allergic transmitter and regulating the permeability of blood vessels. In addition, certain TCM drugs have hormonal effects, i.e., they strengthen their effect through stimulating hypophysis-adrenocortical system, so they can not only suppress immunoreaction, but also remove or reduce pathologic lesion caused by allergic reactions, and have no side effects often found in western medicines. To sum up, according to their suppressive components, TCM drugs fall into three categories: Reticuloendothelial system, cellular immunity, and humoral immunity. Some TCM drugs have two-dimensional regulating effect to immunity, and others have the effects of counteracting against allergic transmitters and non-specific antiinflammation. Well compatibility of drugs in a prescription will bring about the effects of supplementing each other.

Treatment Based on Syndrome Differentiation
• *Insufficiency of the Kidney Yang*

132

Main Symptoms and Signs: Positive result of immunological test, sperm density, sperm mobility being normal, or abnormal, the time of liquefaction of semen being normal, aversion to cold, and cold limbs, pale complexion, dizziness, tinnitus, lassitude in the lumbar area and knees, clear urine not scanty in amount, pale tongue with thin and white coating, deep and thready pulse.

Analysis of the Symptoms and Signs: Insufficiency of Kidney Yang gives rise to hypofunction of sex gland axis and pituitary gland-adrenocortical system, which affects the normal function of organic cellular immunity, humoral immunity and reticuloendothelial system, thus leading to abnormality of immunologic function. aversion to cold, cold limbs, pale complexion, dizziness, clear urine not scanty in amount, pale tongue with white coating, deep and thready pulse indicate insufficiency of Kidney Yang.

Treatment Principles: Warming the Kidney to invigorate Yang; counteracting against immunity and eliminating agglutination.

Prescription: Zini Wenning Tang (Self-made Decoction for Warming Agglutination) Epimedium (Herba Epimeddii) 15g, morinda root (Radix Morindae Officinalis) 9g, dodder seed (Semen Cuscutae) 9g, aconite root (Radix Aconiti Praeparata) 6g, cinnamon bark (Cortex Cinnamomi) 6g, ginseng (Radix Ginseng) 3-6g, Chinese angelica root (Radix Angelicae Sinensis) 9g, astragalus root (Radix Astragali Seu Hedysari) 30g, white peony toot (Radix Paeoniae Alba) 9g, panicled swallowwort root (Radix Cynanchi Paniculati) 9g and dried licorice (Radix Glycyrrhizae) 6g. The above drugs are decocted in water for oral administration, one dose per day, and taking successively over 24-30 doses which constitute for one course of treatment.

Analysis of the Prescription: Epimedium (Herba Epimeddii), morinda root (Radix Morindae officinalis), dodder seed (Semen Cuscutae), aconite root (Radix Aconiti Praeparata) and cinnamon bark (Cortex Cinnamomi) warm and restore Kidney Yang. Ginseng (Radix Ginseng) and astragalus root (Radix Astragali Seu Hedysari) replenish Qi and Blood. Chinese angelica root (Radix Angelicae Sinen-

133

sis) replenishes Blood and activates the circulation of Blood. Chinese angelica root (Radix Angelicae Sinensis) and astragalus root (Radix Astragali Seu Hedysari) used together form Blood-replenishing decoction. White peony root (Radix Paeoniae Alba) astringes Yin and softens the Liver. Panicled swallowwort windy in nature can remove Toxins. Dried licorice (Radix Glycyrrhizae) clears Heat and removes Toxins, and coordinates the effects of other drugs.

TCM holds that strengthening the body resistance to consolidate the constitution means strengthening the immunity. Epimedium (Herba Epimeddii), morinda root (Radix Morindae officinalis), aconite root (Radix Aconiti Praeparata), cinnamon bark (Cortex Cinnamomi), dodder seed (Semen Cuscutae) all can promote the formation or the advanced formation of the antibodies. Ginseng (Radix Ginseng), astragalus root (Radix Astragali Seu Hedysari) can improve non-specific immunologic function. For instance, they can increase lymphocyte transformation rate, or phagocytic function of reticuloendothelial system. Ginseng (Radix Ginseng) can also promote the synthesis of protein, accelerate the formation of immunologic antibodies, regulate cAMP and cGMP of a variety of organs. Astragalus root (Radix Astragali Seu Hedysari) can increase the content of cAMP in plasma, and improve body fluids immunity, increase immunoglobulin content, the plasma agglutinin titer, and improve cell nourishment. Chinese angelica root (Radix Angelicae Sinensis) can promote the circulation of Blood and nourish Blood. When the dose is big, it can activate the the circulation of Blood, when the dose is small, it can nourish Blood. When it promotes the circulation of Blood, it inhibits immunity. When it nourishes Blood, it strengthens immunity. White peony root (Radix Paeoniae Alba) can increase lymphocyte transformation rate. Panicled swallowwort root (Radix Cynanchi Paniculati) is considered to possess antiimmunologic function. Dried licorice (Radix Glycyrrhizae) has the function similar to that of hormones, stimulates hypophysis-adrenal gland system whose function is therefore strengthened.

• *Excessive Consumption of Kidney Yin*

134

Main Symptoms and Signs: Immunologic test being positive, sperm density, sperm vitality being abnormal or normal, or high sperm abnormality rate, or non-liquefaction of seminal fluid; dizziness and tinnitus, dysphoria with feverish sensation in chest, palms and soles, flaccidity of lumbar area and knees, dry mouth and yellowish urine, red tongue with slight tongue coating, feeble and rapid pulse.

Analysis of the Symptoms and Signs: The impairment of Kidney Yin, the abnormality of the body's gonad axis and hyophysis-adrenal gland cortex system can result in hyperim munologic function, and immunologic test is positive. Dizziness, tinnitus, dysphoria with feverish sensation in the lumbar area and knees, dry mouth, tongue and pulse conditions are all signs of excessive consumption of Kidney Yin.

Treatment Principles: Nourishing the Kidney to replenish Essence; inhibiting immunity and relieving agglutination.

Prescription: Zini Xiaoning Tang (Self-made Agglutination-Relieving Decoction)

Dried rehmannia root (Radix Rehmanniae) 12g, ophiopogon root (Radix Ophiopogonis) 9g, figwort root (Radix Scrophulariae) 9g, white peony root (Radix Paeoniae Alba) 9g, glossy privet fruit (Fructus Ligustri Lucidi) 12g, eclipta (Herba Ecliptae) 12g, tortoise plastron (Plastrum Testudinis) 30g, fresh-water turtle shell (Carapax Trionycis) 30g, red peony root (Radix Paeoniae Rubra) 9g, moutan bark (Cortex Moutan Radicis) 9g, red sage root (Radix Salviae Militorrhizae) 30g, panicled swallowwort root (Radix Cynanchi Paniculati) 9g and dried licorice (Radix Glycyrrhizae) 6g. The above drugs are decocted in water for oral administration, one dose daily, and 24-30, doses make up a course of treatment.

Analysis of the Prescription: In the prescription, the first 8 drugs nourish Yin and promote the production of body fluids, remove Heat and cool Blood. Among them, glossy privet fruit (Fructus Ligustri Lucidi) and eclipta (Herba Ecliptae) also have the effect of tonifying and nourishing the Liver and the Kidney. Tortoise plastron (Plastrum Testudinis) and fresh-water turtle shell (Carapax Trionycis) also can nourish Yin and replenish Yang. Red peony root (Radix

135

Paeoniae Rubra), moutan bark (Cortex Moutan Radicis) and red sage root (Radix Salviae Militorrhizae) can also activate the circulation of Blood, and remove Blood Stasis. Panicled swallowwort root (Radix Cynanchi Paniculati) expels Wind and removes Toxins. Dried licorice (Radix Glycyrrhizae) clears Heat and removes Toxins, coordinates the functions of the other drugs.

Such drugs aiming at nourishing Yin and cooling Blood as dried rehmannia root (Radix Rehmanniae), ophiopogon root (Radix Ophiopogonis), figwort root (Radix Scrophulariae), moutan bark (Cortex Moutan Radicis), white peony root (Radix Paeoniae Alba), eclipta (Herba Ecliptae), tortoise plastron and fresh-water turtle shell (Carapax Trionycis) can inhibit hyperim munologic function, and counteract against allergic pathological changes, reduce or relieve the side-effects from the treatment through immunologic inhibitors. Such drugs that activate the circulation of Blood and remove Blood Stasis as moutan bark (Cortex Moutan Radicis), red peony root (Radix Paeoniae Rubra), red sage root (Radix Salviae Militorrhizae), not only have anti-inflammatory effect but also lower capillary permeability, but also reduce exudate from inflammation and promote absorption, but also inhibit cellular immunity and immunity of body fluids. Panicled swallowwort root (Radix Cynanchi Paniculati) has comprehensive immunologic effect. Dried licorice (Radix Glycyrrhizae) has hormonal effect and has the effect similar to that of deoxycorticosterone. It can be used as a suppressant used for antiallergy and anti-inflammation.

• Damp Heat of the Liver Channel

Main Symptoms and Signs: Immunologic test being positive, sperm density, sperm vitality mostly being abnormal, or sperm abnormality rate being high, or non-liquefaction of seminal fluid, stuffiness sensation in chest and palpitation, dizziness and distending head, dry and sticky mouth, thirsty but poor desire to drink, scanty and yellowish urine, red tongue with yellowish and greasy tongue coating, slippery and rapid pulse.

Analysis of the Symptoms and Signs: Damp Heat from the Liver Channel, hyperactivity of body's immune system, or

136

the decrease of the function of reticuloendothelial system result in immunologic abnormality, and positive immunologic test. The downward flow of Damp Heat steaming the sperm-storing organs leads to abnormal spermia, high abnormality rate, or non-liquefaction of seminal fluid. Stuffiness sensation in chest and palpitation, dizziness and distending head, dry and sticky mouth, thirsty but poor desire to drink, scanty and yellowish urine and tongue and pulse condition indicate Damp Heat of the Liver Channel.

Treatment Principles: Clearing Heat and removing Damp; inhibiting immunity to remove agglutination.

Prescription: Zini Chuning Tang (Self-made Decoction for Removing Agglutination)

Gentian root (Radix Gentianae) 9g, coptis root (Rhizoma Coptidis) 3g, scutellaria root (Radix Scutellariae) 9g, prepared rhubarb (Radix et Rhizoma Rhei Praeparata) 3g, dried rehmannia root (Radix Rehmanniae) 12g, moutan bark (Cortex Moutan Radicis) 9g, Chinese angelica root (Radix Angelicae Sinensis) 15g, honeysuckle flower (Flos Lonicerae) 24g, forsythia fruit (Fructus Forsythiae) 12g, dandelion herb (Herba Taraxaci) 18g, oldenlandia (herba Hedyotis Diffusae) 15g and dried licorice (Radix Glycyrrhizae) 6g. The above drugs are decocted in water for oral administration, one dose daily, to be taken successively over 24-30 doses that consist of one course of treatment.

Analysis of the Prescription: The first four drugs and honeysuckle flower (Flos Lonicerae), forsythia fruit (Fructus Forsythiae), dandelion herb (Herba Taraxaci) and oldenlandia (herba Hedyotis Diffusae) clear Heat and remove Toxins, promote diuresis and relieve Heat. Dried rehmannia root (Radix Rehmanniae), moutan bark (Cortex Moutan Radicis) and Chinese angelica root (Radix Angelicae Sinensis) nourish Yin and clear away Heat from Blood, and activate the the circulation of Blood. Dried licorice (Radix Glycyrrhizae) clears Heat and removes toxins, coordinates the functions of all the drugs.

Research results have proved that coptis root (Rhizoma Coptidis), scutellaria root (Radix Scutellariae), dried rehmannia root (Radix Rehmanniae) and honeysuckle flower

137

(Flos Lonicerae), all can increase lymphocyte transformation rate. Coptis root (Rhizoma Coptidis), scutellaria root (Radix Scutellariae), honeysuckle flower (Flos Lonicerae), oldenlandia (herba Hedyotis Diffusae) can strengthen phagocytic function of white cells. Coptis root (Rhizoma Coptidis), oldenlandia (herba Hedyotis Diffusae) can also obviously improve the phagocytic function of the reticuloendothelial system. Gentian root (Radix Gentianae), scutellaria root (Radix Scutellariae), prepared rhubarb (Radix et Rhizoma Rhei Praeparata), coptis root (Rhizoma Coptidis), forsythia fruit (Fructus Forsythiae), moutan bark (Cortex Moutan Radicis), licorice (Radix Glycyrrhizae) can inhibit immunity. Large dose of angelica root promotes the circulation of Blood, and mainly inhibit immunity. The above drugs play their roles through cAMP and cGMP level regulation; therefore, anti-immunity effect is achieved.

138

PART TWO
FEMALE STERILITY

Chapter Four
Diagnosis

Female sterility refers to the non-pregnancy of the woman of reproductive age, with her spouse's reproductive function being normal, living together for over two years without taking any contraceptive measures; or to the non-pregnancy for over two years even if there was history of pregnancy. The former is called primary female sterility, while the latter is called secondary female sterility.

The diagnosis of female sterility includes TCM diagnosis and diagnosis of modern medicine. Like male sterility, the two methods are equally important, and neither side is neglected. TCM diagnosis is based on Four Diagnostic Methods, Syndrome Differentiation according to Eight Principals and Zangfu. In examination of modern medicine, besides careful overall and gynecological examinations, various special examining means are applied to diagnose the actual etiology, such as ovulatory functional disorder, the obstruction in the oviduct, uterine neck factors, immunity factors, and some special diseases that cause female sterility. According to the principle that differentiation of Syndrome and differentiation of diseases are combined, TCM herbal drugs are used for treatment so that long-term best curative effect can be obtained.

TCM Diagnosis of Female Sterility

TCM diagnosis of female sterility is based on Four Diagnostic Methods, and according to woman's physiological and pathologic characteristics, conducted are Syndrome Differentiation in accordance with Eight Principals and Zangfu.

Four Diagnostic Methods
• *Inspection*
Inspection of Complexions: The changes of facial color can reflect the prosperity and decline of visceral Qi and Blood. Inspection of the complexions of the infertile patients are helpful in obtaining the conditions of menstruation and clinical differentiation and syndrome grouping.

Inspection of the Tongue: It includes inspection of the tongue proper and tongue coating. Pale tongue suggests Deficiency of Qi and Blood. It can be observed in the infertile cases caused by bleeding and profuse menstruation. Red tongue is found in the infertile cases caused by Blood Heat or Excess Heat due to Yin Deficiency. Blue purple tongue or tongue with ecchymosis and petechiae in the tip of tongue is seen in the infertile cases caused by stagnation of Qi and Blood Stasis. White greasy tongue coating suggests Damp Syndrome, yellow greasy tongue coating suggests Damp Heat syndrome. Greasy tongue coating suggests accumulation of Phlegm Damp. Gray dark and dry tongue coating suggests Excess Heat. Dark and moist tongue coating suggests Cold due to Kidney Deficiency.

Inspection of General Appearance: After the woman reaches her sexual maturity, the body becomes gradually mature, too. If the age is over 18, but the height is short, muscularly thin, and the breasts are plain, they suggest insufficiency of Kidney Qi. If the woman is short but puffy and the face is as round as a full moon, the skin is rough, they suggest Phlegm Damp in the Interior. The sleek and glossy hair, moderately thick, suggests prosperity of Kidney Qi, and profuse Yin Blood. Trichomadesis, sparse genital hair

142

suggest Deficiency and Decline of Kidney Qi, the insufficiency of Essence and Blood. This can be seen in the infertile cases caused by Kidney Deficiency and Cold Uterine. More hair on the arms and legs or genital area, or the hair distributed in the way of masculinization, even hairs being distributed around the labial mouth suggest the female sterility which is differentiated as Phlegm Damp Syndrome accompanying by Kidney Deficiency. Well-developed vulva, sleek and glossy pubisure suggest normal development. If the appearance of the external genitals is abnormal, such as Luo (spiral vagina), Wen (stricture of vagina), Gu (imperforate hymen), Jiao (horn) which are considered to be congenital abnormalities. Haggard skin of vulva or white pale rough skin suggests Deficiency and Decline of Kidney Qi.

• *Auscultation and Olfaction*

It includes listening to the voice and smelling the odor of the patient. If the infertile patient's voice is low and weak, it suggests Qi Deficiency. Occasional sighing indicates stagnation of Liver Qi. High and strong voice suggests syndrome of Excess Heat Syndrome. If foul-smelling is smelled, it suggests Heat Syndrome. Stinking smell as of rotten fish indicates Cold Damp Syndrome.

• *Interrogation*

It refers to mainly inquiring about the conditions of the patient's sexual life, and menstruation, leukorrhea, pregnancy, and reproduction. Attention should be paid to the ways of interrogation. Too directness is not encouraged, but indirect and reserved ways are suggested.

Interrogation of Age: The infertile patients are closely related to age. If the age is over 35, Kidney Qi is gradually deficient, and endocrine function disorder appears easily. If the age is over 40, Kidney Qi is gradually exhausted, and the Essence and Blood are insufficient, the Chong and Ren Channels are deficient, too. Therefore, the uterine loses nourishment, and pregnancy is impossible.

Interrogation of the History of Menstruation: To infertile women, menarchal age, menstrual cycle lasting period, the condition of the amount, the color, and the nature of menstruation, whether waist or lower abdomen pain and distend-

143

ing nipple exists during menstrual period, etc.—all should be carefully interrogated. If the age of menarche is too young, it is considered to be prematurity; whereas, if the age is too old, it is thought that the genital system develops too slowly. Those patients with regular menstrual cycle, moderate amount of menstruation, with normal color and nature, can be easily treated. Those with forwarded sticky and sticky menstruation with much amount, deep red color or with blood clots are with pathogenic Heat. Those, with forwarded thin menstruation, with much amount, pale color, suffer from Qi Deficiency. Those with delayed menstruation, with little amount, dark color, and small blood clots and pain in the lower abdomen suffer from pathogenic Cold. Those with delayed thin menstruation with little amount, pale color belong to Syndrome of Blood Deficiency. Those with uncertain menstruation, uncertain amount, dark purple color with small blood clots, fullness and distending abdomen suffer from stagnation of Liver Qi. Those, whose menstrual color is purplish red, the amount is great or menstruation does not stop, with too many blood clots and stabbing pain in abdomen, and the pain will be reduced if blood clots are removed out of the body suffer from stagnation of Blood Stasis. Those with tender pain in the lower abdomen during menstrual period or before menstruation belong to Excess Syndrome. If the slight pain in the lower abdomen is relieved by pressing, after the completion of menstrual cycle, the disease belongs to Deficiency Syndrome. During menstruation, Cold and pain in the lower abdomen appear, and are relieved by warmth, then, the disease belongs to Cold Syndrome. Before menstruation, distending pain in the lower abdomen and the pain is greater than distending, it belongs to syndrome of Blood Stasis. Before or during menstruation, distending is greater than pain, it belongs to syndrome of Qi Stagnation. To the above conditions, during treatment, Syndrome Differentiation and treatment are needed. It is more complicated compared with the cases with normal menstruation.

Interrogation of Present Illness State: It includes asking the marriage time, whether contraception is applied, chief diseases the patients once suffered from and what examinations the patient took and the drugs administered.

Interrogation of Pregnancy and Reproduction: It includes asking whether there have been pregnancy, abortion, premature birth, or still birth, and the situation at that time, and whether the development of the uterine is normal.

Interrogation of Leukorrhea History: After the maturity of woman's development, every time before menstruation, intermenstrual period or pregnancy period, leukorrhea is slightly more which is normal physiological phenomenon. If it becomes obviously more, the color is white and it is thin, it suggests Cold Syndrome and Deficiency Syndrome. If the menstruation is yellowish or deep red and sticky, it suggests Heat Syndrome and Excess Syndrome. The amount of leukorrhea is more whose color is as white as mucus of the nose, it suggests Deficiency of the Spleen and Excess of Damp. If the amount of leukorrhea is more and it is as scanty and thin as water, it suggests Deficiency and Decline of Kidney Yang. If leukorrhea is yellow or slightly green with foams, self-feeling of obvious itching in vulva area, most cases suggest downward flow of Damp of the Liver Channel. The amount and the nature of leukorrhea are closely related to cervical sterility.

• *Pulse-feeling and Palpation*

It includes pulse-feeling, palpation of the skin, palpation of the abdominal area.

Pulse-feeling: The woman's pulse is generally weak, but is comparatively vigorous at Chi portion. *Nineteen Difficult Medical Problems*, a chapter of *On Difficult Medical Problems* (*Nan Jing·Shi Jiu Nan*) says, "The male's pulse can be felt up Guan portion, and the female's below Guan portion. That's why the male's Chi portion is always weak, and the female's is always vigorous... A male's pulse like a female's indicates Deficiency Syndrome, while a female's pulse like a man's indicates Excess Syndrome." If menstruation is coming, or menstruation is going on, and the pulse is characteristically slippery, or tense, slippery, and slightly rapid, it is considered to be in normal state. If the pulse is slightly slippery and rapid and full and big and vigorous, it

145

suggests latent heat in the Chong and Ren Channels. It is mostly seen in the cases of preceded menstrual cycle, or profuse menstruation. Deep, slow and thready pulse indicates Yang Deficiency and nterior Colld. It can be found in the cases of preceded menstruation, scanty menstruation. Thready and rapid pulse suggests excessive consumption of the fluid due to Deficiency Heat, the impairment of Yin and insufficiency of Blood. This is mostly seen in the cases of Blood Deficiency and amenorrhea. After pregnancy, Yin the circulation of Bloods downward to nourish the original Qi of fetus. Mostly, the pulse is slippery and rapid, and Chi portion doesn't stop even if pressed. In *On the Differences of Yin and Yang*, a chapter of *Plain Questions* (*Su Wen · Yin Yang Bie Lun*), it says, "The difference of Yin struggling with Yang is called pregnancy. "

Palpation of the Skin : It can know the warmth and coolness, moisture and dry skin. Cool sensation in palms and soles suggest stagnation of Cold Damp, or insufficiency of Yang Qi of the Spleen and the Kidney. Feverish sensation in palms and soles suggest hyperactivity of Fire due to Yin Deficiency.

Palpation of Abdomen : It can help to know whether the abdominal wall is hard, soft, warm or cool, whether pain exists, or whether there are hard lumps and to know their locations, sizes as well. If the abdomen is felt to be soft and the pain is reduced if pressed, and pressing and warming are preferred, it suggests Deficiency Cold type. If pressing leads to a even stabbing pain, it suggests stagnation of Qi and Blood Stasis. If abdomen is felt to be not warm, even cold, it suggests insufficiency of Yang Qi. If it is felt to be hot and painful, it suggests Exces Heat.

Syndrome Differentiation in Accordance with Eight Principal

Syndrome Differentiation of the infertile women in accordance with Eight Principals is based on the analysis and grouping of Yin and Yang, Exterior and interior, Cold and Heat, Deficiency and Excess to find out the nature, and location of the disease. The actual method is generally the same

146

as the one used for other diseases.

• *Yin and Yang*

It is the guideline of Syndrome Differentiation according to Eight Principals: Exterior, Heat and Excess belong to Yang; Interior, Cold and Deficiency belong to Yin. Hyperfunction belongs to Yang, hypofunction belongs to Yin. Yin and Yang are conflicting and unified each other. To some extent, Yin and Yang keeps a dynamic balance. Yin syndrome refers to Deficiency and Decline of Yang Qi in the body, the excessive prosperity of Yin Qi. The disease belongs to Deficiency Syndrome, cold in nature, and the body's reaction is declining. Yang syndrome refers to Yang and Qi Excess, and Vital Qi still exists. The disease symptoms suggest heat, and excessive in nature. The body's functional reaction is excessively prosperous.

• *The Exterior and Interior*

They refer to the location of pathologic changes and the severity of a disease. The symptoms and signs reflected superficially belong to exterior syndrome; and the disease is less severe. The symptoms and signs reflected in the viscera and the pathologic changes deeply located belong to Interior Syndrome, and the disease is severe.

• *The Cold and Heat*

They are two aspects to differentiate the nature of a disease and used to summarize the prosperity and the decline of Yin and Yang. The people in ancient times said, "Excessive Yin leads to Cold, and excessive Yang leads to Heat." "Yin Deficiency produces Heat, and Yang Deficiency produces Cold."

• *The Deficiency and Excess*

They are two aspects to measure the degree, strong or weakness of Vital Qi, and the prosperity and the decline of pathogenic evil. *Classic of Internal Medicine* (*Nei Jing*) says, "Exuberant pathogenic factors lead to Excess Syndrome, and excessive consumption leads to Deficiency Syndrome." Deficiency Syndrome is mostly observed among the patients with lingering diseases or weak body whose Vital Qi is insufficient. It is generally classified into Deficiency of Qi and Blood, Yang or Yin. Excess Syndrome includes Heat

147

Syndrome, pathogenic factors stagnating in the channels and collaterals or in Zangfu or stagnation of Qi and Blood Stasis Syndrome.

Syndrome Differentiating in According with Zangfu

Zangfu theory is also theoretical basis for Syndrome Differentiation and treatment of the infertile patients. Here, only four organs, namely the Kidney, the Liver, the Spleen, the Heart, closely related to female sterility.

• *The Kidney*

The Kidney is crucial to reproductive system. The Kidney is said to be "the source of congenital Essence," "the root of life." The Kidney is divided into Kidney Yang and Kidney Yin. It is the essential material and function of female's reproductive system. The Yin and Yang of the Kidney should be prosperous but also relatively balanced. If Kidney Yang is deficient and declining, or Kidney Yin is impaired and excessively consumed, or Yin is deficient and Yang is excessive, or Yin and Yang are both deficient, then Kidney Qi will be deficient, exhausted, the Essence and Blood will be excessively consumed, and Kidney Yin, the Chong and Ren Channels are malnourished, and female sterility is caused.

• *The Liver*

It stores Blood and governs normal flow of Qi, and has the function to regulate the normal flow of Qi and Blood, coordinate the functions of the viscera. Depression and anger impair the Liver, then Liver Qi will get stagnated; as a result, Blood Stasis will be caused. The stagnation of Liver Qi or Blood Stasis due to stagnation of Liver Qi will cause female sterility.

• *The Spleen*

The Spleen is the source of acquired Essence, and the source of Qi and Blood. Five visceraand six Fu Organs, arms and legs and the bones of the body all depend on its nourishment. Furthermore, the Chong Channel is inferior to Yangming Channel which is the source of much Qi and Blood. The Spleen and the Stomach are healthy and prosperous, and the Essence is abundant, then Qi and Blood will be abundant, and the Chong and Ren Channels will be well nourished.

148

This enables pregnancy possible. If the Spleen suffers from Deficiency, then it will lose the power to acquire Essence, or Spleen Deficiency can not make water and Damp unable to flow smoothly. Damp will stagnate, and it will become Phlegm which obstructs at the Chong and Ren Channels, and obstructs in the uterine. Therefore, irregular menstruation is caused, Essence-acquiring is impossible, and pregnancy is impossible too.

• *The Heart*

It governs Blood Vessles. Qi and Blood are the substances and motivation to maintain the activities of the life. Profuse Qi and Blood lead to smooth circulation of Blood. The insufficiency of Heart Qi leads to stagnation of the circulation of Blood. Deficiency and Decline of Qi and Blood lead to Deficiency of Ren Channel, and the decline and less of Qi in the Chong Channel. Therefore, non-pregnancy is caused.

Diagnosis of Female Sterility by Means of Modern Medicine

The Examinations of Female Sterility due to Ovulatory Dysfunction

• *The Measurement of Basal Body Temperature*

Basal Body Temperature (BBT) refers to the body temperature measured below the tongue after the patient goes to sleep for 6-8 hours and does not do any activities. It is also called resting body temperature, which reflects the body's energy metabolic level in resting condition. The BBT values measured daily are recorded on a temperature form, and the curve formed is called BBT curve.

To a woman whose menstrual cycle is normal, the follicles in the ovary get mature and ovulation begins. After ovulation, corpus luteum formed from the folliculi produces progesterone (also called progestogen). The progesterone exerts its effect not only on the endometrium, but also on temperature regulating centers; therefore, the body temperature goes up slightly. If pregnancy doesn't happen 9 days after ovulation, the corpus luteum begins to degenerate and the production of progesterone will be reduced gradually. Then 4-6 days further later, the body temperature starts to go down. This suggests the coming of menstruation. In most cases, ovulation happens between two menstruations. If a menstrual cycle is 28 days, in 14 days from ovulation to menarche, BBT is higher, generally 36. 8-37℃. From the first day of menarche to the fourteenth day of ovulation, BBT is lower, generally 36. 3-36. 5℃ (It may be even lower during ovulation). The body temperature difference during menstrual cycle is 0. 4-0. 5℃. In BBT form, it appears to be diphasic curve. Generally, it is thought that the patient without ovulatory cycle lacks the effect of heat of progesterone; therefore, BBT will not have the regular change stated above, and in BBT form, BBT appears to be monophasic curve. Through determination of BBT, ovary function can be known indirectly. For example, whether BBT curve is diphasic or monophasic, the length of time of corpus luteum period is long or short, and the range of the increase of the body temperature is large or small, the temperature goes up sharply or in a way of slope, like a flight of stairs, the night temperature phase is stable or fluctuating. Normal corpus luteum period is 12-16 days, and averaged 14 days, but it is not shorter than 11 days (or 10 days). The range of the temperature goes up should be lower than 0. 3℃, and should not appear to be in a stair way, and the night temperature curve should not fluctuate; otherwise, hypoluteoidism happens. Generally, it is believed that the lowest point of the temperature before it goes up is on the day of ovulation, but some of the temperature curves have no lowest point (The curves with the lowest point take up 20-30%). Some lowest points do not appear on the ovulation day, and other aspects should be considered: Cervical mucus becomes transparent, thin, and more, its wiredrawing degree is long, or the effect of vaginal smear changes from minor-moderate degree to moderate-high degree, and plasma LH appears to have peaks through radioimmunoassay (12-24 hours after the peak, ovulation starts), etc. The temperature of some people start to go up 1-2 days before or after ovulation. So, the manifestation of different people are not wholly the same. To sum up,

150

the diphasic ovulatory menstruation is not confirmed clinically through examination of cervical mucus, vaginal cellular smear, the peak of estrogen in the middle stage of menstrual cycle, and LH peak, pregnanediol in the urine or pregnendione in blood, endometrium, etc. In recent years, through endocrine examination, it is found that in the cases of no abnormal ovulation under BBT, many suffer from hypoluteoidism. As far as the etiology is concerned, it is better to say that the egg cell suffers from hypoplasia before ovulation than to say that the forming of the yellow body of ovary is abnormal after ovulation. The BBTs measured of this patients seem to suggest that corpus luteum function is normal; therefore, other examination means should be considered to make accurate analysis.

The determination of BBT changes can be used to guide treatment; what's more, during the treatment and withdrawal period, the curative effects and the effective doses of different drugs can be observed. To those with ovulation and uncertain menstrual cycle, the determination of BBT can help to know the ovulatory period for the purpose of pregnancy. In artificial pregnancy, the determination of BBT is even more needed to know the best time of pregnancy. If BBT high temperature phase is over 20 days, the possibility of pregnancy is over 98%. To the patients with irregular menstruation, two weeks are added before the ovulatory period. It is considered to be the end day of the last menstruation, and it helps to accurately work out the expected date of delivery. Abortion or threatened abortion during the early stage of pregnancy is quite easily diagnosed as irregular menstruation. Correct diagnosis can be achieved through BBT. If complete abortion is suspected, but no fatal sac and villi are found, the decrease of BBT can serve as a reference to rule out ectopic pregnancy. In the early stage of pregnancy, if vaginal bleeding happens, the going down of BBT is helpful to confirm missed abortion, so that timely treatment can be supplied. For the case with habitual abortion, the diagnosis of early stage of pregnancy through BBT is especially important.

The time of BBT determination should be at dawn when

151

the patient just wakes up and doesn't do any things. Put the oral thermometer below the tongue, and ask the patient to close her mouth for more than 5 minutes, and then take out and find out the value, then record it on BBT form, and carefully mark menstruation period, sexual life, drug administration, cold, insomnia, etc. on the paper. For the women who work on three-shift system on the whole have different types of curve and they serve as valuable references (After they sleep for 5-6 hours and record the temperature as soon as they get awake). The determination of BBT must be strict, and must be carried out for three menstrual cycles. At the same time, other examining tools should be used to make correct judgment about ovulation.

• *Endometrial Biopsy*

Endometrium is a special tissue which shows obvious changes under the influence of hypothalamus-hypophysis-ovary secreted hormones. It can reflect the ovary function and hormone level in the body. Examination of endometrium can help to see if such pathologic changes as intimitis, polyp, cancer, etc., happen. It is easy to take tissue sample, and the patients bear it easily. It is a simple and reliable diagnostic method. Diagnostic uterine apoxesis is applied to the infertile patients to find the hormone level in the body and endometrium pathologic changes. To some patients, blood examination shows that progestogen is normal, but the endometrium as the target cell itself is abnormal, it also causes female sterility.

The days of the endometrium tissue in the menstrual cycle can be determined according to the impaired Noyes' Standards for Endometrium Daily Characteristics Changes in Menstrual Cycle (see the following table). Two days lagging behind the standards, the endometrium tissue is considered to be fall-behind matured endometrium.

152

Standards of the Days of Endometrium in Menstrual Cycle

Date	The Characteristics of the Changes of Endometrium
M 15	Occasionally-found vacuoles under the nucleus
M 16	Irregular vacuoles under the nucleus
M 17	The regular and railing vacuoles under the nucleus
M 18	The vacuoles on and below the nucleus
M 19	Light secretion
M 20	Heavy secretion
M 21	Slight interstitial edema
M 22	Heavy interstitial edema
M 23	The interstitial cells around the spiral small arteries are big and round
M 24	The interstitial cells around the spiral small arteries are anterior decidual cells
M 25	The interstitial cells of compact layer near to the surface epithelium are anterior decidual cells and granular cells
M 26	The interstitial cells of the whole compact layer are anterior decidual cells and granular cells
M 27	The white cells exudate and the endometrium is shrunk
M 28	Exudate, dissociation and necrosis

It is reliable to determine the degree of maturity of the endometrium according to Noyes' standards. It has greater clinical, practical value to diagnose corpus luteum insufficiency through endometrium histological changes established according to Noyes' diagnostic standards. The determination of the date of intima of corpus luteum of the first week is based on the changes of glandular epithelium—division, pseudostratification, basal vacuoles. During the second week, it is based on the interstitial changes—edema, anterior decidual changes, division, and the infiltration of lymphocyte cells. According to these, the intima curettage should be conducted 2-3 days before expected menstruation, for the degree of infiltration of interstitial lymphocyte cells and the degree of anterior decidual reaction are the best in-

153

dices to measure the degree of maturity of endometrium. Some people conduct biopsy when menstruation has come, but after the coming of menstruation, the endometrium has lost the morphological change needed to determine the degree of maturity. It can only report that during menstruation whether there is change in secretion period. In actual practice, the endometrium is scraped and obtained from the uterine bottom, front wall or the lower back wall, which has greater diagnostic value. The best specimen should be 2cm, strong tissue which consists of compact layer and spongy layer. There have been reports that through observation of the endometrium of the infertile cases, insufficiency of corpus luteum is divided into three types: Type of slow developmental body of gland, the type of backward developmental interstitial tissue, and the type of developmental disorder of the interstitial tissue of the body of gland. Among the three types, the first is quite common.

• *The Determination of Internal Secretion*

It mainly refers to the determination of blood, urine hormone. Especially, radioimmunoassay, which has better correctness, is helpful to diagnose female sterility.

The Total Amount of Estrogen in Plasma (E_2): E_2 is one of the most sensitive indices to measure ovary function, pregnancy period, and ovulation. It also can reflect the start and the end of the function of the yellow body of ovary. During follicle period, E_2 increases from 1-5pg/ml to 100-400pg/ml, one day before ovulation, but on the day of ovulation, it decreases to 70-100pg/ml, and in the middle stage, it again rises to 100-200pg/ml. According to the fluctuating condition of the curve, the development condition and the normality of corpus luteum can be diagnosed. Generally, the value of E_2 is over 300pg/ml (250-400pg/ml).

The Determination of Plasma Progesterone (P): The determination of progesterone in plasma can help to know the condition of the formation and the function of corpus luteum. During normal cycle, 3-9 days after ovulation, P rises from 1ng/ml to 10-20ng/ml, and goes down during the dissolving period of corpus luteum (12 ± 2 days after ovula-

154

tion). The increase of P means that the reaction to the sharp increase LH is slightly earlier than ovulation period. It is the latest test to determine ovulation. When determination is finished, it is the end of ovulation. From the level of P and the period lasting, the function of corpus luteum can be judged. If P level can not increase to 5-7ng/ml, or it lowers after 8 days after ovulation, then any fertilized ovum can not implant, and will die. So, though to use P to determine ovulation is not better than LH and E_2, it can help to observe and correct the function of the yellow body of ovary and improve pregnancy rate.

There is still controversial over the standards of blood progesterone level of insufficiency of corpus luteum. Israel reported that blood progesterone content during the middle stage of the corpus luteum is larger or equal to 3ng/ml which signals ovulation. Ross regarded 5ng/ml, the value of blood progesterone content in the middle stage of corpus luteum as the normal lower limit of ovulation. Raclavanska and Snyer put forward 10ng/ml, the value of blood progesterone content, as the dividing line to measure whether corpus luteum function is normal or abnormal. Abraham regarded the total value of blood progesterone measured 3 times 11-4 days before menstruation, being larger than 15ng/ml, as the normal value. It is reliable compared with only one time of measurement (Gu Meili, et al, 1988). The diagnosis and treatment standard of female sterility with TCM in combination with Western medicine in China should be that the total value of plasma progester is greater than 10ng/ml in successive 2 times 6 days after ovulation. However, the measure of plasma progesterone radioimmunoassay is limited by the conditions of technology, equipment, etc. It is difficult to use it widely in clinic.

In recent years, many experts, both home and abroad, compared plasma progesterone determination with endometrium biopsy, used to evaluate the function of the yellow body of ovary. Jones holds that plasma progesterone content is consistent with endometrium reaction. The endometrium 2 days before menstruation can completely reflect the state of function of progesterone and the reaction of tar-

155

get organ to the hormone. Shepard and Senturia found that the cases that the endometrium histologic stages are consistent with plasma progesterone take up 75%. Goldstein reported that the cases that two aspects are consistent took up 51%. Rosenfeld found that though the plasma progesterone content of normal endometrium is higher than that of the endometrium of backward maturity, it has no statistical significance. What's more, the contents of progesterone of the groups have a lot of overlaps, and it is held that to diagnose the insufficiency of the corpus luteum, endometrium biopsy is more important. Many scholars point out that the disconsistency between plasma progesterone and the endometrium histological changes is related to the progesterone receptor content of the endometrium. Some people compared the progesterone receptor content of cytoplasm of endometrium cells of 22 cases (including 13 cases with P peak being larger than 15ng/ml) with backward development of endometrium and 9 cases with normal endometrium development. They found that of the former is obviously lower than that of the latter. The progesterone peak value of 13 cases is normal. But because of insufficiency of progesterone receptor content, endometrium may also show backward development. Keller regarded this phenomenon as "pseudoinsufficiency of corpus luteum." It suggests that those with normal P peak value lack progesterone receptors, endometrium may also suffer from maldevelopment (Zhang Liwei, et al, 1990).

The Determination of Gonadotropic Hormone (FSH, LH): FSH directly stimulates the growth of follicles. Because the fluctuation of FSH in menstrual cycle is greater, it is not used. It is a common way to use LH to observe ovulation, but LH is controlled by LHRH. The release of LHRH is like pulse, and the degradation of it in blood is influenced by exterior factors, like food, drugs and psychologic factors. So successive specimen-taking has diagnostic significance. Most people select blood specimen, and it can also be determined through urine. The peak of LH can only be measured out in the middle stage of menstruation, and in the rest of time, it fluctuates slightly. So it can be used as a reference for the process of follicle growth. However, when LH

156

peak is determined, it is too late to perform fertilization. At present, the commonest method is to determine FSH and LH levels by means of blood radioimmunoassay. If FSH in blood is greater than 40mIu/ml, LH is greater than 25mIu/ml, the patient suffers from hyperfunction of hypophysis. If FSH is normal or slightly lower, but LH is higher, polycystic ovary syndrome may be considered with the overall condition being considered. Being used to determine ovulation, the peak of LH in blood, and measured one day before ovulation should be greater than 40mIu/ml. In recent years, there have been reports of the application of RIA determination to measure LH in urine. The peak of LH in urine in place of LH peak in blood can be used to predict ovulation. It's simple to take urine specimen, and repeated tests can be made. At home, Liu Ping and others reported LH 150mIu/ml as LH-RIA peak in urine.

LH in Urine Determined by Enzyme Immunoassay (EIA): In 1983, EIA began to be used abroad to measure LH in urine. In 1985, Knee reported monoclonal antibody EIA being used to measure LH in urine. Liu Ping and others at home used monoclonal antibody EIA to measure LH in urine. The quantity determination of EIA showed the basal level of LH in urine during follicle stage and corpus luteum stage was 20mIu/ml, and the peak value was 40mIu/ml, LH in urine was between 20-40mIu/ml. Then it may be considered that LH peak is coming. At the same time, RIA was used to measure the value of LH in blood and urine. The result showed that urine EIA can be used to determine the peak value of LH before ovulation. EIA to determine LH in urine is simple and reliable, and the results can be obtained visually directly. One time of determination takes only 30 minutes. It is practical and it's easy to take urine specimen and repeated measurements can be conducted. What should be stressed is that whether LHRIA or LHEIA, the menstrual cycles without LH peak mostly belongs to ovulation; on the other hand, there is LH peak but no ovulation unnecessarily, and the normal function of corpus luteum, LUFS sometimes happens.

The Determination of Progesterone in Saliva by Means of Radioimmunoassay: In the past, the determination of pro-

157

gesterone mostly used blood specimen; but blood steroid hormones have circadian fluctuating rhythms, and the statistics obtained from only one time of determination can not accurately show the dynamic changes of the hormones in the body. In recent years, a lot of data have shown that salivary progesterone (SP) can be used as the reliable index to evaluate the function of the yellow body of ovary. The collection of saliva is non-damaging, and it can be collected many times for the purpose of dynamic observation, and easy storage and doesn't affect the subject's daily life. Generally, enough specimen amount 3-5ml can be obtained in a short time and can be kept for 6-9 months under $-20\,^{\circ}\text{C}$. The concentration has no obvious changes. So, the subject can collect specimen at home, and keep in the refrigerator and collect together and send it to the laboratory for determination.

The purpose of body progesterone determination is to monitor ovulation. In the past, plasma progesterone (PP) value is used to judge ovulation. Generally, PP>30 nmol/l means menstrual cycle of ovulation. PP<10 nmol/L means less ovulation, but PP fluctuates day and night greatly. One time of determination may cause missed diagnosis. Compared with blood progesterone, fluctuation of SP is small. It can accurately reflect the state of ovary function. In normal menstrual cycle, the regular patterns of SP fluctuation are: In 1-12 days of menstrual cycle, SP is usually lower than 56pmol/L or not over 100pmol/L. From the 12th day to the twenty-first day, it goes up rapidly. On the twenty-first, it can reach its peak value (The range is 230-550pmol/L). Later, it gradually decreases. In menstrual cycle without ovulation, SP doesn't increase and its value is less than 56pmol/ml. Though SP and PP have menstrual cyclic changes, SP has no circadian fluctuating rhythms.

In addition to the function of monitoring ovulation, SP also has guiding value in ovulation-inducing treatment and the determination of early stage pregnancy. In the process of ovulation-inducing drug treatment, to the infertile patients, SP determination can help to accurately learn the dynamic changes of the hormones in the body, and it can timely guide and regulate treatment plan. In pregnant corpus luteum

158

stage, SP may decrease slightly, then, increase rapidly. On the eleventh day of ovulation, there are obvious differences in SP between the non-pregnant and pregnant women. The former's decreases to the level of proliferative stage, and the latter increases steadily. If great early abortion happens, SP will rapidly decrease to the level of proliferative stage. The content of salivary steriod doesn't exceed 10% plasma, and SP is only 1% or so of PP. In this low concentration determination, if there is no strict quality control, it will lead to great error. So, in the test, the requirement of radioimmune quality control and the determination of salivary specimen should be acquired, and the experiment conditions should be strictly controlled to reduce operating errors.

• *The Examination of Cervical Mucus*

With the fluctuation of sexual hormone level in menstrual cycle, there are different changes to cervical mucus in its amount, nature, viscosity, the type of mucus crystals. Observing these changes can indirectly find out the ovary function. Under the influence of estrogen, the water content in cervical mucus increases. The nearer it is to ovulatory stage, the thinner the mucus will be, the higher the ductility will be. When ovulatory stage comes, the cervical mucus is clear and crystal, like the egg white and the wiredrawing length can be 10cm or so. After ovulation, cervical mucus becomes sticky, turbid, like jelly, and ductility becomes lower, the wiredrawing length is only 1-2cm. From the 7th day or so of the menstrual cycle, cervical mucus gradually appears to be fernlike crystals. After ovulation, the fernlike crystals disappear gradually and oval crystals remain.

Cervical scoring (CS) is often used as one of the means to monitor ovulation. From the 1-2 days after completion of the menstrual cycle to the fourth day when BBT goes up, uterus neck is examined every day, and 2 times every week during corpus luteum stage. Examine cervical mucus' amount, nature, wiredrawing degree, the width of the uterine mouth opening, do cervical mucus smear, and observe the form of crystals under low-magnification microscope. The scoring is conducted according to improved Insler's Scoring Standards:

159

Cervical Scoring Standards

Score	Mucus Amount & Color	Uterine Mouth	Wiredrawing	Fernlike Crystal
0	no; yellow, intransparent	closed	negative	negative
1	little; milky	slightly loose	2-3cm	very little more cells
2	moderate in amount; thin	1-1.5mm, probe can be inserted	4-8cm	thin trunk, slightly soft tops of the branches, sometimes similar to the after-snow tree branches
3	much in amount; thin	2-3mm wide open	more than 10cm	rough, strong trunk, long bran-ches

Ovulation often occurs when scores are 10-12.

• B-Ultrasound Scanning Used to Monitor Ovulation

Since 1972, Kratochwil and others reported for the first time to use B-ultrasound to show follicles, now, "B-ultrasound" scanning has become an effective, often used, method to monitor ovulation. The method brings high accuracy, no injury to human body, no pain, and it is simple and fast to operate. Through dynamically observing the changes of follicle ultrasonic pictures can monitor many indices of follicle development and ovulation. Its advantages not only surpass those of BBT, cervical mucus examination, but also are even better than determination of blood hormone level and abdominoscopy.

The earlier time of follicle ultrasound developing may be on the 7th day of menstrual cycle, and the shortest diameter showed is 5mm. 4-5 days before ovulation, the main follicle diameter grows at a speed of 2-3mm per day. Just before ovulation, the follicles grow mature. The matured follicles appear to be round or oval, whose diameters are 15-30mm, and there are no echoing area opaca, but there are good transparency, and clear borders. One day before ovulation, cumulus oophorus picture can be seen in 20% of the matured follicles; and most of the pictures appear in the matured fol-

160

licles whose diameter is longer than 18mm. This predicts that ovulation will happen in 24 hours. Most reports hold that when the diameter of the follicles is between 18-25mm, the chance of pregnancy is great. If the diameter is smaller than 18mm, it's hard to get pregnant.

Female sterility which is caused by ovulatory disturbance takes up 15-25% among the total infertile cases. In the women with regular menstrual cycle, diphasic BBT, through ultrasound examination, the development and ovulation of 13-44% of the follicles in the cycle are abnormal. The ultrasound reflects that no follicle development or the follicle diameter shorter than 14mm means anovulatory cycle. The follicle diameter longer than 14mm, but shorter than 18mm means it is ovulatory cycle of the little follicles. The follicle diameter shorter than 30mm means it is the ovulatory cycle of the big follicles. LUFS has three ultrasound manifestations: ① On the expected ovulation day, the volume of the follicles remain unchanged, and the crystal wall grows thick gradually. 2-4 days later, a lot of light spots occur inside the follicles, and gradually disappear. ② On the expected ovulatory day, the volume of follicles remain unchanged, and the inside echoing becomes strong gradually. 2-4 days later, a lot of light spots occur inside the follicles and gradually disappear. ③ On the expected ovulation day, the volume of follicles rapidly increases to 30-50mm, or even greater, and continues to exist until the end of the cycle or the beginning of the next cycle or even longer.

LUFS refers to that though the follicular cells can not be ejected from the matured follicles, the patients have regular menstruation and normal corpus luteum function. The occurrence rate takes certain proportion among the infertile women. Because these women's menstrual cycle is regular, BBT is diphasic, it causes difficulties to clinical diagnosis. In the past, abdominos-copy was applied 2-4 days after ovulation to confirm this disease whether ovulation spots exist. In recent years, B-ultrasound examination has become the first choice of the method to diagnose LUFS.

The follicle rupture observed by "B-ultrasound examination" signals ovulation, which takes place in 24 hours after

161

LH peak value. In most cycles, LH peak value, the largest follicle diameter, much amount of cervical mucus, the most typical crystals, the lowest point of BBT occur on the same day, that is one day before ovulation.

To monitor ovulation, B-ultrasound examination is a reliable and simple method, especially in the diagnosis of the disease of follicle development and ovulation. It overrides all other clinical indices. However, it also has its shortcomings. For example, it has difficulties in observing some diseases in oviduct, endometriosis, abnormal ovum position, and the follicles of obesity patients. With the development of ultrasound technology, the appearing of vaginal probe remedies this shortcoming.

Vaginal ultrasound examination need not fill the urinary bladder, and has no feeling of uncomfort, and has a high resolving power, and is especially for corpulent patients. Some people compared abdominal ultrasound examination and vaginal ultrasound examination, and thought the latter is superior to the former. They also thought vaginal ultrasound can direct follicle puncture in place of the many cases which follicles are taken through abdominoscopy, for puncture guided by vaginal ultrasound has the advantages of little danger, low cost, and easy to operate. What's more, it was found that when the diameter of the pregnant cyst during early stage of pregnancy is 2mm, it can be recognized. When the concentration of β-HCG reaches 141mIu/ml, the pregnant cyst during early stage of pregnancy can be recognized. This suggests that vaginal ultrasound examination can diagnose pregnancy earlier than abdominal ultrasound examination. There have been reports that vaginal ultrasound examination can help to raise the diagnostic rate of ectopic pregnancy, and abdominal ultrasound examination can help diagnose out 50% of the adnexal lumps. Many medical workers have already used the method of obtaining follicles through the guidance of vaginal ultrasound to do IVF-EF in place of abdominoscopy. However, when it reaches the middle stage of pregnancy, the uterus enlarges day by day, and the position of the fetus raises day after day, and is getting further and further from the vagina. It is hard to detect by means of vaginal ultrasound technique.

• *Five Indexes Used to Monitor Ovulation Comprehensively*

The five indices include BBT, cervical mucus scoring (CS), plasma E_2, RIA, ultrasonic scanning (USS). The purpose of comprehensively monitoring ovulation is to improve the accuracy of the diagnosis. Though BBT enables a patient to obtain a curve of a cycle through self-monitoring so that she can roughly retrospectively judge whether follicle development exists according to this curve; however, it is easily affected by many factors. Plasma E_2 and LH are closely related. It is accurate and reliable to use them to predict ovulation, but it is restrained by test conditions, and it is not fit to popularize. USS can directly help to learn the condition of follicle development and diagnose ovulation, especially to directly observe LUFS. This is superior to any of the examining tools. But USS can not help to know the endocrine condition of the follicles. It is reliable to predict ovulation through CS. Generally, CS can reflect the condition of follicle growth, and endocrine function; what's more, it is easy and simple to practice CS, and has the value to popularize.

• *Ovulation Prediction Through Intimal Cells Smear*

In 1981, Affandi held that smear cytologic examination of intima suction used to predict ovulation is a simple, safe, accurate method. In 1986, Chen Jixia used uterus sprayer to take specimen to study the possibility of cytology in the application of intima stages determination, and put forward the standards of intima stages determination. Under the condition that the specimen is taken by endometrium cell sample-taker with digroove and sheath, the accuracy of cytological determining ovulation is 97.5%. It suggests that cytological determining ovulation is a simple, safe, reliable method. Though it can not determine the time of ovulation, it can accurately reflect whether ovulation has already taken place during the third week of the cycle. It has certain clinical value to the study of infertile patients.

• *Vaginal Cell Smear Examination*

Vaginal cell smear examination can be used in the understanding of ovary function, the level of estrogen and whether

163

ovulation exists. It has certain practical value as indication of endocrine treatment, the examination of curative effect, and the evaluation of prediction.

According to the different conditions of ovary function, different pictures may appear in vaginal smear. Usually, keratinized cells count is used to classify estrogen levels. The diagnostic standards are: ① The proportion of Keratinized cells or the cells of compact nuclear superficial layer affected slightly is under 20%; ② The proportion of Keratinized cells or the cells of compact nuclear superficial layer affected moderately is 20-60%; ③ That affected highly is 60-90%.

Under the influence of estrogen, in smear, usually there are no basal layer cells. When ovary function is low, such as climacterium, lactation, or amenorrhea, there are few superficial cells but there are basal layer cells. Therefore, the number of basal layer cells appearing can be used to judge the degree of the downcast of ovary function. The diagnostic standards are: ① The slight downcast refers to that the cells of basal layer are below 20%. ② The moderate downcast refers to that the cells of basal layer are between 20-40%. ③ The high downcast refers to that of the underlayer cells are above 40%.

• *The Comparison of Various Methods of Predicting Ovulation*

BBT is at present a commonly-used method to monitor ovulation. It is generally thought that the increase of temperature happens one day after ovulation; however, in clinical retrospective practice, 3-day-in-a-row-going-up temperature should be observed so that the ovulation day can be confirmed, so it can only be considered as the end of retrospective reference pregnancy period (FP). What's more, in measuring temperature, the mental fluctuation, the disturbance of infection, the factors in the exterior, etc. all can affect body temperature. But, at present, BBT is still a simple method. In recent years, the temperature of the urine excreted the first time in the morning is considered to be BBT. The observation of cervical mucus and the periodic changes of the nature is one of the methods to predict ovulation.

But, cervical mucus can only reflect estrogen level, and can not confirm whether there is ovulation. Also, the reactions of cervical glands to estrogen are different. Some show good reaction in low-level estrogen, but a few people show insufficient reaction in normal estrogen level. Also, in some cases of delayed or scanty LH secretion, mucus secretion lasts, and the later appearance of oval corpuscles affect the prediction of ovulation. Cervical scoring is one of the methods used to monitor ovulation. It is used to regularly examine cervical mucus, mucus nature, wiredrawing, and the opening degree of uterus mouth, and to do cervical mucus crystallizing examination, and to score according to the improved Insler's scoring standards. Endometrium biopsy is a simple and reliable means to diagnose ovulation and corpus luteum function if specimen-taking time is correctly chosen, and histological diagnosis made according to Noyes' diagnostic standards. Estrogen (E_2) is one of the most sensitive indices in examining ovary function, pregnancy period, and ovulation. E_2 and LH RIA all can reliably predict whether ovulation occur in 1-2 days. Plasma progesterone (P) assay can help to observe the formation period and the function of corpus luteum. It can also be used to judge whether corpus luteum function is sufficient. However, these endocrine RIAs are limited by equipment conditions and the patients sufferings. Enzyme immunoassay (EIA) of urine LH and salivary progesterone (SP) assay can get rid of the pain of blood taking. B-ultrasonic scanning has become an effective method at present in monitoring evaluation. This method has a high accuracy, brings no injuries to the body, no sufferings, and is easy, simple and rapid to practice. Through dynamic observation of the changes of follicle ultrasound pictures, follicle development and ovulation indices can be monitored, especially has special value in the diagnosis of LUFS. It is superior to the rest of the indices. Vaginal ultrasonic examination need not fill the Bladder, brings no uncomfortable feelings, has high resolving rate, fit for the patients with obesity, and especially fit for ovulation monitoring, early stage pregnancy diagnosis, the diagnosis of ectopic pregnancy, abdominal masses and the guidance in follicle puncturing in

165

place of follicle-taking through abdominoscopy. However, B-ultrasonic scanning (USS) can not help to learn the follicle endocrine condition. For the principle of rapidness, accuracy, simplicity, a comprehensive ovulation monitoring of the five indices—BBT, CS, E_2, LH, and USS—is an even accurate, feasible way. Intimal cells smear monitoring ovulation is a simple, safe, reliable method. Though it can not determine the exact time when ovulation happens, during the third week of the cycle, it can accurately reflect whether ovulation has already taken place. Vaginal cell examination can help to learn ovary function, and the level of estrogen, to judge whether there's ovulation. It has certain practical value as an indication of endocrine treatment, effect test and prediction evaluation.

Examination of Tubal Sterility
To detect whether or not the fallopian tuber is unobstructed or not is an important method in searching for the etiological factors in infertile cases. The commonly used methods include tubal ventilation test, tubal solution perfusion test, tubal pigment perfusion method, the uterus tubal meglucamine diatrizonate roentgenography, tubal acoustic holography, tubal liquid perfusion under endoscope, etc. Besides the application of these methods in diagnosis, they are also used to deroppilate slightly tubal adhesion, and tubal obstruction. The above methods have their own properties, and are chosen for use according to the actual condition. Liquid perfusion method is the primary selection to clinical patients, and the various kinds of roentgenography are used for further examination or the comparison between the conditions before and after the treatment. To the patients with the exterior and internal genital, trichomonal or mycotic inflammation, severe cervicitis, severe cervical erosion, uterus bleeding, severe heart and lung and other overall diseases; or having a history of sexual intercourse in 3 days, the examinations listed above are avoided. Traditionally, the examination is conducted 3-7 days after completion of the menstrual cycle. Now, many hospitals have broken the taboo. In principle, the examination can be conducted

any time after the ending of menstruation. Sometimes, for reducing operating process, benefiting the patients, one operation is carried out to conduct tubal liquid perfusion test, and endometrium biopsy, but it should be done several days before menstruation, tubal liquid perfusion test first, and endometrium biopsy next.

• *Tubal Solution Perfusion Examination*

Solution perfusion examination is one of the basic methods to test the unobstruction of the oviduct. The liquid used here is mainly physiological saline. Some use 0. 25-0. 5% novocaine solution to prevent tubal spasm. The perfusion rate is 5ml per minute with a total volume of 30-40ml. If there are no resistance, external leaking, reflux, it suggests the unobstructed oviduct. If great resistance, a reflux of more than 10ml are observed, it indicates that the oviduct is obstructed. If solution can still be perfused into it after pressure is given, but there is certain resistance or little reflux, it suggests that the oviduct is open, but it is not smooth. If the solution is gradually perfused in the process of perfusion pushing after pressure is supplied, it indicates that inside the lumen or fimbrial end, there is adhesion, which is pushed aside by solution. Solution perfusion examination is simple and easy for the patient to accept, and is used for comparison between the conditions before and after treatment.

• *Salpingography of Uterus*

The contrast medium is perfused into the uterus and reaches the oviduct. It can directly show the position, size, appearance, whether normal or not, and bore conditions of the oviduct. Contrast examination not only helps to examine whether the oviduct is unobstructed or not, but also helps to learn the length and curvature of the fallopian tube, the range of pathologic changes, the location of adhesion or obstruction, whether there are exterior pressing pathologic changes, etc. , in the tube, and can also diagnose stenosis of cervix or laxation of cervix, chronic endometritis, tuberculosis of uterus, dysplasia of uterus, abnormality of uterus, uterine polyp, uterine hysteromyoma and uterine carcinoma, etc.

The contrast medium used the earliest was 40% iodized

oil. Before operation, iodine allergic test is conducted. The contrast time is usually fixed at 3-7 days after the completion of menstrual cycle. The volume of iodized oil is 6-10ml at a time, and it should be perfused in slowly, and the pushing force should not be great. If resistance is observed, or the patient suffers from pain, injection is stopped. For avoiding tubal spasm, a subcutaneous injection of 0.5mg atropine or an intramuscular injection of 10mg valine, or puncturing at Hegu (LI 4), and Neiguan (PC 6) is applied. The obstructed parts may be located at the oviduct's interstitial area, isthmus, ampullae, and fimbriae. Tubal adhesion is manifested as sactosalpinx, adhesion of tubal fimbria, or peripheral adhesion of tubal fimbria end. To the patients with partially tubal adhesion, though their oviduct can eject drug liquid, there is adhesion in peripheral fimbria end to the varying degree, which makes the contrast medium unable to flow smoothly through the oviduct and to spread to pelvic cavity; so in the pelvic cavity, there is spread contrast medium, and there is restricted liquid drug accumulation in the oviduct. Tubal tuberculosis is characterized by miliary transparent spot shadows, narrowed, stiff lumen with villi peripherally, or multiple tubal stricture with various degrees of thickness, zigzagging borders like cooked noodles made from bean or sweet potato starch, or thinned, stiffened interrupted (intermittent) lumen like the rusty fine iron thread with its obstructed end restricted and enlarged whose shape is like flower bud. These patients of tubal tuberculosis also usually suffer from at the same time calcification of pelvic cavity.

Recently, for lack of 40% iodized oil contrast medium, 76% or 60% meglucamine diatrizonate ejectio is applied to carry out uterus salpingography, which leads to good result. Meglucamine diatrizonate is water soluble iodine preparations with little adhesion, fast flowing rate. If uterus development is normal, and the oviduct is unobstructed, on the fluorescent screen, the contrast medium can be seen overflowing from the fimbria of the fallopian tube to the pelvic cavity while diffusion is good, take the first picture and diagnosis can be gained from it. 20 minutes later, fluoroscopy is conducted or the second picture is taken. The volume of

168

meglucamine diatrizonate is 10ml; and when necessary, it can be added. Iodine allergic test should be made before operation.

• *Acoustic Salpingography*

Acoustic salpingography, another method to diagnose whether fallopian tube is unobstructed or not, is simple, efficient, direct, and safe to operate. First of all, slowly inject 20ml of normal saline water into uterine cavity; then, change to use an injection springe with 20ml of 20% hydrogen dioxide solution absorbed. First, perfuse 10ml, use the probe to press the left side lightly, and observe the right side of the fallopian tube. Then, perfuse the remained 10ml into the uterine cavity. Acoustic salpingography diagnoses whether the fallopian tube is unobstructed or not according to the flowing condition of oxygen bubbles in pelvic cavity and fallopian tube through an injection of normal saline water into the pelvic cavity which is then dilated, which then results in the formation of a sound-penetrating window with 2% hydrogen dioxide solution being injected. When the fallopian tuber is normal, the oxygen bubbles move across the tube into the abdominal cavity through fimbria end. If fallopian tube is obstructed, the oxygen bubbles flow back, and are shown clearly on the ultrasonic screen. What's more, when the fallopian tube is unobstructed, after the perfusion of hydrogen dioxide solution, the patient experiences light nausea, dizziness, distending pain in abdominal area, etc. If the oviduct is obstructed, or slightly obstructed, there will be no this reaction or the reaction is light. But acoustic salpingography has its shortcomings. It can not show at the same time the uterus and the two appendixes. So one side must be checked, then the other side. What's more, it is hard to show in the screen whether the uterus is one-side leaned, or the run of the oviduct and the uterus cavity are on the same plane.

• *Abdominoscopy*

If the fallopian tube is obstructed because of inflammatory adhesion, part of the patients may suffer from adhesion to the varying degree about the fallopian tube, ovary or the uterus. It is hard to help confirmation by the commonly used tubal solution-perfusion test, phenol red test, and uterus iodized oil salpingography, and to be clear about these pathologic changes has great significance in working out therapeutic plan. Abdominoscopic examination has the following advantages: ① Under direct observation, whether or not adhesion between fallopian tube, ovary, or the uterus and the pelvic wall, and degree of adhesion can be determined according to range of adhesion and the width and thickness of furnicular fiber, or lysis is carried out under the abdominoscope. ② When carrying out the operation, inject methylene blue solution to the uterus cavity. To observe the condition of methylene blue solution overflowing from fimbria can accurately judge whether the fallopian tube is unobstructed. For the patients with tubal obstruction, it can help to determine the obstructed location and its degree.

• *Comparison Between Uterus Salpingography and Abdominoscopy*

Beijing Xiehe Hospital, China Institute of Medical Science, treated 122 cases of female sterility between March, 1979 and October, 1986 through uterus salpingography together with Caesarean operation or abdominoscopy. 97 cases experienced Caesarean operation after contrast. The coincidence of the two was 79. 7%. 52 cases experienced abdominoscopy after contrast, the coincidence of the two was 66. 3%. It was held that the uncoincidence was because of technical factors and tubal spasm. The patients with obstruction at the corner of the uterus revealed through contrast were advised to receive abdominoscopy. Salpingography and abdominoscopy are two important methods in the examination of female sterility. The documental literature reported that the coincidence of the tubal examination results from the two methods was 46-89%. The uncoincidence of the two was because of the two cases. ① Technical Factors: During contrast, the perfusion of iodized oil is not enough which is mistaken for non-opening. The iodized oil flowing into the oviduct causing ovary cysts with adhesion is mistaken for non-opening. ② Spasm: The patients are nervous, the perfusion rate of contrast medium is too big, or the contrast medium temperature is too low. This can cause tubal spasm.

170

Spasm occurs in most cases at the corner of the uterus. The x-ray photos of the corner of the uterus of tubal spasm mostly show as a round shape, or as sharp angle. Before operation, the injection of atopine and other spasm-relieving drugs can be helpful in relieving spasm, but the effect is not certain. This group of cases of one year all received routine injection of atropine before salpingography and abdominoscopy, but the oviduct of four patients still experienced spasm. Snowden recommended to use 10mg of glucagon through intramuscular injection as spasm-relieving medium from the oviduct. The curative effect was 80% (Sun Aide, et al, 1988).

Through HSG retrospective analysis and comparison examination by endoscope of 231 cases, Rice JP (1986) found that it has little value to use HSG to diagnose the unobstruction of fallopian tube. Among 100 cases found to have abnormal changes in fallopian tube through HSG diagnosis, pseudonegative rate was 14.9%, pseudopositive rate was 15.9%, similar to 8-24% and 6-24% reported in literature and reports. Misdiagnosis of obstruction at proximal end of fallopian tube is in most cases related to spasm contraction of the uterus corner. Misdiagnosis of tubal distal obstruction is caused by higher viscosity of the contrast medium in the fallopian tube compared with methylene blue. The accuracy of HSG examination of the condition of the uterus cavity is higher; so it can be used to select the patients with abnormal uterus. However, abdominoscope examination not only can confirm whether the fallopian tube is unobstructed but also can discover other pathogenic problems that affect reproduction, such as endometriosis, adhesion, etc. So, in examining the uterine factors in female sterility, HSG can be used; however, in examining the factors outside the uterus, abdominoscope examination has greater significance and is safer.

• *Salpingoscopy*

Many of pathogenic changes of tubal mucus can not be detected through salpingography and abdominoscopy. It is the main reason of female sterility after microsurgical restoring operation on fallopian tube. Salpingoscope is a hard light

171

conducting fiber telescope whose diameter is 3mm. It is inserted into fallopian tube when abdominoscope examination is conducted. It can help to observe and study directly the local mucus. Brosens, et al (1987) examined 44 cases of infertile patients. Among 27 infertile patients whose salpingoscopy showed normal, seven were found to have plica abnormality, such as cohesion or adhesion, four were diagnosed to have pathogenic damage at interstitial area or isthmus area through salpingoscope or abdominoscope examination. 13 were found to have one-sided or two-sided hydrosalpinx through uterine salpingography. After examination, it was confirmed that two had no hydrosalpinx, among which one's adhesive membrane plicae on infundibular part were normal, the big plicae at ampullar region were enlarged, and the small ones became flat. The tubal wall became thin and transparent. These suggested tubal myo-architectonic abnormality. The other 11 cases with hydrosalpinx experienced examination on mucus pathogenic changes after the fallopian tube was cut open.

The results showed that salpingoscope examination is a necessary supplementary method of pelvioscopy. It can help to find the lumen pathologic changes. Their range and degree which can not be discovered through uterine salpingography and abdominoscope examination. It can supply reliable basis for diagnosis of tubal sterility, selection of curative ways and judgment of prediction.

Examination of Sterility due to Cervical Factors

Among female infertile cases, 5-10% are caused by cervical abnormality and secretory abnormality. In normal cases, during sexual intercourse, about 100-150 millions sperms accumulate outside the external orifice of uterus and in vaginal vault. After ejaculation, the sperma agglutinates immediately, and the movement of spermia is restricted, but they immediately liquefy through proteaselytic effect, immediately pass cervical mucus, enter cervical cavity, and move up to be fertilized. If cervical mucus stops the coming through of the sperms, it can cause female sterility.

Cervical mucus is mainly produced by secretory cells of

172

cervical endometrium. The main element is a hydrogel, rich in carbohydrate, and formed by mucin of glucoprotein. This determines the main physical properties of cervical mucus. External researchers suggest that the movement of spermia is related to glucose level in cervical mucus. In the cervical mucus of some infertile patients, glucose concentration was indeed found to decrease. Ovary hormones regulate secretion of cervical mucus. Estrogen stimulates the neck of uterus to produce a great deal of water mucus, thin and clear transparent, favorable to the penetration of sperms. Progesterone inhibits secretory activity of cervical epithelial cells; therefore, cervical mucus becomes less and sticky which is unfavorable to the penetration of spermia. In normal cases, the penetrating power of spermia to cervical mucus increases gradually from the ninth day of menstrual cycle, and reaches a peak until ovulation period, and is inhibited 1-2 days after ovulation. For the cases with chronic cervicitis, cervical epithelial secretion increases. Cervical mucus becomes sticky, unfavorable to the penetration of spermia, containing a great many of white cells phagocytizing sperms. Seminal serum contains a number of proteins which enter female's genital duct as antigens absorbed by cervical epithelia, causing immune reaction. In recent years, the incidence of antisperm antibodies is high in cervical mucus of the infertile patients. The antibodies of this kind exert agglutinating and braking effect on spermia. This is also one of the causes of female sterility.

Scoring must be made to the following examinations as far as female sterility caused by cervical mucus problems is concerned.

• *Analysis of seminal fluid and examination of cervical mucus*

Analysis of seminal fluid includes seminal volume, nature and time period for liquefaction, sperm number, sperm survival rate, and sperm mobility, sperm abnormality rate, sperm penetrating power, averaged sperm moving rate, staining examination, whether having pyocytes and agglutination, etc. (see Chapter One). The performance of cervical mucus affects sperm activity and penetrating power. The

173

method of collecting cervical mucus is to use tuberculin springe connected with sterile plastic tube to push 1cm deep into the neck of uterus to absorb clean mucus. If it can absorb 0.4-0.6ml, it suggests normal development of follicles. Before or during ovulation cycle, the amount of cervical mucus is great, thin, and clear, and whose wiredrawing is $\geqslant$ 10cm, the fernlike crystal is "卅" with no cells, and pH being higher than 7-8.2, showing alkaline, which can neutralize the acid of genital duct, and is most fit for the penetration of sperms.

• *Huhner's Test*

The test should be conducted during the predicted ovulatory period. Before the test, 5 days of avoiding sexual activities is needed. 206 hours after sexual intercourse, cavascope is used to expose the neck of uterus. Take vaginal posterior fornix mucus first, and examine whether moving spermia exist. If there are, it suggests success of sexual intercourse, then suck the seminal fluid at the lower part of cervical tube, and place it on a glass slide, and covers it with a coverglass. Under high power lens, in every field of view, there are more than or as many as 20 active spermia, it suggests abnormality, and that the spermia can penetrate cervical mucus. On the other hand, in every field of view, if there are fewer than or as many as 5 sperms whose mobility is low, or the spermia are dead ones, it suggests oligospermia or cervical mucus abnormality, or problem of immunity. Patients with cervical or vaginal inflammation must be treated first, then undergo the test.

• *Penetrating Test of Spermia in Vitro*

Take one drop of cervical mucus of ovulatory period of the sterile female, and a drop of fresh seminal fluid of the husband. Place them on a glassslide, which are spaced between 2-3mm. Use a coverglass to slightly cover them to enable them to contact. Observe them under a microscope. If sperm's penetration of cervical mucus shows positive, it suggests normality of sperm mobility and cervical mucus. In mucus, there are no antisperm antibodies.

• *Cross Test of Seminal Fluid and Cervical Mucus*

To the sterile patients whose sperms can not penetrate cer-

174

vical mucus, proved through penetrating test of sperm in vitro, they must undergo seminal fluid-cervical mucus crossing test. The method is to use seminal fluid of the sterile male and cervical mucus of normal female; and cervical mucus of sterile female and seminal fluid of normal male to respectively carry out spermia in vitro penetrating test to determine that the causes that prevent spermia from penetrating cervical mucus are of seminal problems or problems of cervical mucus.

In the patients of cervical sterility, anatomical factors should not be neglected, such as cervical canal narrowness, adhesion, laceration, atresia, septum, double cervix, dysplasia, inflammation, erosion, etc. These etiological factors can to the varying degree prevent the spermia from entering cervical canal or change the physiochemical properties and volume of secretion of cervical mucus; therefore, it causes difficulty to the penetration of sperms and finally results in female sterility.

Examination of Sterility due to Immune Factors
If a married couple can not achieve the wish of having a baby for a long period of time, and their reproductive organs are not found to suffer from organic or functional diseases, they are usually called "the patient of female sterility due to unknown reasons." To these, the possibility of female sterility due to immune factors should be considered. Immune female sterility can be defined in a broad sense and a narrow one. Broadly, it means that because the body produces self-immunity to testis, ovary and its germinal cells. The self-immunity manifests in male as abnormal seminal fluid after routine examination, such as oligospermia, asthenospermia or azoospermatism, and in female as functional ovulatory disorder, such as ovary senilism or anergy ovary syndrome. By narrow definition is meant that the examination of the husband's seminal fluid is normal, too, and that there are proofs of antireproduction immunity. These couples have no clear organic diseases in reproductive system. The male can produce antibodies to his own spermia and cause the spermia to agglutinate and brake. This is called self-immunity. The

175

female can produce antibodies to the sperms, and cause the sperms to lose mobility in vaginal duct, or lose the power to penetrate the neck of uterus. Furthermore, the female can produce self-immunity to the organs of self-reproductive system.

The female's vaginal duct can produce local immune reaction to the outcoming antigens like bacteria, fungus, viruses, sperms, antigens of blood of type A, B, O and in secretory material of the neck of uterus, cervical cavity and vaginal duct, the reaction produces the corresponding antigens like IgG and IgA. These immunoglobin are combined and secreted by lymphacytic tissues with immune activity. Besides the locally secreted materials similar to plasma IgA which is called secreted immunoglobin A (SIgA), it is also found that some infertile patients have antisperm antibodies in microcirculation, but there are no antibodies in cervical mucus. It is proved clinically that the positive rate and the titer of sterile female's cervical mucus containing antisperm antibodies are higher than those of blood serum. The reason that women produce antisperm antibodies is because that in sexual intercourse, sperm antigens contact the vaginal duct, and uterus and immune reaction is caused. But, there are also some women who produce antisperm antibodies without having had sexual intercourse.

At present, the following ways are used to examine immune female sterility.

• *Huhner's Test*

See the previous part of this chapter. Some people encourage to preliminarily use it to determine whether there are antibodies. Some people researched the relationship between sperm and antibodies and Huhner's test. 127 cases of sterile women due to unknown causes underwent examination of antisperm antibodies of cervical canal mucus, blood serum, and sperm serum, and compared with Huhner's test. It was found that the antibody positive rate of the bad group of Huhner's test was 67.5%, but that of the normal group was 21.4%.

• *Sperm-Cervical Mucus Penetrating Test*

The method is simple. Suck the cervical mucus before

176

ovulation into a capillary and place it in the seminal fluid (husband's or sperm supplier's), and keep it for one hour at 37℃. Observe the farthest distance of the sperms penetrating under a low power lens. The distance shorter than 5mm is considered to have no penetrating power, that between 6-19mm is considered to have moderate penetrating power, and that longer than 20mm is considered to have good penetrating power.

• *Sperm-Cervical Mucus Contacting Test*

Drop one drop of seminal fluid on each end of a glass slide. One drop is added with the same size of cervical mucus, and the other drop is used for contrast. Keep them at 37℃ for 15-20 minutes and observe the sperm mobility under a microscope. In the sperm specimen with mucus, if fibrous or fine wire-like materials occur, and the sperms can not move forward, and shake about at the same place, it is considered to be positive. This method can be used for selective diagnosis of immune female sterility.

• *Enzyme Linked Immunosorbent Assay (ELISA)*

In October, 1986, the Second Academic Conference of Gynecology and Obstetrics Specialized Committee of China TCM and Western Medicine Combined Research Institute established the diagnostic standards for immune female sterility: ① The female sterility caused not by the factors other than the common ones excluded by clinical and other various examinations. ② Blood serum or cervical mucus antisperm antibodies are positive, or antioval zona pellucida antibodies are positive (This point can be confirmed). ③ Huhner's Test, in 2 hours before ovulation and after sexual intercourse, every field of view of high power lens, the number of actively-forwarding sperms in cervical mucus is less than 5. ④ Sperm-cervical mucus contacting test: Preovulation test shows that the sperms on the contacting surface with cervical mucus are "shivering," not moving, or moving slowly, observed under the lens.

Examination of Sterility due to Intrauterine Adhesion

Intrauterine Adhesion (IUA) is caused by uterine wall adhesion which leads to partial or complete metratresia or adhesion of internal orifice of uterus, thus causing menstrual disorder. It is often manifested as amenorrhea or scanty menstruation or sterility, and sometimes habitual abortion or gynecological complications. Any factor that damages endometrium can lead to IUA. Artificial absorption causes exposition of basis of endometrium, the degeneration and fibrosis of velocity left over by incomplete uterine curettage, or retention of placenta in missed abortion causes the activity of fibroblast to increase, Adhesion after placenta is removed, repeated uterine curettage in the condition of hydatidiform mole—all of this can cause uterus to suffer from IUA. Furthermore, endometritis, salpingitis, and tuberculosis of endometrium also can cause IUA. Pharmacological examination shows, except for endometrium, there are still fibrous tissue, smooth muscle, and degenerated villi. Menstruation disorder and sterility are chief clinical symptoms. If intrauterine adhesion area is larger, menstruation decreases obviously. The patients with adhesion of orifice of uterus may encounter amenorrhea. For the patients with endometriosis, pelvic examination shows adnexa tenderness, or uterine tenderness. Hysterosal-pingography (HSG) shows filling defect of uterine cavity, twisted and deformed uterine cavity. Mostly, fallopian tube is normal. The patients with fibrosis of uterine cavity has no filling defect, but uterine defect is irregular, the edges are stiff. Under uteroscope, there is threadlike fibrous adhesion on the thin layer of endometrium.

In diagnosing this disease, besides asking in details the related case history of diseases, gynecological examination, HSG and uteroscope examination are indispensable. Through uteroscope examination, it can help to know degree of adhesion, and to take endometrium for biopsy. For the patients with adhesion of orifice of uterus, it must be detected by using uterine cavity probe which is also used to separate adhesion. After operation, contraceptive device is placed inside uterus to prevent adhesion the second time. The actual incidence of sterility caused by intrauterine adhesion is not low, and calls for attention.

Soules, et al (1982) held that among sterility of gynecolo-

178

gy and obstetrics, about 15-20% are caused by tubal or o-
vary adhesion. Luciano, et al (1983) held that except for severe uterine appendage injuries, after gynecological operation, pelvic adhesion is the main reason of sterility, and also
the direct factor of the failure after sterile operation.

Examinations of Sterility due to Endometriosis

Endometriosis is a gynecological disease because of the
endometrium grows at any location outside uterine cavity.
The common locations are listed here: Ovary, utero-sacral
ligaments, seroa of posterior wall of lower uterine segment,
Douglas' culde-sac, and pelvic peritoneum of sigmoid
colon, etc. Most experts reported that the incidence of female sterility caused by endometriosis reaches high up to 30-
40%. Sterility due to endometriosis is caused by multiple
factors. The ectopic endometrium in abdominal cavity forms
local chronic inflammation. This stimulates the function of
acrophages, which damages sperms or fertilized follicles.
The ectopic endometrium also can trigger autoimmune reaction which produces antiovary and antien-dometrium antibodies.

The former affects corpus luteum function, and the latter
can change endometrium which is unfavorable to fertilization
of follicles. The ectopic endometrium and acrophages all can
cause the increase of prostagladin (PG) in abdominal cavity.
The high concentration PG affects ovulation and the function
of corpus luteum. For example, it is manifested as endocrine
disorders, diseases of FSH, the increase of PRL, and the decrease of LH receptors of follicular cells. These all can become the obstacles to follicle maturity and ovulation function, and can cause the withering of corpus luteum, etc. So,
the actual reasons of female sterility due to en-dometriosis
are complicated.

Before wide application of abdominoscope, the cases with
light or moderate endometriosis, chest-open examination
can make clear and correct diagnosis possible. In recent
years, under abdominoscope, the ectopic focus can be seen
directly. Under the direct observation, the ectopic focus usually appears to be purplish blue, brown or black implanted

179

focus. The pathologic changes mostly involve utero-sacral ligament, ovary, retrouterine excavation, and the peritoneum of the folded part of bladder. Furthermore, there is also adhesion in pelvic cavity. Attention must be given to the range and degree of adhesion: Whether it is loose or compact adhesion. Severe adhesion can cause retrouterine excavation to disappear, or the ovary to adhere to retrouterine excavation and broad ligament posterior lobe. The typical endometrium is retroversion of uterus accompanying irregular nodes on retrouterine excavation. When uterus is lifted up, ovary is seen to adhere to retrouterine excavation. Sometimes ovary becomes big but capsule becomes thick, and the surface of ovary is still smooth. If other ectopic endometrium implantation focuses exist, it is hard to confirm only by direct observation of abdominoscope. Then, at this point, cyst wall puncture should be applied. If what is sucked out is chocolate sticky liquid, then ovary endometriosis can be diagnosed with confirmation. In abdominoscope examination, if possible, it is better to supply biopsy to focus part. The most suitable period for abdominoscope examination is the early stage of corpus luteum. At this time, it is easy to see the ectopic implantation focus. When abdominoscope examination is applied to the patients with endometriosis, usually, methylene blue liquid should be perfused into uterine cavity to observe if oviduct is unobstructed.

In October, 1986, on the Second Academic Conference of Gynecology and Obstetrics Committee of China TCM and Western Medicine Combined Research Institute, the following diagnostic standards were established:

Pathological Standards: The section has the following proofs: ① Endometrium glands, ② Endometrium interstitium, ③ Having histobleeding proof, red blood cells, containing ferric xanthematin, local connective tissue proliferation. In this case, confirmed diagnosis is made.

Abdominoscopy Diagnosis: ① A number of purplish blue spots in retrouterine excavation, posterior peritoneum, accompanied by increased abdominal liquid growth (usually bloody). ② Uterosacral ligament is thick, appearing to gray

180

nodes, accompanied by loose adhesion, and the oviduct is mostly unobstructed. ③ Ovary capsule is thickened. The surface is not smooth, adhesive, and often seen to have brown old bleeding plaques. ④ Ovary adhesion is slightly larger, and oviduct is mostly unobstructed. *Clinical Diagnosis*: ① Progressing dysmenorrhea. ② Progressingly worsening discomfort in lower abdomen and lumbosacral portion. ③ Periodical irritative symptom of rectum, progressingly worsening. ④ Tender nodes on posterior fornix, utero-sacral ligament, or isthmus. ⑤ Appendage adhesive lumps accompanied by capsule node feeling, oviduct is unobstructive. ⑥ The above lumps on appendages before and after the completion of menstrual cycle have obvious changes in size (No anti-inflammation is applied). If one of the above points A, B and C, and one of the points D, E and F, exist at the same time, this disease can be diagnosed.

Abdominoscope examination has not been used widely; however, B-ultrasonic picture examination has actual significance to the diagnosis of this disease. Endometriosis is divided into ectopic endometrium in myometrium and the organs and tissues outside uterus. The ectopic endometrium in myometrium causes syndrome of myogland. It can lead to the homogenous enlargement of the volume of uterus, the echoing of myometrium increases with scattered spotty streak coarse echoing, liquid area opaca is larger than 1cm. The signs and symptoms are even obvious after menstrual cycle. Endometrium loses its normal appearance, and the ectopic endometrium in other organs often include ectopic endometrium in ovary and peritoneum, retrouterine excavation, etc. Because of cyclic bleeding, ovary is enlarged in which there are liquid round area opacae with large volume, in which there are scattered concentrated light reflections. The repeated bleeding makes oviduct, ovary adhere to other organs. The pulling and position change alter the anatomical relations between tubal fimbria end and ovary. These changes have their own image characteristics.

181

Examination of Sterility due to Leuteinized Unruptured Follicle Syndrome

Leuteinized unruptured follicle syndrome (LUFS) refers to a group of symptoms and signs manifested as the following: The menstrual cycle is regular, and it is supposed to have ovulation, but actually the follicles are unruptured, and there's no ovulation during the middle stage of menstruation. It is one of the important reasons of female sterility due to unknown causes. Among the infertile patients, the incidence of LUFS determined by abdominoscope examination was reportedly to be 6-79%. Clinically, patients with LUFS are also diagnosed to be sterile patients due to unknown causes, dysplasia of corpus luteum, endometriosis or pelvicitis. For the sterile patients with ovulatory dysfunction after the success of induction of ovulation should be considered to have the possibility to suffer from this disease. Besides the manifestations of the above-mentioned diseases, the patient has no other symptoms and signs. In the examinations, it may be found that the patient has regular menstruation and diphasic BBT. Endometrium of diagnostic uterine curettage before menstruation shows secretory stage changes. Estrogenmia, progesterone may be in normal ranges after BBT increases. No stigma in ovary is observed under abdominoscope 2-4 days after the going up of BBT. It needs successive observation of 2-3 cycles.

Serial B-ultrasonic examination in monitoring the growth and development of ovary and follicles have the following advantages: Convenience, simplicity, no damage, successive observation possible and follow-up study. For the convenience of evaluation of the growth and development of follicle in ovary, serial B-ultrasonic examination should be conducted in menstrual cycle; that is, in 4 days before predicted ovulation till the 3 days after blood LH peak, once a day, and in the rest of the days, once every 2-3 days. Normally, there are B-ultrasound signs. Before ovulation, follicle diameter is 21.5 ± 0.5mm. After ovulation, the advantageous follicles are small or the borders are unclear, folded with small sparse light spots in area apaca without tensile force. 1-2 days later, it can be seen that the corpus luteum forms

182

light beam. The whole ovary is a low echoing area, and there are hydrops in retrorectal excavation. LUFS examination shows no signs of ovulation stated above. After LH peak, follicle value continuously becomes big. The averaged diameter is 33.5mm. There are no light beam and hydrops.

Chapter Five
Treatment Methods

Main Points for Treatment Principles Based on Syndrome Differentiation

The treatment of female sterility should be conducted as a whole. On the basis of Syndrome Differentiation, such principles should be followed as "searching for the primary cause of disease in treatment," "Deficiency Syndrome should be treated with the method of tonification, while Excess Syndrome should be treated by purgation and reduction," "Treating Cold Syndrome with hot-natured drugs, while treating Heat Syndrome with cold-natured drugs." However, in actual treatment, ways of treatment, different pathogenesis of different syndromes should be considered to work out a therapy, to conduct therapy, to be in compatibility of medicines in a prescription, and get the medicine remedy. Though female sterility has more etiological factors, there are no more than two Syndromes: Deficiency and Excess. Deficiency Syndrome of female sterility includes Kidney and Blood Deficiency; Excess Syndrome of female sterility includes stagnation of Liver Qi, Blood Stasis and Phlegm Damp. *The Rules for Treating Women's Diseases*, a chapter of *Complete Works of Zhang Jingyue (Jing Yue Quan Shu · Fu Ren Gui)*, says, "The importance of woman is blood which can produce Essence. Thus pregnancy can be realized. If desiring to observe her disease, a doctor should see the condition of menstruation. If desiring to treat her disease, a doctor should try to regulate her menstruation." So, the

184

main points of Syndrome Differentiation are based on Syndrome Differentiation of menstruation diseases. Among disorders of menstruation and blood is considered to be a main factor; and the cycle, amount, color, nature, smell, and other changes of menstruation are taken as the properties of Syndrome Differentiation. The preceded menstrual cycles [Early] suggest Blood Heat or Qi Deficiency. The delayed menstrual cycles indicate Blood Deficiency or Blood Cold. The men- [Late] struation in big amount is mainly seen in the cases of Blood Heat or Qi Deficiency. The menstruation in little amount is mainly seen in the cases of Blood Deficiency or Blood Cold. The bright red or purplish red color of menstruation suggests Heat Syndrome; dark red, Cold Syndrome; light red, Deficiency Syndrome; sticky menstruation, Deficiency Cold Syndrome; more blood clots in menstruation, Blood Stasis Syndrome. As for pain in lower abdomen, if it is reduced by pressing, it suggests Deficiency Syndrome; intolerant to pressing, Excess Syndrome; relieved by warmth, Cold Syndrome; aggravated by warmth, Heat Syndrome; occurring before menstruation or in menstrual period, Excess Syndrome; occurring after the completion of menstrual cycle, Deficiency Syndrome. During the latter stage of menstruation, Kidney Deficiency is referred to if there are following signs: Menstruation is less in amount and dark in color, thin in nature with thin and clear leukorrhea, pain in lower abdomen, soreness in lumbar area; Blood Stasis is referred to if menstruation is less or more in amount, pain in lower abdomen and lumbar area, purplish black in color. Before and during menstruation, the pain is worsening, and intolerant to pressing. The uncertain menstruation, the more or less amount of it, depressed mental states, restlessness suggest stagnation of Liver Qi. More leukorrhea, sticky in nature, fat body and white face suggest Phlegm Damp.

The key to treating female sterility is to regulate menstruation and search for the primary causes of the disease. Lou Quanshan says in *Detailed Outline of Medicine (Yi Xue Gang Mu)*, "The method of pregnancy all is to regulate menstruation first," which is called "method of regulating menstruation to get pregnant." So the treatment should regard

185

promoting Kidney Qi, benefiting Essence and Blood, nourishing the Chong and Ren Channels, regulating menstruation
as the general rules. Through regulation and tonification of
Zangfu organs, Qi and Blood are regulated, and the Chong
and Ren Channels are regulated and solidified. Among
them, regulating and tonifying Zangfu organs is an important rule in the treatment of female sterility. Regulating and
tonifying Zangfu organs includes restoring the Kidney,
soothing the Liver, and reinforcing the Spleen. *Menstruation Regulation*, a chapter of *Fu Qingzhu's Gynecology and
Obstetrics (Fu Qing Zhu Nu Ke · Tiao Jing)*, says, "Menstruation comes from the Kidney." So the primary place of
regulating menstruation is the Kidney. Through Kidney-
restoring, Yang and Yin are balanced. According to the condition of the diseases, the following methods can be chosen:
Restoring the Kidney to support Yang, nourishing the Kidney to benefit Yin, tonifying and benefiting Kidney Qi, tonifying both Yin and Yang. Soothing the Liver is to regulate
the Liver's function of governing the normal flow of Qi. The
dysfunction of the Liver in governing normal flow of Qi may
lead to stagnation of Liver Qi, Heat Syndrome due to stagnation of Liver Qi, insufficiency of the Liver Blood, the impairment and excessive consumption of Liver Yin, etc. And
finally, they will lead to dysfunction of the Chong and Ren
Channels and the disease is resulted in. The method of treatment is to soothe the Liver to remove stagnation of Liver Qi,
purpge the Liver of pathogenic Fire, nourish Blood to soften
the Liver, etc. The Spleen and Stomach are the sources of
acquired Essence, the places where Qi and Blood are produced, and which govern the storing and obtaining and di-
gesting food, transporting materials to the whole body. If
the functions of the Spleen and Stomach are normal, the Sea
of Blood is full and menstruation comes on time, and pregnancy is no of problem; otherwise, the dysfunction of the
Spleen and Stomach leads to insufficiency of nutrients, or to
the malfunction of food digestion and nutrients transportation, or accumulation of water and Damp, which damages
the Chong and Ren Channels to result in female sterility. So
the treatment of strengthening the Spleen and regulating the

function of the Stomach should be conducted. The common methods include reinforcing the Spleen to benefit Qi, reinforcing the Spleen to remove Damp, tonifying the Spleen to restore normal function, warming and tonifying the Spleen Yang.

Qi, Blood, woman's menstruation and pregnancy are closely related. The derangement of Qi and Blood usually leads to irregular menstruation and sterility. So regulation of Qi and Blood is also one of the chief methods in the treatment of female sterility. In Syndrome Differentiation, it should be clear whether the disease is because of Qi or Blood, Deficiency or Excess, Cold or Heat. Regulating Qi includes tonifying Qi and regulating the normal flow of Qi. Blood regulation includes invigorating Blood and nourishing Blood, removing Heat and cooling Blood, activating the the circulation of Blood to remove Blood Stasis, warming the channels and nourishing Blood. For the cases with diseases of both Qi and Blood, such methods of treatment as tonifying Qi to benefit Blood, invigorating Blood to benefit Qi, tonifying both Qi and Blood, or activating Qi flow to promote the circulation of Blood, or promoting the circulation of Blood to remove Blood Stasis, etc. should be taken after we differentiate what is primary and what's secondary pathogenic changes of Qi and Blood. Proper method should be chosen according to different conditions in Syndrome Differentiation in clinic.

To sum up, the above-mentioned are the general rules of treatment of female sterility. Flexibility should be applied in clinical application and should not be done letter to letter. As what is said in *The Rules for Treating Women's Diseases*, a chapter of *Complete Works of Zhang Jingyue* (*Jing Yue Quan Shu · Fu Ren Gui*), "Getting pregnant has no fixed methods. Different people need different drugs which benefit accordingly. So the case of Cold Syndrome needs drugs, warm in nature. For the case of Heat Syndrome, drugs cool in nature are needed. For the cases with habitual abortion, drugs astringent in nature are supplied, and for the cases of Deficiency Syndrome, drugs for tonification are used. Treating what is the main problem will result in balance be-

187

tween Yin and Yang and normal digestion of nutrients transportation. "

TCM Treatment Principles and Pathology of Western Medicine

Principles of treatment of TCM and etiopathogenesis of modern medicine have certain inner relations. Especially, the research of the inner relationship between the Kidney and regulation of human's reproductive physiological function indicates that the Kidney regulates the productive function through the axis system of the brain—the Kidney—the Chong and Ren Channels-uterus. This is similar to modern concept of modern medicine that reproductive physiological function is regulated by the axis of cerebral cortex-hypothalamus-hypophysis-ovary.

Ovulatory Dysfunction and Invigorating the Kidney to Soothe Liver

Ovulatory dysfunction is an important reason of sterility. The dysfunction of the axis system of hypothalamus-hypophysis-ovary often leads to obstruction to ovulation function. The periodical change of the level of estrogen in Blood (Mainly E_2) is the key to regulating ovulation cycle. If E_2 level is not high enough to stimulate the peak of LH secretion before ovulation, ovulatory dysfunction occurs. By using examinations of BBT crystallization of cervical mucus, vaginal cytological smear, etc. , estrogen level in the Interior and its periodical changes can be learned. If crystallization of cervical mucus suggests delayed ovulation or no ovulation, low estrogen level, clinically, the disease is accompanied by obvious symptoms indicating Stomach Deficiency. Furthermore, estrogen level and balance of Kidney Yin and Yang has certain relationship; that is, the estrogen level of patients with Deficiency of Kidney Yin is slightly higher, and most of their eosin indices of exfoliative cytoscopy of vagina are low. Also, part of the patients' crystallization

188

examination of cervical mucus or exfoliative cytoscopy of vagina suggests no ovulation but with high estrogen level, clinically, the disease is accompanied by symptoms of stagnation of Liver Qi. So, drugs that regulate Kidney Yin and Kidney Yang and soothe the Liver are often used to treat obstruction in ovulatory function. Generally, the patients with low estrogen level are supplied with the method of Kidney-restoring; the patients with continuous high estrogen level are supplied with the method of Liver-soothing. As far as the patients with Kidney Deficiency are concerned, for the patients with Deficiency of Kidney Yin with high estrogen level, nourishing Kidney Yin is considered to be the main factor. Patients of Deficiency of Kidney Yang with low estrogen level are supplied with warming Kidney Yang as a main factor. Therefore, ovulatory dysfunction is closely related to the Kidney and the Liver. Invigorating the Kidney and soothing the Liver are the important methods of treating ovulatory dysfunction.

Obstruction of Fallopian Tube and Method of Promoting Blood Flow by Removing Obstruction

Obstruction of fallopian tube is mostly caused by acute, chronic salpingitis, or chronic pelvicitis, tuberculosis of fallopian tube, or adnexa adhesion after pelvic operation, or endometriosis, etc. Inflammation causes local tubal hyperemia, edema, inflammatory exudate, fibrous tissue growth—all of this leads to obstruction. Drugs that promote the circulation of Blood to remove Blood Stasis can improve local blood microcirculation, promote the increase of macrophagocytes and activate their function, and effectively loosen the adhered tissues, thus benefiting unobstruction of fallopian tube. If edema of fallopian tube occurs, drugs that reinforce the Spleen to induce diuresis, reduce exudate and remove Damp are added, the therapeutic effects of which are proved clinically.

189

Application of TCM Artificial Cyclic Therapy Through Syndrome Differentiation

"TCM Artificial Cycle," on the basis of the method of restoring the Kidney, uses the drugs by intimating the physiological change of woman's menstrual cycle. Generally, TCM artificial cycle improves the function of sexual gland through regulating the balance of "the Kidney-the Chong and Ren Channel-menstruation-uterus," that is, it gives full play to curative effect through the improvement of the function of "hypothalamus-hypophysis-ovary axis." In the inter-regulating relationship of hypothalamus-hypophysis-ovary axis, large doses of estrogen show negative feedback inhibiting effect, but small doses of estrogen show active feedback effect; that is, it stimulates hypothalamus-hypophysis-ovary axis, induces LH peak, promotes restoration of menstruation and ovulation. Clinical research has proved that TCM artificial cycle has the effect similar to that of small dose estrogen. It doesn't exert substitute effect in the treatment of menstruation and ovulatory dysfunction, but plays a regulative effect. Artificial cyclic therapy, on the basis of the four stages of menstrual cycle, respectively invigorates the Kidney and nourishes Yin at latter stage of menstruation, reinforces the Kidney to remove obstruction from the collaterals during intermenstrual period, warms the Kidney to strengthen Yang before menstruation, and promotes the circulation of Blood to remove obstruction from the channels during menstruation period.

Invigorating the Kidney and nourishing Yin at the latter stage of menstruation

4-14 days in menstrual cycle is considered to be the latter stage of menstruation, i. e., proliferative stage. This stage prepares for ovulation with the development of follicles, gradual increase of estrogen secretion, growth and restoration of endometrium. TCM holds that this stage is the restoring and vegetative stage of Yin and Blood. Under the effect of Kidney Qi, the uterus is filled with Essence and Blood, Qi and Blood are well coordinated. Cu Luanpao Tang (Decoction for Promoting Follicle Development) is used to invigorate the Kidney and nourish Yin. The prescription is formed by prepared rehmannia root (Radix Rehmanniae Praeparata), dried human placenta (Placenta Hominis), Chinese yam (Rhizoma Dioscoreae), glossy privet fruit (Fructus Ligustri Lucidi), wolfberry fruit (Fructus Lycii), curculigo rhizome (Rhizoma Curculiginis), epimedium (Herba Epimedii), fleece-flower root (Radix Polygoni Multiflori), dipsacus root (Radix Dipsaci), dodder seed (Semen Cuscutae) and Chinese angelica root (Radix Angelicae Sinensis).

Invigorating the Kidney and Activating the Collaterals during Intermenstrual Period

Approximately the 14th day of menstrual cycle is considered to be intermenstrual period, i. e. , ovulatory period. With the development and maturity of follicles, estrogen secretion reaches a peak; therefore, hypophysis is stimulated to secrete a great deal of luteotropic hormones (LH) and preovulation peak is formed which leads to the rupture of the matured follicles and finally ovulation. TCM holds that during this period, Yin Essence of the Kidney is furthermore enriched and transformed under the effect of Kidney Yang. One-sided pain in lower abdomen, sensation of distending pain of breasts, leukorrhea with thin and transparent in nature, and good wiredrawing and increase of BBT. This is the key stage when TCM drugs are used to regulate artificial cycle. In about 3 days before ovulation (i. e. , the 11-14th day of menstrual cycle), Cu Pailuan Tang (Decoction for Promoting Ovulation) is given to invigorate the Kidney and remove obstruction from the collaterals and to promote ovulation. The drugs in the prescription include curculigo rhizome (Rhizoma Curculiginis), epimedium (Herba Epimedii), red peony root (Radix Paeoniae Rubra), Chinese angelica root (Radix Angelicae Sinensis), chuanxiong rhizome (Rhizoma Ligustici Chuanxiong), cyperus tuber (Rhizoma Cyperi), safflower (Flos Carthami), motherwort (Herba Leonuri),

191

Herba Lycopi, achyranthes root (Radix Achyranthis Bidentatae), vaccaria seed (Semen Vaccariae), sweetgum fruit (Fructus Liquidambaris) and peach kernel (Semen Persicae).

Warming Yang and Invigorating the Kidney During Premenstruation

The period from ovulation to the coming of menstruation is called premenstruation, i. e., secretion period. This is a stage when corpus luteum gets mature, and degenerates. Under the influence of endocrine hormones, endometrium gets successively thick to adapt pregnancy and fertilization. TCM holds that during this period, Yin is sufficient, and Yang gradually waxes, of Kidney Qi gradually gets prosperous and the uterus is warm, pregnancy will be possible. During intermenstrual period, the coition of the sperms and the follicles gets relieved. Then, Qi and Blood of Zangfu Organs accumulate at the Chong and Ren Channels under the effect of Kidney Yang, and nourish the fetus. Otherwise, if there is no pregnancy, Qi and Blood of Zangfu Organs flow downward to the Sea of Blood to enable menstruation to come out on time. After ovulation, BBT increases. Diphasic BBT is considered to be the guide of Syndrome Differentiation of the wax of Yang. Therefore, the principle of treatment for the period is warming Yang and restoring the Kidney. Cu Huangti Tang (Decoction for Promoting the Development of Corpus Luteum) restores the Kidney and warms Yang, benefits Qi and nourishes Blood to promote maturity of corpus luteum, and forms excellent material basis for pregnancy or the coming of next menstruation. The drugs of the prescription include prepared rehmannia root (Radix Rehmanniae Praeparata), curculigo rhizome (Rhizoma Curculiginis), epimedium (Herba Epimedii), cinnamon bark (Cortex Cinnamomi), Chinese angelica root (Radix Angelicae Sinensis), desertliving cistanche (Herba Cistachis), dodder seed (Semen Cuscutae), raspberry (Fructus Rubi), Chinese yam (Rhizoma Dioscoreae), dangshen rhizome (Radix Codonopsis Pilosulae) and prepared licorice (Radix Glycyrrhizae Praeparata).

192

Promoting Blood Flow and Removing Obstruction from the Channels

The coming of menstruation symbolizes the beginning of a new menstrual cycle. During this period, because of the sharp decrease of sexual hormone in the body, endometrium, necrosis, exfoliation occur, and menstruation is formed. TCM thinks during this period, Yang is too much and excessive Yang changes to Yin. Because of gradual prosperity of Yang Qi day after day, the Sea of Blood gets filled regularly. Under the effect of Kidney Yang, those materials are transported out, and menstruation comes, and a new menstrual cycle begins. The key of whether menstruation can be drained out is "unobstruction." The usual menstruation is not drained, new menstruation can not be produced. Therefore, the key point of treatment during this period is regulating menstruation by activating the flow of Qi and promoting the circulation of Blood. Qiao Jing Tang (Decoction for Regulating Menstruation) is applied. Herbal drugs include Chinese angelica root (Radix Angelicae Sinensis), red peony root (Radix Paeoniae Rubra), prepared rehmannia root (Radix Rehmanniae Praeparata), chuanxiong rhizome (Rhizoma Ligustici Chuanxiong), peach kernel (Semen Persicae), safflower (Flos Carthami), cyperus tuber (Rhizoma Cyperi), green tangerine orange peel (Pericarpium Citri Reticulatae Viride), tangerine peel (Pericarpium Citri Reticulatae), Herba Lycopi, achyranthes root (Radix Achyranthis Bidentatae) and motherwort (Herba Leonuri) (Xu Jingsheng, 1988).

From 1963 to 1985, the Second People's Hospital of Jiangxi Province treated 154 cases of female sterility due to ovulatory dysfunction by way of TCM Artificial Cycle, acupuncture, acupuncture combined with TCM artificial cycle, and simplified TCM artificial cycle triple therapy (including simplified TCM artificial cyclic therapy, Villus Decoction therapy, sperm-giving therapy by enlarging the uterus). Among the total cases, 121 were cured, 10 were treated effectively, and 23 failed to respond to the medical treatment. The pregnancy rate was 78.57%. 131 were pregnant by inducing method (including two groups: Recovery

193

and effectiveness). The total ovulatory rate was 85.06%.
Methods of Treatment: ①TCM Artificial Cyclic Therapy:
according to the four stages of ovary cycle changes, a corre-
sponding cyclic legislative formula is taken: restoring the
Kidney—promoting the circulation of Blood to remove Blood
Stasis—restoring the Kidney—promoting the circulation of
Blood to regulate menstruation, and the following medicines
are correspondingly used as sequential therapy: Cu Luanpao
Tang (Decoction for Promoting Follicle Development), Cu
Pailuan Tang (Decoction for Promoting Ovulation), Cu
Huangti Tang (Decoction for Promoting the Development of
Corpus Luteum), Huo Xue Qiao Jing Tang (Decoction for
Promoting Blood Flow and Regulating Menstruation). The
patients were classified into two types: ① The Kidney Yang
of Deficiency Type: Cu Luanpao Tang (Decoction for Promoting Follicle Development): The drugs in the prescription
include curculigo rhizome (Rhizoma Curculiginis), epimedium (Herba Epimedii), Chinese angelica root (Radix Angelicae Sinensis), Chinese yam (Rhizoma Dioscoreae), dodder
seed (Semen Cuscutae), morinda root (Radix Morindae Officinalis), desertliving cistanche (Herba Cistachis), prepared rehmannia root (Radix Rehmanniae Praeparata), 10g
for each drug. Drugs in the prescription Decoction for Promoting Ovulation include Chinese angelica root (Radix Angelicae Sinensis), red sage root (Radix Salviae Miltiorrhizae), motherwort (Herba Leonuri), peach kernel (Semen
Persicae), safflower (Flos Carthami), spatholobus stem
(Caulis Spatholobi) and dipsacus root (Radix Dipsaci), 10g
respectively; cyperus tuber (Rhizoma Cyperi) 6g, cinnamon
twig (Ramulus Cinnamomi) 3g; Decoction for Promoting
Corpus luteum Development include donkey-hide gelatin
(Colla Corii Asini), tortoise-plastron glue (Colla Plastri
Testudinis), Chinese angelica root (Radix Angelicae Sinen-
sis), prepared rehmannia root (Radix Rehmanniae
Praeparata), dodder seed (Semen Cuscutae), prepared
fleece-flower root (Radix Polygoni Multiflori Praeparata),
dipsacus root (Radix Dipsaci) and Chinese yam (Rhizoma
Dioscoreae), 10g respectively. Decoction for Promoting
Blood Flow and Regulating Menstruation: Chinese angelica

194

root (Radix Angelicae Sinensis), prepared rehmannia root (Radix Rehmanniae Praeparata), red sage root (Radix Salviae Miltiorrhizae), red peony root (Radix Paeoniae Rubra), Herba lycopi, motherwort (Herba Leonuri), 10g respectively, cyperus tuber (Rhizoma Cyperi) 6g. ② Deficiency of Kidney Yin: The drugs included in the first decoction are glossy privet fruit (Fructus Ligustri Lucidi), eclipta (Herba Ecliptae), red sage root (Radix Salviae Miltiorrhizae), Chinese yam (Rhizoma Dioscoreae), dodder seed (Semen Cuscutae), prepared rehmannia root (Radix Rehmanniae Praeparata), desertliving cistanche (Herba Cistachis) and prepared fleece-flower root, 10g respectively. The drugs included in the second prescription are red sage root (Radix Salviae Miltiorrhizae), red peony root (Radix Paeoniae Rubra), Herba lycopi, prepared rehmannia root (Radix Rehmanniae Praeparata), wolfberry fruit (Fructus Lycii), 10g respectively; safflower (Flos Carthami), peach kernel (Semen Persicae) and cyperus tuber (Rhizoma Cyperi), 4g respectively; coix seed (Semen Coicis) 15g. The drugs included in the third prescription are moutan bark, tortoise plastron (Plastrum Testudinis), wolfberry fruit (Fructus Lycii), glossy privet fruit (Fructus Ligustri Lucidi), eclipta (Herba Ecliptae), prepared rehmannia root (Radix Rehmanniae Praeparata), prepared fleece-flower root (Radix Polygoni Multiflori), desertliving cistanche (Herba Cistachis) and dodder seed (Semen Cuscutae), 10g respectively. The drugs included in the last prescription are red sage root (Radix Salviae Miltiorrhizae), red peony root (Radix Paeoniae Rubra), Herba lycopi, prepared rehmannia root (Radix Rehmanniae Praeparata), poria (Poria) and motherwort (Herba Leonuri), 10g respectively. 4-6 doses of Cu Luanpao Tang (Decoction for Promoting Follicle Development) is taken since the competion of menstruation. 4 does of the second decoction is taken before ovulation, 6-9 does of the third is taken after ovulation, and 3-5 doses of the last decoction is taken before menstruation. ② Therapy of Promoting Ovulation by Acupuncture: On 11-16th days of menstrual cycle, acupuncture and moxibustion of the acupoints are applied. Selection of the Acupoints: Sanyinjiao

195

(SP 6), Guanyuan (REN 4), Diji (SP 8) and Shuidao (ST 28) in Group I. Guilai (ST 29), Dahe (KID 12), Qugu (REN 2) and Xuehai (SP 1) in Group II. Shuidao (ST 28), Zhongji (REN 3), Guilai (ST 29) and Sanyinjiao (SP 6) in Group III. The points of the three groups were needled in turn, one group daily, successively over 4-6 days, with uniform reinforcing-reducing method. The needles were retained for 30 minutes with moxibustion. (3) Acupuncture Therapy Combined with TCM Artificial Cyclic Therapy: The drugs were administered according to TCM artificial cyclic therapy, and acupuncture was added to promote ovulation while the patient takes decoction for promoting ovulation (The acupoints were the same as the acupunctured group). (4) Triple Therapy: It refers to a combined therapy of simplified TCM artificial cycle, Villus Decoction therapy, sperm-giving therapy by enlarging the uterus. ① Simplified TCM Artificial Cyclic therapy is used for two types: Deficiency of Kidney Yang and Deficiency of Kidney Yin. To the first type, Jianhua Cu Luanpao Tang (Simplified Decoction for Follicle Development): Curculigo rhizome (Rhizoma Curculiginis) 10g, epimedium (Herba Epimedii) 10g, Chinese angelica root (Radix Angelicae Sinensis) 10g and cyperus tuber (Rhizoma Cyperi) 6g. Simplified Decoction for Promoting Ovulation: Chinese angelica root (Radix Angelicae Sinensis) 10g, cyperus tuber (Rhizoma Cyperi) 6g, peach kernel (Semen Persicae) 10g, safflower (Flos Carthami) 8g, Simplified Decoction for Promoting the Development of Corpus Luteum: Morinda root (Radix Morindae Officinalis) 10g, dodder seed (Semen Cuscutae) 12g, Chinese angelica root (Radix Angelicae Sinensis) 10g and argyi leaf (Folium Artemisiae Argyi) 4g. Simplifeelica root (Radix Angelicae Sinensis) 10g, cyperus tuber (Rhizoma Cyperi) 6g, chuanxiong rhizome (Rhizoma Ligustici Chuanxiong) 6g and Herba lycopi 10g. For the second type: The first decoction includes glossy privet fruit (Fructus Ligustri Lucidi) 10g, eclipta (Herba Ecliptae) 10g, dipsacus root (Radix Dipsaci) 10g and dodder seed (Semen Cuscutae) 10g. The second decoction is composed of red sage root (Radix Salviae Miltiorrhizae) 10g, cyperus tuber (Rhizoma Cyperi) 6g, peach kernel (Semen

Persicae) 6g and safflower (Flos Carthami) 6g. The third decoction has drugs of prepared rehmannia root (Radix Rehmanniae Praeparata) 15g, desertliving cistanche (Herba Cistachis) 10g, dodder seed (Semen Cuscutae) 10g and prepared fleece-flower root (Radix Polygoni Multiflori) 15g. The fourth decoction is comprises of red sage root (Radix Salviae Miltiorrhizae) 10g, cyperus tuber (Rhizoma ˙Cyperi) 6g, red peony root (Radix Paeoniae Rubra) 10g and Herba lycopi 10g. Administration is the same as the previous one. ② Villus Decoction Therapy: When taking decoction for promoting follicles, the patients take additionally one villus extracted from artificial abortion (i. e. , the complete pregnancy material is uterine cavity extracted during artificial abortion). Observe the influence of villus decoction in raising estrogen level. ③ Sperm-giving Therapy by enlarging the Uterus: It is done on the first day of predicted ovulation and postovulation.

TCM artificial cyclic therapy, on the basis of restoring the Kidney, regulates the balance between Kidney Yin and Kidney Yang. Reinforcing the Kidney to support Yang stimulates ovary function. It not only has gained curative effect in the clinical treatment of female sterility due to anovulation, but also has been proved to be effective in basic experiment research. According to research, such drugs that restore the Kidney as morinda root (Radix Morindae Officinalis), dodder seed (Semen Cuscutae), desertliving cistanche (Herba Cistachis) enable the weights of hypophysis and ovary of the experimental grown-up rats to increase, increase the response of hypophysis to LH-RH, and enable it to secrete more LH and strengthen HCG/LH receptor function of ovary. As a result, it improves inner nervous endocrine regulative mechanism. This is the basis for inducing ovulation. Promoting the circulation of Blood to remove Blood Stasis is another therapy in TCM artificial cyclic therapy. It can be used only when follicles develop and get mature to a certain degree; that is, when index of Keratinized cells reaches above 40%. Therefore, it should be used in the middle of menstrual cycle, i. e. , on the basis of restoring the Kidney. Basic experiments have proved that promoting the circula-

197

tion of Blood to remove Blood Stasis can promote ovulation; that is, the combined use of peach kernel (Semen Persicae) and safflower (Flos Carthami) in decoction for promoting ovulation can obviously increase the content of $PGF_{2\alpha}$ in ventricle blood of the big rat's ovary-uterus. This is one reason of inducing the mature follicles to ovulate. Method of acupuncture promoting ovulation refers to that acupuncture is used to influence "hypothalamus-hypophysis-ovary axis" through vegetative nervous system, therefore, to regulate their functions. Villus is the remains of Essence and Blood. It restores the congenital Essence, and has obvious effect in raising estrogen level, and makes up for the slowness of estrogen level increase by decoction for promoting follicles. So when Rongmao Tang Jia Cu Luanpao Tang (Villus Decoction and Decoction for Promoting Follicle Development) are used in combination. It can strengthen the effect of Cu Pailuan Tang (Decoction for Promoting Ovulation) in restoring the Kidney, therefore, speed up and promote the development and maturity of the follicles, and provide basic condition for promoting the circulation of Blood to remove Blood Stasis or acupuncture used to promote ovulation. In addition, it is hard to determine the pregnancy rate of the patients, sexual intercourse negative by TCM artificial cyclic therapy, but sperm-giving therapy by enlarging the uterus makes up for this shortcoming. To sum up, the reason of TCM artificial cyclic therapy in promoting ovulation and treating anovulatory female sterility may be improving "hypothalamus-hypophysis-ovary" functions through the regulation of the functions of "the Kidney-sexual function—the Chong and Ren Channels-uterus," but not substitute for the hormones in the body (Lin Zhijun, 1987).

The influences of "TCM artificial Cyclic Therapy" on human hypothalamus-hypophysis-ovary axis: Research has shown TCM artificial cyclic therapy regulates the functions of hypothalamus and hypophysis two-dimensionally, therefore, keeps the body's endocrine state balanced. The significance of it lies in the improvement of the body's regulative mechanism. Through regulation, the functions of hypothalamus-hypophysis are tending towards normality. TCM artificial cycle can change the reaction peak phases of LH-RH-A stimulation test. When FSH, LH secretions are slightly lower, compared with the condition before treatment, the reactivity of LH-RH-A stimulation test goes up markedly after the treatment. The reactive peak may be delayed to 120 minutes. If hypersecretion of FSH and LH occurs, the reactivity of LH-RH-A stimulation test lowers after the treatment compared with that before the treatment, and reactive peak may be forwarded. This is related to TCM artificial cycle's changing synthetic and storing abilities of the hypothalamus and the sensitivity of hypothalamus. The Influences of TCM Artificial Cycle on Ovary are discussed below. For the group with high LH, low or normal FSH, E_2 increases obviously after TCM artificial cycle treatment. This is related to the following facts: After the treatment, the ratio of LH/FSH is regulated. The increase of FSH can strengthen the activity of aromatized enzyme of ovary, and enable the granular cells to transform more androgenic hormone into estrogen. Because of this, ovary function has been improved. Trace estrogen effects of TCM artificial cyclic therapy. For the group of high FSH and LH, after the treatment through TCM artificial cyclic therapy, self-feeling symptoms have been improved, vaginal secretion increases, and sexual desire is improved, with no obvious increase of plasma E_2. It suggests TCM artificial cyclic therapy can play trace estrogen effect in the body, improve the symptoms of lack of estrogen. In one word, the treatment of TCM artificial cyclic therapy has two-dimensional effect, i. e. , TCM artificial cycle doesn't solely exert exciting or inhibiting effect to hypothalamus— hypophysis—ovary axis, but has regulative effect. What's more, it has multiple effects, i. e. , TCM artificial cyclic therapy can influence various levels of sexual gland, and have effect of the functions of hypophysis, and ovary (Wang Qin, et al. , 1989).

Treatment Based on Syndrome Differentiation of Sterility due to Disorders of Fallopian Tube

Diseases of fallopian tube are important reasons of female sterility. Fallopian tube has sophisticated physiological effects. It plays an important role in ovum absorption, fertilization of ova, and rupture, maturity and transportation of the fertilized ovum. Diseases of fallopian tube are caused mainly by acute, chronic salpingitis, or tuberculosis of fallopian tube, endometriosis, adnexa adhesion after pelvic operation, etc. These diseases cause such pathologic changes as hyperemia of fallopian tube, edema, inflammatory infiltration, empyema, hydrops, growth of granulation, etc. All this finally leads to obstruction of fallopian tube or unobstructed-but-not-smooth fallopian tube. This affects the conjugation of ovum and sperm which leads to the impossibility of pregnancy. According to statistics data, about 30-40% of the infertile woman patients are caused by diseases of fallopian tube.

There are no special statements about obstruction of fallopian tube in TCM. The symptoms of it are found here and there in such accounts as "On No Pregnancy," "Infertility," "Irregular Menstruation," "Mass in the Abdomen," "Leukorrhea," etc.

Etiology and Pathogenesis
• *Blood Stasis due to Stagnation of Qi*

During menstruation period and stegmonth, neglect of hygiene and absorption of nourishment, attack of pathogenic factors, combining with residual Blood which stagnates in the uterus; or the seven emotions damage the Zangfu organs in the Interior lead to stagnation of Qi, and then to unsmoothness of the circulation of Blood, to the obstruction of Blood Stasis in the channels and collaterals, and finally to obstruction of fallopian tube.

• *Accumulation of Cold and Damp*

200

Vegetarian diet causes Yang Deficiency, then Cold is produced in the Interior, and Yang Qi can not warm the limbs, can not help to digest food and steam water. The functions of Zangfu Organs are in poor state; or Cold in the Exterior attacks the body, and it accumulates in the uterus, and Blood Stasis occurs due to Cold, or Deficiency of the Spleen leads to its failure to digest food, transport nutrients to the whole body and to help in water metabolism. As a result, retention of water occurs, and Cold Damp accumulate, which obstructs the channels and collaterals. Finally, obstruction of fallopian tube is induced.

• *Damp Heat Stagnation*

Because the patient is attacked by pathogenic Damp Heat, or because of hyperactivity of Liver Fire, Heat accumulates in Blood, and Damp Heat obstruct the channels and collaterals. Finally, obstruction of fallopian tube is caused.

Main Points of Diagnosis

Such examinations of unobstruction of fallopian tube as tubal liquid-perfusion, salpin-gography, etc. are the basis for the diagnosis of this disease. Syndromes can be determined by differentiating Cold and Heat in combination with the local and overall manifestations of Blood Stasis due to Qi Stagnation.

Treatment Based on Syndrome Differentiation

• *Blood Stasis due to Stagnation of Qi*

Main Symptoms and Signs : Obstruction of fallopian tube or unobstructed-but-not-smooth fallopian tube. The coming of menstruation is not certain, and menstruation is not smooth, whose color is purplish dark with blood clots, pain in lower abdomen or distending pain of breasts before menstruation, restlessness, and usually lower abdominal indistinct pain or stabbing pain. Purplish dark tongue with ecchymosis and petechiae, pale tongue coating, tense and thready pulse. Gynecological examination shows the adnexae on the two sides become thick or are tender; and tender nodes can be found in vaginal posterior fornix and sacral ligament.

Analysis of the Symptoms and Signs : The Interior damage

201

by seven emotions, stagnation of Qi obstruction of the circulation of Blood, or the channels and collaterals of uterus attacked by pathogenic factors, conjugated with remaining Blood—all can obstruct the channels and collaterals and finally it leads to obstruction of fallopian tube or unobstructed-but-not-smooth fallopian tube. Liver Qi does not flow smoothly, and the Liver fails to govern normal flow of Qi, disturbance of the Chong Channel is caused. As a result, the coming of menstruation is not certain. Blood Stasis due to stagnation of Qi causes unsmoothness of menstruation. Stagnation of Liver Qi due to accumulation of Qi leads to obstruction of channels. This is why pain in lower abdomen and distending pain of breasts occur before menstruation. Blood Stasis accumulates in collaterals of uterus, so pain is caused due to obstruction. This is the reason of lower abdominal indistinct pain or stabbing pain. Tongue and pulse conditions indicate Blood Stasis.

Treatment Principles: Promoting the circulation of Blood to remove Blood Stasis; resolving lumps to make fallopian tube unobstructed.

Prescription: Tong Guan Tang (Decoction for Removing Obstruction from Fallopian Tube) (Prescription based on the clinical experience of the author)

Parched pangolin scales (Squama Manitis) 9g, Chinese honey locus (Spina Gleditsiae) 15g, burreed tuber (Rhizoma Sparganii) 9g, zedoary (Rhizoma Zedoariae) 9g, prepared frankincense (Resina Olibani Praeparata) 9g, prepared myrrh (Myrrha Praeparata) 9g, Japanese sea tangle (Thallus Laminariae) 9g, sargassum (Sargassum) 9g, red peony root (Radix Paeoniae Rubra) 9g, red sage root (Radix Salviae Miltiorrhizae) 30g, peach kernel (Semen Persicae) 9g, motherwort (Herba Leonuri) 30g, prunella spike (Spica Prunellae) 9g and sweetgum fruit (Fructus Liquidambaris) 15g. All the drugs above are decocted in water for oral administration, one dose per day, and taking continuously over 2-6 months (stop taking it during menstruation period).

Analysis of the Prescription: Parched pangolin scales (Squama Manitis) and Chinese honey locus (Spina Gleditsiae) remove Blood Stasis and resolve lumps, regulate men-

202

struation and remove obstruction from the collaterals. Burreed tuber (Rhizoma Sparganii) and zedoary (Rhizoma Zedoariae) remove Blood Stasis, promote the normal flow of Qi and alleviate pain. Frankincense (Resina Olibani) and myrrh (Myrrha) activate the circulation of Blood and alleviate pain and swelling, and promote muscle formation. Japanese sea tangle (Thallus Laminariae) and seaweed resolve hard lumps. Red peony root (Radix Paeoniae Rubra), red sage root (Radix Salviae Miltiorrhizae), peach kernel (Semen Persicae) and motherwort (Herba Leonuri) promote the circulation of Blood and remove Blood Stasis, cool Blood and remove Toxins. Sprunella spike (Spica Prunellae) removes Fire and dissolves lumps. Sweetgum fruit (Fructus Liquidambaris) removes obstruction from the channels and collaterals. The whole prescription promotes the circulation of Blood and removes Blood Stasis, resolves lumps, promotes the normal flow of Qi by removing obstruction from the collaterals. It can not only improve the local blood transportation and blood rheology of fallopian tube, but also promote the loosening and assimilation of adhesion of fallopian tube to remove obstruction from the lumen of fallopian tube.

• *Retention of Cold and Damp*

Main Symptoms and Signs: Fallopian tube is obstructed or unobstructed but not smooth, delayed menstruation with less amount, dark color with blood clots, thin and cold leukorrhea, cold limbs, pain in lower abdomen relieved with warming and pressing, thin and more urination, loose stool, pale tongue with white greasy tongue coating, deep thready or deep slippery pulse, and no other unusual has been found in gynecological urination.

Analysis of the Symptoms and Signs: Cold Damp accumulate in the channels and Blood Stasis stagnates in uterus, and the channels and collaterals are obstructed. So fallopian tube is obstructed or unobstructed but not smooth. Blood Stasis occurs because of Cold, or insufficiency of Yang Qi causes hyperactivity of Yin Cold; therefore, the circulation of Blood is not smooth. So, menstruation is delayed with less amount, dark color. Pathogenic Cold and Damp accumulate

203

in the uterus and conjugate with blood; so, when menstruation is coming, there are blood clots and pain in lower abdomen due to Cold, which is reduced by warming and pressing. Cold is pathogenic Yin which damages Yang Qi which can not reach the surface of the body. So, limbs are cold. Thin and more urination, loose stool and signs of pulse are signs of Cold and Damp.

Treatment Principles: Promoting the circulation of Blood to remove Blood Stasis; warming the channels and removing obstruction from the collaterals.

Prescription: Wen Guan Tang (Decoction for Warming Fallopian Tube) (Prescription based on the clinical experience of the author)

Parched pangolin scales (Squama Manitis) 9g, Chinese honey locus (Spina Gleditsiae) 15g, burreed tuber (Rhizoma Sparganii) 9g, zedoary (Rhizoma Zedoariae) 9g, prepared myrrh (Myrrha Praeparata) 9g, red peony root (Radix Paeoniae Rubra) 9g, red sage root (Radix Salviae Miltiorrhizae) 30g, peach kernel (Semen Persicae) 9g, sweetgum fruit (Fructus Liquidambaris) 15g, Chinese angelica root (Radix Angelicae Sinensis) 9g, prepared aconite root (Radix Aconiti Praeparata) 6g, cinnamon bark (Cortex Cinnamomi) 6g, common fennel fruit (Fructus Foenicuii) 6g, poria (Poria) 9g, epimedium (Herba Epimedii) 15g, amethyst (Fluorite) 30g and centipedefern (Scolopendra) 3g. The above drugs are decocted in water for oral administration, one dose daily, to be taken successively over 2-6 months.

Analysis of the Prescription: The effects of the first nine drugs are the same as the explanations given previously. Chinese angelica root (Radix Angelicae Sinensis), pungent in taste and warm in nature, nourishes Blood and promotes the circulation of Blood. Aconite root, cinnamon bark (Cortex Cinnamomi), epimedium (Herba Epimedii) and amethyst (Fluorite) warm the Kidney and remove obstruction from the collaterals. Common fennel fruit (Fructus Foenicuii) warms Kidney Yang to help remove obstruction. Poria (Poria) removes exudate and water. Centipedefern (Scolopendra), salty in taste and warm in nature, removes

Toxins and relieves spasm, removes obstruction from the collaterals and dissolve lumps. The whole prescription promotes the circulation of Blood and removes Blood Stasis, warms the channels and removes obstruction from the collaterals, and promotes the opening of fallopian tube.

• *Retention of Damp Heat*

Main Symptoms and Signs: Obstruction of fallopian tube, or unobstruction but unsmooth ness of fallopian tube, forwarded menstruation, more in amount, sticky in nature, bright red or purplish red in color, with blood clots, yellowish leukorrhea, pain in lower abdomen, intolerance to pressing, red face and hot body, dry throat with a bitter taste, dark urine, dry stool, red tongue with yellow or yellow greasy tongue coating, slippery rapid pulse. Gynecological examination shows a larger uterus with pain if pressing, and the adnexae on the two sides may become thick with pain if pressed.

Analysis of the Symptoms and Signs: Retention of Damp Heat obstructs the channels and collaterals of uterus, so fallopian tube is obstructed or unobstructed but not smooth. The pathogenic Heat accumulates in the Chong and Ren Channels, and it forces blood to flow, so menstruation is forwarded with more amount. The menstruation is bright red in color or purplish red and sticky in nature if there is Heat in Blood. Menstruation gets stagnated, so it has blood clots. Damp Heat damages the Ren Channel, so the color of leukorrhea is yellowish. Damp Heat steams uterus, so it is damaged and Damp Heat accumulates in the channels and collaterals, so pain in lower abdomen occurs, which is intolerable to pressing. The other signs and symptoms suggest Damp Heat.

Treatment Principles: Promoting the circulation of Blood to remove Blood Stasis; clearing Heat to remove obstruction from the collaterals.

Prescription: Qing Guan Tang (Decoction for Removing Heat from Fallopian Tube) (Prescription based on the clinical experiences of the author)

Parched pangolin scales (Squama Manitis) 9g, Chinese honey locus (Spina Gleditsiae) 15g, burreed tuber (Rhizoma

205

Sparganii) 9g, zedoary (Rhizoma Zedoariae) 9g, prepared myrrh (Myrrha Praeparata) 9g, red peony root (Radix Paeoniae Rubra) 9g, red sage root (Radix Salviae Miltiorrhizae) 30g, peach kernel (Semen Persicae) 9g, motherwort (Herba Leonuri) 30g, prunella spike (Spica Prunellae) 9g, sweetgum fruit (Fructus Liquidambaris) 15g, moutan bark (Cortex Moutan Radicis) 9g, phellodendron bark (Cortex Phellodendri) 9g, honeysuckle flower (Flos Lonicerae) 30g, forsythia fruit (Fructus Forsythiae) 15g, dandelion herb (Herba Taraxaci) 18g and patrinia (Herba Patriniae) 24g. The above drugs are decocted in water for oral administration, one dose per day, and taking successively over 2-6 months.

Analysis of the Prescription: The effects of the first 11 drugs in the prescription are the same as the explanations given previously. Moutan bark (Cortex Moutan Radicis) and phellodendron bark (Cortex Phellodendri) clear Heat and cool Blood, remove Toxins and promote diuresis. Honeysuckle flower (Flos Lonicerae), dandelion herb (Herba Taraxaci), forsythia fruit (Fructus Forsythiae) clear Heat and promote diuresis, remove Toxins and resolve lumps. The whole prescription promotes the circulation of Blood and removes Blood Stasis, clears Heat and removes obstruction from the collaterals and finally opens fallopian tube.

Besides the above three types, clinically, Blood Stasis due to Qi Deficiency, accumulation of Phlegm Damp, Blood Stasis due to Kidney Deficiency can be found in clinic, and be treated according to Qi Deficiency, Kidney Deficiency and accumulation of Phlegm Damp by using the drugs with modifications, and thus better curative effect can be obtained.

Current Research
1. A report of Tong Guan Tang (Decoction for Removing Obstruction from Fallopian Tube) used to treat 108 cases of female sterility due to obstruction of fallopian tube revealed that among the total cases, 72 received uterotubal iodized oil roentgenography or uterotubal meglucamine diatrizonate roentgenography, and 36 received uterotubal solution-perfusion test. Among the 72 cases given salpingography, 8 suf-

fered from bilateral interstitial obstruction; 10, bilateral isthmic obstruction; 16, obstruction of bilateral ampullar region; 23, bilateral fimbria obstruction; 15, mixed obstruction, among which 8 also were complicated with hydrops. These patients were treated with Jiajian Tong Guan Tang (Modified Decoction for Removing Obstruction from Fallopian Tube) (The drugs of the prescription are the same as Syndrome Differentiation and treatment Type of Blood Stasis due to Qi Stagnation). The drugs were decocted in water, and taking one dose per day. Modifications of the Prescription: For the cases of Qi Deficiency, dangshen (Radix Codonopsis Pilosulae) and astragalus root (Radix Astragali Seu Hedysari) were added; for the patients with stagnation of Liver Qi, bupleurum root (Radix Bupleuri), green tangerine peel (Pericarpium Citri Reticulatae Viride) and tangerine peel (Pericarpium Citri Reticulatae); for the patients of Cold accumulation, aconite root, cinnamon bark (Cortex Cinnamomi), lindera root (Radix Linderae) and common fennel (Fructus Foeniculi); for the patients with hydrops, umbellate pore fungus (Polyporus Umbellatus), poria (Poria) peel, Herba Lycopi and coix seed (Semen Coicis); for the patients with appendicitis, patrinia (Herba Patriniae), sargentgloryvine (Caulis Sargentodoxae), dandelion herb (Herba Taraxaci) and diding (Herba Violae); for the patients with tuberculosis, stemona root (Radix Stemonae) and Chinese mahonia leaf (Folium Mahoniae); for the patients with severe pain in lower abdomen, corydalis tuber (Rhizoma Coptidis), cat-tail pollen (Pollen Typhae) and baked lucid ganodermia (Gaboderma Lucidum). One treatment course is over 2 months. After the course of treatment, salpingography or tubal solution-perfusion were used. The patients who failed to respond to the treatment again took the drugs for 1-2 courses of treatment, and the longest course of treatment can be 6 months. Most of the patients gained effects after they took the medicine for 1-2 courses of treatment. After the treatment, the total effective cases were 97 (89.8%). 92 were cured completely (including pregnant and tubal-open-again cases), with a recovery rate of 85.2%. Among them, 22 were pregnant, with a pregnancy rate of 20.

207

4%. 11 cases failed to respond to the treatment, with an ineffective rate of 10.2%. Because among the total effective cases, 8 suffered from anovulation, 12 had problem of dysplasia of corpus luteum, 16 had problem of their male's seminal being abnormal which obviously affected pregnancy rate (Jin Weixin, et al, 1991).

Animal experiments have proved that the toxicity of Decoction for Removing Obstruction from Fallopian Tube is quite low. After the young rat was perfused 40ml/kg of the decoction (equal to 120g/kg of herbal drug), there was no toxic reaction observed. From this, it can be calculated that no acute toxic reaction can be found if a grown-up takes orally 6000ml of the decoction a time. Subacute toxic experiments have shown that after the young rate was perfused 0.2ml/10g of the decoction successively for 45 days, there were no derangement, necrosis, hyperemia, edema, inflammatory cellular infiltration, etc. in rat's organs. Abnormality experiments also showed no bad influence from the decoction on the fetus rat. This provides basis of safety for clinical application of the decoction.

In experiment, local tissue edema caused by the increase of permeability of blood vessels due to carrageenin and croton oil was also observed. Decoction for Removing Obstruction from Fallopian Tube can inhibit the hind toe edema of the young rat caused by carrageenin ($P<0.01$), and also inhibit the young rat's auricular inflammation caused by croton oil. It suggests that the decoction can inhibit the increase of permeability of blood vessels caused by carrageenin and croton oil, inhibit edema of focus tissues, and possess certain antiinflammation effect. The decoction remarkably decreases the rat's number of times of body twisting caused by acetic acid ejection into the abdominal cavity ($P<0.01$), because acetic acid can cause everlasting pain stimulation in deep and large area of the abdominal cavity, and causes acute inflammation, and the decoction can counteract against the inflammation caused by acetic acid. This of course suggests that the decoction possesses inflammation-inhibiting effect. This is consistent with the facts that the decoction can inhibit the rat's auricular inflammation caused by croton oil

208

and the rat's hind toe inflammation caused by carrageenin. The perfusion of the decoction through rat's stomach also remarkably decreases the specific viscosity of the whole blood ($P < 0.05$), but affects little about the specific viscosity of plasma. This may be related to the following facts. The increase of the number of electric charges on the surface of red cells makes Zeta potential increase; therefore, the repelling force among the red cells becomes big, and this inhibits the clustering of the red cells; as a result, the specific viscosity of the whole blood is reduced. The same, the increase of the metamorphotic ability of the red cells enables them to go through Blood Vessels smaller than their own diameter (The diameter of the red cells is 7-8μm). On the other hand, the loss of this ability causes the specific viscosity of the red cells in the movement of blood microflow. Therefore, the increase of red cell's metamorphotic ability correspondingly decreases the viscosity of the whole blood, and improves microcirculation. In the experiment, it was observed that the decoction can inhibit the young rat's microcirculation disturbance caused by hypophysis posterior pituitary hormones ($P < 0.01$). Hypophysis posterior pituitary hormones cause contraction of blood vessels, and influence microcirculation greatly. Normal saline water control group is manifested as arteriole spasm, small vein blood stagnation, unclear vascular bed, slow the circulation of Blood, purple blood, and red cell clustering, unhomogenous the circulation of Blood, blood clots in blood vessels to these severe cases. However, the rats receiving Decoction for Removing Obstruction from Fallopian Tube showed unchange of the appearances of arterioles, venules, such as diameter, color, etc., and the rate of the circulation of Blood obviously became quicker compared with the control group ($P < 0.01$), and there was no blood coagulation in microvessels of blood. This suggests that the decoction can counteract against blood vessel contraction caused by hypophysis posterior pituitary hormones, speed up the rate of blood microflow, and improve microcirculation. Arachidonic acid is an important precursor material in the synthesis of prostaglandin (PG) material. Under the effect of epoxy en-

209

zyme, arachidonic acid forms peroxide in prostaglandin, and then under the effect of the enzyme it is synthesized into prostaglandin E, F, D, A, etc. And it may also be synthesized into PGI_2 and TX_2 under the effect of prostacyclin synthesis enzyme, thrombosysthesis enzyme, and then later is disintegrated to 6-K-$PGF_{1\alpha}$ and TXB_2. Prostacyclin can prevent adhesion of platelet to wall of blood vessels, and possess great effect of inhibiting platelet coagulation, enlarge Blood Vessels. But the physiological effect of TXA_2 is just opposite against the above material. It can cause contraction of blood vessels, strong coagulation of platelet. From this, it can be seen that PGI_2 and TXA_2 in blood have important effect in regulating mechanism's blood circulation. Because the physiological half-life period of PGI_2 and TXA_2 are quite short, to determine the content of 6-K-$PGF_{1\alpha}$ and TXB_2 to represent the level of each of their precursor material. The results of experiments have shown that Decoction for Removing Obstruction from Fallopian Tube can decrease TXB_2 level in plasma of the rat ($P < 0.01$), increase 6-K-$PGF_{1\alpha}$ gement of blood cells, and it also decreases the specific viscosity of the whole blood, benefits the improvement of microcirculation disturbance caused by inflammation, favors nourishment supply to the tissues, improves histological plastics and tissue regeneration ability. The above results have shown the decoction's effect of promoting the circulation of Blood and removing Blood Stasis, improving microcirculation, decreasing inflammatory exudate and improving assimilation, and anti-inflammation. TCM thinks obstruction causes pain. The decoction's effect of promoting the circulation of Blood and removing Blood Stasis improves blood microcirculation, reduces pain. It actually shows the principle that the pain is removed if the tube is unobstructed. In Decoction for Removing Obstruction from Fallopian Tube, Chuanxiong rhizome (Rhizoma Ligustici Chuanxiong), red sage root (Radix Salviae Miltiorrhizae), red peony root (Radix Paeoniae Rubra) and peach kernel (Semen Persicae) have certain antibacterial and removing inflammation and anti-analgetic effects. This is consistent with the following facts: The decoction inhibits the young rat's auricular inflammation caused by croton oil and the hind toe inflammation caused by carrageenin and the decrease of the number of times of body twisting caused by acetic acid injection to abdominal cavity. The decoction's effect of promoting the circulation of Blood and removing Blood Stasis in helping decreasing the whole blood's specific viscosity, increasing the content of plasma 6-K-PGF$_{1\alpha}$ lowering TXB$_2$ and T/6 ratio, counteracting against microcirculation disturbance caused by hyophysis posterior pituitary hormones may be the important reason of improving the plastic and regeneration of fallopian tube and improving transformation and assimilation of proliferative pathogenic changes. At the same time, Japanese sea tangle (Thallus Laminariae), sea-weed, parched pangolin scales (Squama Manitis), Chinese honey locus (Spina Gleditsiae) and sweetgum fruit (Fructus Liquidambaris)—having the effect of softening and resolving lumps and removing obstruction from the collateralssupplement the effect of promoting the circulation of Blood and removing Blood Stasis, benefits the removal of inflammation of fallopian tube, and the re-opening of tubal canal. The decoction can diastolize uterus, soothe muscle of fallopian tube. This benefits the removal of tubal inflammation and histoplastics, the removal and assimilation of foreign body in fallopian tube, and finally favors unobstruction of fallopian tube. In addition, the patients with tubal inflammation also often suffer from abdominal uncomfort feeling, or pain, and Decoction for Removing Obstruction from fallopian Tube can relieve these clinical symptoms and signs. Also, the non-specific antipain effect of the prescription is also related to its effect on loosening smooth muscle.

Decoction for Removing Obstruction from Fallopian Tube slightly excites the animal's endocrine axis system, which is manifested as the growth of uterus of the young rat ($P < 0.01$), and slight increase of ovary weight ($P > 0.05$), slight increase of the times of follicle ovulation ($P > 0.05$) and slight increase of the contents of estradiol, FSH, and LH ($P > 0.05$), and almost unchange of progesterone in plasma. So, the effects of part of the herbal drugs may be presented

211

through influencing animal's reproductive endocrine axis system. That the decoction can slightly excite the animal's reproductive endocrine axis system is the result of the comprehensive effect of this prescription (Wang Shurong, et al, 1990).

2. Report of 87 cases of obstruction of fallopian tube treated by TCM herbal drugs reported that removing Blood Stasis was taken as the main method of treatment. According to clinical manifestations, the patients were divided into 5 types: Blood Stasis due to Qi Stagnation, accumulation of Phlegm Damp, accumulation of Cold Damp, Blood Stasis due to Qi Deficiency, hyperactivity of Heat due to Blood Stasis. ① Blood Stasis due to Qi Stagnation: Used was the method of promoting the circulation of Blood by activating the normal flow of Qi, removing Blood Stasis to remove obstruction from the collaterals. The drugs commonly used were Chinese angelica root (Radix Angelicae Sinensis), spatholobus stem (Caulis Spatholobi), bupleurum root (Radix Bupleuri), bighead atractylodes rhizome (Rhizoma Atractylodis Macrocephalae), moutan bark (Cortex Moutan Radicis), cyperus tuber (Rhizoma Cyperi), white peony root (Radix Paeoniae Alba), Herba Lycopi, lindera root (Radix Linderae), aucklandia root (Radix Aucklandiae), tangerine leaf (Folium Citri Reticulatae), sappan wood (Lignum Sappan), pangolin scales (Squama Manitis), sweetgum fruit (Fructus Liquidambaris), etc. ② Accumulation of Cold Damp: Used was the method of warming the channels to remove Cold, promoting the circulation of Blood to remove obstruction from the collaterals. The drugs commonly used are spatholobus stem (Caulis Spatholobi), Chinese angelica root (Radix Angelicae Sinensis), aconite root (Radix Aconiti Praeparata), cinnamon bark (Cortex Cinnamomi), dodder seed (Semen Cuscutae), epimedium (Herba Epimedii), cynomorium (Herba Cynomorii), amethyst (Fluorite), cyperus tuber (Rhizoma Cyperi), burreed tuber (Rhizoma Sparganii), zedoary (Rhizoma Zedoariae), baked ginger, etc. ③ Accumulation of Phlegm Damp: Used was the method of removing Phlegm and Blood Stasis and regulating menstruation. The drugs often used include fritillary

212

bulb (Bulbus Fritillariae), atractylodes rhizome (Rhizoma Atractylodis Macrocephalae), dried oyster shell (Concha Ostreae), airpotato yam (Rhizoma Dioscoreae Bulbiferae), Chinese honey locus (Spina Gleditsiae), Japanese sea tangle (Thallus Laminariae), sprunella spike (Spica Prunellae), sea pumice (Pumex), red sage root (Radix Salviae Miltiorrhizae), red peony root (Radix Paeoniae Rubra), pangolin scales (Squama Manitis), sweetgum fruit (Fructus Liquidambaris), Chinese angelica root (Radix Angelicae Sinensis), etc. ④ Blood Stasis due to Qi Deficiency: Used was the method of benefiting Qi to replenish Blood, promoting the circulation of Blood to remove Blood Stasis. The drugs often used include dangshen (Radix Codonopsis Pilosulae) rhizome (Radix Codonopsis Pilosulae), astragalus root (Radix Astragali Seu Hedysari), bighead atractylodes rhizome (Rhizoma Atractylodis Macrocephalae), poria (Poria), Chinese yam (Rhizoma Dioscoreae), red peony root (Radix Paeoniae Rubra), tangerine peel (Pericarpium Citri Reticulatae), Chinese angelica root (Radix Angelicae Sinensis), chuanxiong rhizome (Rhizoma Ligustici Chuanxiong), peach kernel (Semen Persicae), red sage root (Radix Salviae Miltiorrhizae), spatholobus stem (Caulis Spatholobi), pangolin scales (Squama Manitis), sweetgum fruit (Fructus Liquidambaris), etc. ⑤ Hyperactivity of Heat due to Blood Stasis: The method of clearing Heat to cool Blood, removing Blood Stasis and resolving lumps are used. The drugs often used include sargentgloryvine (Caulis Sargentodoxae), patrinia (Herba Patriniae), dandelion herb (Herba Taraxaci), barbat skullcap (Herba Scutellariae Barbatae), astragalus root (Radix Astragali Seu Hedysari), phellodendron bark (Cortex Phellodendri), moutan bark (Cortex Moutan Radicis), red peony root (Radix Paeoniae Rubra), burreed tuber (Rhizoma Sparganii), zedoary (Rhizoma Zedoariae), ground beetle (Eupolyphage sinensis), etc.

To the patients with such pathogenic changes as occasional pain in lower abdomen, or severe dysmenorrhea, accompanied by salpingitis, extensive adhesion of pelvic adhesive tissues, often external treatment is applied to help treatment. ① Enema Method: Promoting the circulation of Blood to re-

213

move Blood Stasis and resolving lumps are taken as the main method. The drugs often used include burreed tuber (Rhizoma Sparganii), zedoary (Rhizoma Zedoariae), sappan wood (Lignum Sappan), hornet nest (Nidus Vespae), Chinese honey locus (Spina Gleditsiae), etc. According to the situation of the tissue, the drugs were used with modification. The drugs were decocted in water to 150ml and an enema springe was used to enemate the liquid into anus, one time a night, and stop using during menstruation. ② Iontophoresis Method: Take 50ml of the decoction of the above-discussed syndromes or of enema decoction, to pour on a piece of gauze and lay on the affected area of lower abdomen and differentions in the decoction were enemated into the pelvic cavity through the application of iontophoresis physiotherapy apparatus. This method can help and improve cure effects. ③ External Application Method: Add 30g vinegar into dregs of decoction, bake it hot in the iron pot, wrap it with a gauze bag, and lay it hot on the affected area.

The patients with obstruction of fallopian tube are mostly differentiated as Blood Stasis Syndrome and Excess Syndrome, and drugs aiming at elimination are used in most cases. Therefore, 2 months later after the treatment, it is better to add the drug benefiting Qi, the commonly used drugs include dangshen rhizome (Radix Codonopsis Pilosulae), astragalus root (Radix Astragali Seu Hedysari), big-head atractylodes rhizome (Rhizoma Atractylodis Macrocephalae), Chinese yam (Rhizoma Dioscoreae), etc. For the purpose of supporting Vital Qi and improving cure effect. For the patients with irregular menstruation, drugs for regulating menstruation should be added according to Syndrome Differentiation.

The results of treatment: 20 patients (23%) were cured in 3 months; 29, in 3-6 months, 33.3%; 35, in 6-12 months, 40.2%; 3, in one year, 3.5%. After the treatment, 75 got pregnant, with a pregnancy rate of 86.2%. The 12 patients, not pregnant, were given tubal iodized oil roentgenography, and it showed that the fallopian tubes of them were all unobstructed. Follow-up found among the 44 pregnant recovered patients, since birth giving, the children developed normal-

214

ly, and intelligence was also normal (Li Xiangyun, 1989).

3. A clinical analysis of 121 cases with female sterility due to tubal diseases through TCM and western medicine combined was done.

Chinese herbal medicine: Most of the patients' illness conditions were differentiated as Syndrome of Blood Stasis and marked by pain in lower abdomen, and took "promoting the circulation of Blood to remove Blood Stasis" as the chief principle. The drugs were used with modifications in combination with differentiation of diseases and Syndromes. Prescription: Tail of Chinese angelica root (Radix Angelicae Sinensis) 30g, red peony root (Radix Paeoniae Rubra) 20g, peach kernel (Semen Persicae) 15g, safflower (Flos Carthami) 15g, Eupolyphage 15g, pangolin scales (Squama Manitis) 10g, Sichuan chinaberry (Fructus Meliae Toosendan) 15g, citron fruit (Fructus Aurantii) 12g, corydalis tuber (Rhizoma Coptidis) 20g, giant knotweed (Rhizoma Polygoni Cuspidati) 30g. Modifications: For the patients with tubal tuberculosis, the following drugs are added such as burreed tuber (Rhizoma Sparganii) 10g, zedoary (Rhizoma Zedoariae) 10g, stellaria root (Radix Stellariae) 20g and wolfberry bark (Cortex Lycii Radicis) 30g. For the patients accompanying by tubal hydrops, added were additionally tetrandra root (Radix Stephaniae Tetrandrae) 15g, Herba Lycopi 15g and red bean (Semen Phaseoli) 30g to remove obstruction from collaterals and eliminate water. For the patients with adnexa thickening and pain if pressed, revealed through gynecological examination, added additionally were burreed tuber (Rhizoma Sparganii) 10g, zedoary (Rhizoma Zedoariae) 10g, diding (Herba Violae) 30g and patrinia (Herba Patriniae) 30g to strengthen the effect of softening hardness, remove swelling, clear Heat, and eliminate Toxins. For the patients with vegetarian body accompanied by shortness of breath, acratia, sweating, astragalus root (Radix Astragali Seu Hedysari) 30g and dangshen rhizome (Radix Codonopsis Pilosulae) 15g are added. The drugs were decocted in water for oral administration, one dose per day.

Treatment by Western Medicine: Intrauterine injection can be used. For the case with obstruction of fallopian tube

215

caused by common bacterial inflammatory adhesion, given were an injection of α-chymotrypsin and an injection of gentamicin (80,000U) added with normal saline water to dilute to 30ml. For the case with tuberculosis obstruction of fallopian tube, change gentamicin to kanamycin injection 0.5g. From the third day after the completion of menstrual cycle, every 2-3 days, an injection was given, and it was not stopped until the day before ovulation period, which consisted of one course of treatment. The number of times of treatment was up to disease condition. For the case with obstruction of fallopian tube accompanied by anovulation, after fallopian tube was unobstructed, 50mg clomiphine was administered orally once a day, beginning from the fifth day of menstruation onset, and successively for 5 days.

Effects of Treatment: After the treatment, getting pregnant in 2 years was considered to be recovered. Among 121 patients, 80 became pregnant, (among them, 3 patients experienced natural abortion, and got pregnant again later). 42 had already given births to child, and all were natural births. The babies developed normally. It is thought that interuterine injection method brings a faster cure rate in removing obstruction from fallopian tube compared with TCM treatment, but it is inferior to TCM in the treatment of cicatricial contracture of fallopian tube, tubal stiffness, epithelial adhesion of fallopian tube, or withering change of tubal mucus to restore peristalsis function (Jia Kefu, et al, 1988).

4. A summary report of 115 cases of obstruction of fallopian tube treated by Sini San Jiawei (Modified Decoction for Resuscitation) regards that this syndrome mostly have manifes tations of stagnation of Liver Qi to the varying degree, such as, mammary swelling, pain in lower abdomen, abdominal pain before menstruation, etc. So, Modified Decoction for Resuscitation was used. At the same time, from what was revealed by salpingography, for the cases with tubal adhesion and obstruction, added were additionally red sage root (Radix Salviae Miltiorrhizae), notoginseng to remove Blood Stasis, loosen adhesion in favor of reopening of fallopian tube. Also, pangolin scales (Squama Manitis), Chinese honey locus (Spina Gleditsiae), sweetgum fruit

(Fructus Liquidambaris), etc. were used to remove obstruction from fallopian tube. Ophiopogon root was added to nourish Yin and promote body fluids. The author held that it is also important to administer drugs in reference of menstrual cycle. For the patients complicated with hypoplasia of corpus luteum, added additionally were the drugs restoring the Kidney and supporting Yang in the middle stage of menstruation (Deglued antler powder, cinnamon bark (Cortex Cinnamomi), dried human placenta (Placenta Hominis), etc.) to improve the function of corpus luteum. Drugs promoting the circulation of Blood and removing Blood Stasis were used in large doses to the cases with hyperactivity of Qi and Blood several days before menstruation. For the case of Qi Deficiency after the completion of menstrual cycle, drugs tonifying and nourishing were added. Regulating menstrual cycle not only benefits regulating or maintaining menstrual cycle, but also favors removing obstruction from fallopian tube, but also improves clinical cure effect. For making up for the shortcomings of internal treatment, the author often selected drugs promoting the normal flow of Qi to activate the circulation of Blood, resolving lumps and removing Blood Stasis as the main method, supplemented with the drugs with good taste and flavor, removing obstruction from the channels and collaterals, causing resuscitation, softening adhesion to form enema prescription, hot pressing prescription, to improve cure effect.

Prescription for oral use: Bupleurum root (Radix Bupleuri) 10g, bitter orange (Fructus Aurantii) 12g, red peony root (Radix Paeoniae Rubra) 12g, dried licorice (Radix Glycyrrhizae) 3g, red sage root (Radix Salviae Miltiorrhizae) 30g, notoginseng (Radix Notoginseng) powder 3g (to swallow in different times), pangolin scales (Squama Manitis) 20g, ophiopogon root (Radix Ophiopogon is), Chinese honey locus (Spina Gleditsiae) and sweetgum fruit (Fructus Liquidambaris) 10g respectively. The drugs were taken one dose daily, and stopped using during menstruation. For the case with pain in lower abdomen, leukorrhea, yellow in color, sticky in nature, and fetid in swelling, black nightshade and mockstrawberry were used; for the case with distending

217

pain of breasts before menstruation, hornet nest (Nidus Vespae) and litchi seed (Semen Litchi); for the cases with pain in lower abdomen or more leukorrhea, thin, and fishy in smell during menstruation, delayed antler powder (Cornu Cervi Degelatinatum), cinnamon bark (Cortex Cinnamomi); for the case with tubal hydrops, knoxia root (Radix Knoxiae), ground beetle (Eupolyphage sinensis), epimedium (Herba Epimedii) and Herba Lycopi; for the case with tubal tuberculosis, sprunella spike (Spica Prunellae) and centipedefern (Scolopendra); for the case with uterine maldevelopment, dogwood fruit (Fructus Corni) and dried human placenta (Placenta Hominis); for the case with white face and pale tongue, Chinese angelica root (Radix Angelicae Sinensis) and astragalus root (Radix Astragali Seu Hedysari).

Prescription for hot compressing: Herba Gaultheriae 30g, Sichuan aconite root (Radix Aconiti) 10g, clematis root 20g, cinnamon bark (Cortex Cinnamomi) 10g, frankincense (Resina Olibani) 20g, myrrh (Myrrha) 20g, Chinese angelica root (Radix Angelicae Sinensis) 20g, safflower (Flos Carthami) 10g, red sage root (Radix Salviae Miltiorrhizae) 30g, red peony root (Radix Paeoniae Rubra) 15g. The above drugs were made into granules like red beans (Semen Phaseoli), and put into a cloth bag, and some wine was dripped into it, and they were steamed for 40 minutes, and used for hot pressing in lower abdomen. A hot-water bag was used to keep warm and keep the temperature at 40°C for about 40-60 minutes, one time per day, and change a bag every 2 days. The treatment was stopped during menstruation.

Prescription for enema: Red sage root (Radix Salviae Miltiorrhizae) 30g, red peony root (Radix Paeoniae Rubra) 30g, burreed tuber (Rhizoma Sparganii) 15g, zedoary (Rhizoma Zedoariae) 15g, bitter orange (Fructus Aurantii) 15g, Chinese honey locus (Spina Gleditsiae) 15g, Chinese angelica root (Radix Angelicae Sinensis) 15g, frankincense (Resina Olibani) 10g, myrrh (Myrrha) 10g and Herba Gaultheriae 15g. The above drugs were decocted in water and concentrated to 200ml, to be taken one dose every

218

night, keep for enema. The appropriate temperature was about 39℃. After the decoction was taken for 10 times, the patient should rest for 3-4 days. The treatment was not used during menstrual period. 115 cases in average needed 4 courses of treatment (One menstrual cycle is equal to one course of treatment). 63 (54.78%) were recovered; 27 (23.47%) responded effectively to the treatment; and 25 cases (21.73%) failed to respond to the treatment (Xu Runsan, 1987).

5. Clinical observation report of female sterility caused by obstruction of fallopian tube treated by TCM herbal drugs injection into uterine cavity showed that satisfactory effects were obtained by using TCM mixed liquid for intrauterine injection. For comparing the cure effects, 95 cases were divided into two groups. 30 cases in TCM Group, 65 cases in Western Medicine Group. Western Medicine Group was treated by choosing 1-2 antibiotics (penicillin, gentamicin, kanamycin, or streptomycin) added with hydroprednisone acetate 5mg, or R-chymotrypsin for a few patients; then 12-15ml of injection water was added. TCM Group was given isatis root injection 4ml, compound red sage root (Radix Salviae Miltiorrhizae) injection 4ml, 20% placenta tissue liquid 4ml, which were used in combination. The two groups started the treatment 2-3 days after the completion of menstrual cycle, and injection was given every 2 days until menstruation period. It could be used successively for 3 menstrual cycles (i.e., one course of treatment). Later, the groups were observed for 2 months. Unobstruction test of fallopian tube was given to the non-pregnant patients to observe the progress of treatment.

Therapeutic effects: That those among the 95 cases receiving intrauterine injection got pregnant was considered to be successful in treatment. The total effective rate was 21%. Among the 20 pregnant cases, except for 3 cases experiencing natural abortion, all had term births. Among them, 7 of 30 cases (23.3%) of TCM Group got pregnant. 13 of 65 cases (20%) of western medicine group got pregnant. The difference of the pregnancy rate of the two hydrops were not significant. It suggests that TCM intrauterine injection therapy

219

is the same as western medicine. The author thinks that western medicine intrauterine injection has a long history, but many people were allergic to antibiotics, then, TCM injection needs no allergy test, brings no reaction. Therefore, it has certain advantages and clinical application significance (Lu Haonian, 1988).

Female Sterility Treated by Means of Acupuncture and Moxibustion

Acupuncture, a special way for menstrual regulation and pregnancy, can not only regulate menstruation, but also induce ovulation. In recent years, the study of female sterility treated with acupuncture has gained satisfactory progress.

Mechanism of Acupuncture Treating Female Sterility by Inducing Ovulation

Menstruation and pregnancy are interrelated to the channels and collaterals of the Kidney, the Liver, the Spleen and other Zangfu Organs. The Kidney Channel of Foot Shaoyin controls congenital Essence. From acupoint Yongquan (KID 1) to acupoint Shufu (KID 27), there are 27 acupoints, among which, one-third are interrelated to irregular menstruation and pregnancy. The Spleen Channel of Foot Taiyin controls acquired Essence. There are 21 acupoints from Yinbai (SP 1) to Dabao (SP 21), among which one-fourth are interrelated to irregular menstruation and pregnancy. The Liver Channel of Foot Jueyin controls Qi and Blood regulation. There are 14 acupoints from Dadun (LIV 1) to Qimen (LIV 14), among which, half are interrelated to irregular menstruation and pregnancy. Therefore, that acupuncture can promote ovulation and thus treat female sterility has a close interrelation with the channels and collaterals of the Kidney, the Liver, the Spleen and other Zangfu Organs.

The three different channels: The Chong Channel (Vital Channel), the Ren Channel (Anterior Midline Channel) and the Du Channel stretch out from one place, and multiple abscess each other. "the Chong Channel, the Sea of Blood,"

220

through Qichong (ST 30), crosses and converges with the Foot Shaoyin and merges into the Kidney Channel and supported by congenital Kidney Qi. The Chong Channel also crosses and converges with Qichong (ST 30) of the Stomach Channel of Foot Yangming, receiving the nourishment of acquired essential substances from foodstuff. The congenital Essence and acquired essential substances from foodstuff all accumulate in the Chong Channel. This plays an important role in menstrual regulation and ovulation.

"The Ren Channel, controlling the growth of fetus," through the channels and collaterals, crosses and converges with overall Yin Channels at Shanzhong (REN 17), and controls Yin channels of the whole body, thus it is the Sea of Yin Channels. Essence, Blood and Body Fluid all are controlled by the Ren Channel. It is also the fundamental of pregnancy. If Qi of the Ren Channel can flow smoothly, menarche and fertilization can be normal. If the Ren Channel suffers from excessive consumption and Deficiency, then a-menorrhea happens, and thus configuration and constitution of a human body fails. Thus, pregnancy can not result.

"The Du Channel, the Sea of the Yang Channels," can hold together all Essence of the body because it penetrates the whole spinal cord and belongs to the Kidney. The Ren Channel and the Du Channel cross and converge at Yinjiao (DU 28), circulate and move back and forth, and thus keep the comparative balance of Qi of Yin Channels and Qi of Yang Channels, and regulate menstruation so that menarche comes normally. If the Du Channel suffers from certain illness, pregnancy will not happen.

Commonly Used Acupoints in the Treatment of Sterility Through Ovulation Promotion

• Guanyuan (REN 4)

The Chong Channel originates beneath Guanyuan (REN 4) where female sterility is treated. The patient lies supine. Guanyuan (REN 4) is located 3 cun below the navel and in the median line of the abdomen. The patient should be instructed to urinate prior the treatment. Insert the needle obliquely at the depth of 2-3 cun until the patient experi-

221

ences a feeling of aching and distendtion which extends to the external genitals. The needle is maintained at this depth for 15-30 minutes. Alternately moxibustion of 3-7 moxa-cones may be applied to this point for 20-30 minutes.

• *Zhongji (REN 3)*

The Ren Channel originates from beneath the Ren Channel. To use this acupoint can treat female sterility. The patient lies supine. Zhongji (REN 3) is located along the median line of the abdomen 4 *cun* below the navel. The patient should be instructed to urinate prior the treatment. Insert the needle obliquely at the depth of 2-3 *cun* until the patient experiences a feeling of aching and distendtion which extends to the external genitals. The needle is maintained at this depth for 15-30 minutes. Alternately moxibustion of 3-7 moxa-cones may be applied to this point for 20-30 minutes.

• *Qihai (REN 6)*

This acupoint controls diseases of urogenital system, and can treat female sterility. The patient lies supine. Qihai (REN 6) is located 1.5 *cun* below the navel at the central point of the line between the navel and Guanyuan (REN 4). The patient should be instructed to urinate prior the treatment. Insert the needle obliquely at the depth of 2-3 *cun* until the patient experiences a feeling of aching and distendtion which extends to the external genitals. The needle is maintained at this depth for 15-30 minutes. Alternately moxibustion of 3-7 moxa-cones may be applied to this point for 20-30 minutes.

• *Zigong (Extra)*

This acupoint is to treat female non-pregnancy over a long period of time. The patient lies supine. Zigong (Extra) is located 3 *cun* beside Zhongji (REN 3). The patient should be instructed to urinate prior the treatment. Insert the needle obliquely at the depth of 1.5-3 *cun* until the patient experiences a feeling of aching and distendtion which extends to the external genitals. The needle is maintained at this depth for 15-30 minutes. Alternately moxibustion of 3-7 moxa-cones may be applied to this point for 20-30 minutes.

• *Sanyinjiao (SP 6)*

It is an acupoint where the Kidney, the Spleen and the

Liver Channels meet. It governs diseases of urogenital system and Yin Blood in female. The patient sits upright with falling feet or lie supine. The acupoint is located directly 3 *cun* up the tip of medial malleolus and at the back edge of tibia. The patient should be instructed to urinate prior the treatment. Insert the needle obliquely at the depth of 1-1.5 *cun* until the patient experiences a feeling of aching and distendtion which extends to the external genitals. The needle is maintained at this depth for 15-30 minutes. Alternately moxibustion of 3-7 moxa-cones may be applied to this point for 20-30 minutes.

Acupuncture in the Treatment of Sterility Through Promoting Ovulation

At first, the patient should be instructed to measure his BBT according to a menstrual period consisting of 28 days from the 12th to 14th day of menarche. One treatment a day, and continuously over 3 days. For better curative effect, the patient can be given acupuncture therapy from the 8th to 12th day of menarche one time every other day. From the 12th to 14th day, the patient changes to be given acupuncture therapy one time per day. Alternately, moxibustion is given.

The practitioner may choose 2-3 points among the "ones most in use" and supply acupuncture therapy alternately. Long needle may be chosen for Zigong (Extra) and is inserted down for 3-4 *cun*, to prickle directly the area where ovary is located at until ovary function is stimulated. To the patient whose menstruation is delayed, according to the days of the menstrual period, the number of times of needling may be determined. Three menstrual cycles make one course of treatment. When treating the patient, pay attention to De Qi (needling sensation) or "response" in order to improve curative effect. BBT is a main indicator of the therapeutic effect, and also the treating effect can be measured through such ways of measuring ovulation as continuous measurement of follicle growth by B-ultrasonic sound or through radioimmunoassay (RIA) of endocrine hormones, so that systematic observation can be carried out and curative

223

effect can be judged.

Current Research

"A Clinical Study of Promoting Ovulation by Electric Acupuncture" observed the curative effect of acupuncture in 55 patients with irregular menstruation and without ovulation. 55 patients all underwent history-taking, gynecological examination, BBT examination, vaginal exfoliative smear cytological examination, cervical examination, pelvic ultrasonic examination, and urinary FSH measurement. 25 of them also received peritoneoscopy and radioimmunoassay of FSH, LH, PRI in blood. After those examinations, it was found that 42 suffered from polycystic ovary syndrome, 9 with amenia due to dysfunction of hypothalamus—pituitary, 3 with dysfunctional uterine bleeding, 1 with infrequent menstruation. Among them, 15 had problem of female sterility. Guanyuan (REN 4), Zhongji (REN 3), Zigong (Extra) and Sanyinjiao (SP 6) were chosen for the treatment. The stimulating method was uniform reinforcing-reducing or mild electrotherapy (3Hz < 5mA) to produce warm, slight distending response in lower abdomen to make Qi and Blood circulate. Each treatment is over 30 minutes every day since the 14th or 16th of menstruation. Curative Effect: After the above therapy, in the first month, diphasic BBT appeared in 31 patients, and four were pregnant. This indicates that acupuncture therapy can promote ovulation. After comparing 50 courses of treatment of vaginal exfoliative cytologic smear examination before and after acupuncture therapy, it was found that the method was effective in 50% of the patients with EI>81%. Among that, the group of the patients with EI > 70% showed a decrease in EI and in the group of the patients with EI< 30%, those who showed an increase in EI also showed an increase in the cases of ovulation ($P < 0.05$). This indicates that acupuncture can cause estrogen change in 50% of the patients. To study the interrelationship between the effect of acupuncture promoting ovulation and the changes of sympathetic nerve activity, the changes of skin temperature of the hands were observed after acupuncture therapy. The results were that 35 showed an increase in

224

skin temperature of the hand, among whom, biphasic BBT appeared in 29 patients. 20 showed a decrease in skin temperature of the hands, among whom, biphasic BBT only happened in 2 patients after the treatment ($P < 0.05$). The results above showed that after needling, the result of acupuncture promoting ovulation was better to those whose sympathetic nerve system activity was restrained. This not only offers one indication of acupuncture therapy promoting ovulation, but also may suggest that etiology is interrelated to disturbed central nerves. To confirm this, at the same time of observing the changes of skin temperature, the changes of β-EPIS (β-endarphin like immunoreactive substance) level in blood was measured. The result suggested that while acupuncture therapy regulated the activities of sympathetic nervous system, hypophysis also regulated β-EPIS release function; what's more, these changes were related to the effects of acupuncture therapy promoting ovulation. Through blood FSH and LH assay, the mean value of blood FSH and LH and pulse frequency in the group of acupuncture promoting ovulation all increased. Before needling, the follicular diameter was 6.50 ± 0.58mm. After needling with the increase of FSH and LH levels, follicles grew large rapidly and then were ovulated. In the group with no ovulation, before needling, the follicular diameter was 10.40 ± 3.21mm; after needling, after the diameter reached 14-16mm, it began to grow smaller. All the above suggests that electric needling could have a better result under the condition that patient's sympathetic nerve activities and adrenal axis are relatively constrained. This could be understood that after needling, the patients of this kind have smoothly Qi and Blood circulation. This also suggests that needling can regulate hypothalamus-pituitary function; therefore, ovulation is promoted. For instance, those whose hypothalamus-hypophysis can normally secrete gonadotropic hormone may have a problem of poor ovary response, which causes a poor result in acupuncture promoting ovulation or no obvious response (Yu Jin, et al, 1990).

"A Clinical Observation of Acupuncture Therapy to Induce Ovulation" reported that acupuncture therapy was used to

225

treat 34 cases with female sterility and 7 cases with pubertal amenorrhea. The patients were treated 3 times each month comprised one course of treatment. The patients were needled on the 12th, the 13th, and the 14th day of the menstrual cycle, one treatment per day, for three consecutive days using moderate stimulation. Selection of acupoints: On the first day, Guanyuan (REN 4), Guilai (ST 29) and Sanyinjiao (SP 6) were needled. On the second day, Zhongji (REN 3), Qichong (ST 30) and Zusanli (ST 36) were selected. On the third day, Mingmen (DU 4), Chengjiang (REN 24) and Xuehai (SP 1) were stimulated. Therapeutic effects: Among 34 patients with female sterility, 8 became pregnant after one course of treatment. 6 became pregnant after two courses of treatment. 8 became pregnant after three courses of treatment. 3 became pregnant after six courses of treatment. Altogether 25 (73.52%) were cured. 9 failed to respond to the treatment. As for 7 patients with pubertal amenorrhea, 2 started to have menstrual period after two courses of treatment, and 4 started to have menstrual period after three courses of treatment. The curative rate was 85.7%. 1 patient did not response to the treatment. There is certain relationship between body response to acupuncture and curative result. Because of the individual differences, the response was divided into three types: Strong, moderate and weak. The patients with strong response showed a better curative result in a shorter course of treatment. The patients with weak response showed a poor curative result, in a longer course of treatment (Liu Jizhang, 1987).

"Ovulation Induced by A Combination of Acupuncture Therapy and TCM—An Observation of 59 Cases" reported an observation of the short-term curative effect of 59 patients with menoxenia of non-ovulation treated mainly with electropuncture coordinated with treatment based on overall Syndrome Differentiation, the cause, nature, location of the illness, and the patient's physical condition according to the basic theory of TCM. Through pneumoperitoneography and pelvic pneumography, abdominoscope or B-ultrasonic scanning examination, it was found that 3 suffers from polycystic ovary syndrome, 7 suffers from dysfunctional bleeding of anovulation, and 22 suffers from scanty menstruation. Based on Syndrome Differentiation, it was found that 31 are identified as Kidney Deficiency Syndrome, and 14, Syndrome of Spleen-Kidney Yang Deficiency. Therapeutic methods: Select Guanyuan (REN 4), Zhongji (REN 3), Zigong (Extra) and Sanyinjiao (SP 6). Since the 14th day of menstruation, electropuncture was used one time, and altogether for 3 days. Stimulating intensity was 3Hz, electric current intensity was within 5mA, and the stimulation was lasted for 30 minutes. Later, the patients were observed for one week. If BBT didn't go up, electropuncture was applied one time more. One menstrual cycle was considered to be one course of treatment. With electropuncture treatment, the patients feel warm in lower abdomen. 59 patients received electropuncture treatment first for 3 months. If there was no ovulation, the treatment with materia medica was added for two months. The course of treatment was 1-5 months. BBT in the patients should be biphasic, or the patients got pregnant. After the application of electropuncture for three months, among the 59 patients, 20 (33.9%) had ovulation in two months. Then 11 of them had ovulation with a ovulatory rate of 52.5%. However, there was no clear difference between the effect of acupuncture plus materia medica and the effect of solely acupuncture ($P > 0.01$). There was also no clear difference among the effect of the types of the diseases or Syndrome Differentiation ($P > 0.01$). The report held that acupuncture therapy and herbal medicine treatment supplement each other (Zhu Xiudu, et al, 1987).

Thread embedding therapy was used to treat 18 patients with sterility because of non-ovulation and 6 patients with secondary amenorrhea. In 3-7 days after completion of the menstrual cycle in infertile patients. The patients with amenorrhea didn't have ovulation. 2cm of size "0" surgical catgut was inserted down into Sanyinjiao (SP 6) for 1cun with a needle with stylet. After De Qi, push the stylet and bury the surgical catgut there. After thread burying, if BBT was biphasic, but luteal function was not normal enough, then, after the second menstrual cycle, an intramuscular injection of 1000u HCG was given 2 times a week. After the

227

going up of BBT, the injection was changed to 1,000u per day, and given continuously over 4 days to keep the function of the yellow body of ovary. As a result, except for two cases who were not followed up, 20 patients had their menstrual cycles, and 18 had ovulation, 4 patients had no ovulation because they suffered from secondary amenorrhea. 16 became pregnant, among whom, 7 didn't use HCG. This method has the function of inducing ovulation, and has no side effects. One time of thread embedding therapy could regulate ovary function over a long period of time, and it is an ideal ovulation promoting method (Chen Deyong, 1984).

Treatment Based on Syndrome Differentiation

Main Points of Diagnosis
Those who have got married for over 2 years, having been living together with their spouses, whose reproductive functions are normal, and who can not get pregnant though contraception measures are not used or who once had given births to children, but can not get pregnant any more over two years, are considered to be patients with sterility. During diagnosis, both the wife and husband should go through certain examinations to make sure the causes of sterility.

Treatment Based on Syndrome Differentiation
• *Female Sterility due to Kidney Deficiency*

Main Symptoms and Signs: No pregnancy over a long period of time after marriage. Less menstruation with dull color during the late period of menstruation, or scanty menstruation or amenia; dark and gloomy face, with soreness and weakness along spinal column, cold sensation and dragging feeling in lower abdomen, hyposexuality, clearness and thinness of leukorrhea, profuse clear urine, loose stool, pale tongue with slight white tongue coating, deep or slow pulse.

Analysis of the Symptoms and Signs: Kidney stores congenital Essence. Because of Kidney Deficiency, the Chong and Ren Channels loose their sources for nourishment, and

228

the Sea of Blood is not sufficient, causing female sterility though the patient has married for a long period of time, less menstruation with dull color during the late period of menstruation, or infrequent menstruation or amenorrhea. Because of insufficiency of Kidney Yang, decline of Fire from the Gate of Life and retention of Cold in the uterus result. As a result, the patient's face is dark and gloomy, soreness and weakness along spinal column, cold sensation in lower abdomen, indifference to sexual activities and scanty whites. Because of Deficiency of Kidney Yang, to the upper part, it can not warm Spleen Yang, and to the lower part, it can not warm the Bladder, thus causing loose stools, and profuse clear urine. Pale tongue and white tongue coating, deep or slow pulse are all symptoms and signs of the decline and Deficiency of Kidney Yang.

Treatment Principles: Restoring the Kidney to warm the uterus; nourishing Blood to regulate menstruation.

Prescription: Yulin Zhu Jiajian (Modified Chinese Unicorn Pill) (Prescription from *Complete Works of Zhang Jingyue*)

Ginseng (Radix Ginseng) 3g, Chinese yam (Rhizoma Dioscoreae) 9g, poria (Poria) 9g, prepared rehmannia root (Radix Rehmanniae) 12g, Chinese angelica root (Radix Angelicae Sinensis) 9g, white peony root (Radix Paeoniae Alba) 9g, Chuangxiong rhezome (Rhizoma Ligustici Chuangxiong) 6g, dodder seed (Semen Cuscutae) 9g, eucommia bark (Cortex Eucommiae) 9g, deglued antler powder (Cornu Cervi Degelation) 9g, pricklyash peel (Pericarpium Zanthoxyli) 2g and prepared licorice (Radix Glycyrrhizae) 6g. The above drugs are decocted in water for oral administration, one dose daily, and 6-9 doses successively after completion of the menstrual cycle.

Analysis of the Prescription: In the prescription, Si Jun Zi Tang (Decoction of Four Noble Drugs) strengthens the Spleen and replenishes Qi. Si Wu Tang (Decoction of Four Ingredients) enriches Blood. Dodder seed (Semen Cuscutae), eucommia bark (Cortex Eucommiae), deglued antler powder (Cornu Cervi Degelation) warm and nourish the Liver and the Kidney, nourish the acupoint the Chong and Ren

Channels. Pricklyash warms the Du Channel to support Yang. The whole prescription can not only warm and nourish congenital Kidney Qi to produce Vital Essence, but also tonify the Spleen and Stomach to produce Blood, and regulate Blood and Channels to enrich Essence and Blood, and nourish the Chong and Ren Channels, and then pregnancy could be achieved.

Modifications of the Prescription: For the case with lower abdomen feeling cold, and with severe pain in lumbar area, the following herbal drugs are added to the above prescription: Prepared aconite root (Radix Aconiti) 6g, morinda root (Radix Morindae Officinalis) 9g, common fennel fruit (Fructus Foeniculi) 6g, argyi leaf (Folium Artemisiae Argyi) 6g, amethyst (Fluorite) 30g, epimedium (Herba Epimedii) 15g, curculigo rhizome (Rhizoma Curculiginis) 9g, desertliving cistanche (Herba Cistachi) 15g, dipsacus root (Radix Dipsaci) 15g, antler glue (Colla Cornus Cervi, baked) 9g and dried human placenta (Placenta Hominis) powder 6g (to be taken with boiling water). For the case with less amount of menstruation during later period of menstruation, the above prescription is added with wolfberry fruit (Fructus Lycii) 15g, fleece-flower root (Radix Polygoni Multiflori) 15g, astragalus root (Radix Astragali Seu Hedysari) 30g, cyperus tuber (Rhizoma Cyperi) 9g, red sage root (Radix Salviae Miltiorrhizae) 30g, peach kernel (Semen Persicae) 9g, safflower (Flos Carthami) 9g, cyathula root (Radix Cyathulae) 12g, spatholobus stem (Caulis Spatholobi) 15g, dried hawthorn fruit (Fructus Crataegi) 30g, Herba Siphonoste 9g and chicken's gizzard-skin (Endothelium Corneum Gigeriae Galli) 9g. For the case with insufficiency of Yin producing Heat, the above prescription is added with glossy privet fruit (Fructus Ligustri Lucidi) 12g, eclipta (Herba Ecliptae) 12g, dried rehmannia root (Radix Rehmanniae) 12g, moutan bark (Cortex Moutan Radicis) 9g, wolfberry fruit (Fructus Lycii) 15g, mulberry (Fructus Mori) 15g, dogwood fruit (Fructus Corni) 9g and tortoise plastron (Plastrum Testudinis) 15g. For the case with stagnation of Liver Qi, the above prescription is added with bupleurum root (Radix Bupleuri) 9g, cyperus tuber (Rhizoma

230

Cyperi) 9g, moutan bark (Cortex Moutan Radicis) 9g, curcuma root (Radix Curcumae) 9g and lindera root (Radix
Linderae) 9g. For the case with stagnation of Blood, the
above prescription is added with peach kernel (Semen Persicae) 9g, safflower (Flos Carthami) 9g, moutan bark (Cortex
Moutan Radicis) 9g, cyathula root (Radix Cyathulae) 12g,
Herba Lycopi 9g, motherwort (Herba Leonuri) 30g, dried
cat-tail pollen (Pollen Typhae) 9g, parched lucid ganoderma (Gaboderma Lucidium) 9g, corydalis tuber (Rhizoma
Corydalis) 9g, myrrh (Myrrha) 9g, burreed tuber (Rhizoma
Sparganii) 9g and zedoary (Rhizoma Zedoariae) 9g.

• *Female Sterility due to Stagnation of Liver Qi*

Main Symptoms and Signs: No pregnancy over a long period of time after marriage, and uncertainty of the delay or
advancement of menstrual cycles, pain in lumbar area during menstrual period, with menstruation in abnormal
amount, distending pain at sternocostal part or breast, mental depression, dysphoria and irritation, normal or dark red
tongue with slight white tongue coating and tense pulse.

Analysis of the Symptoms and Signs: Stagnation of Liver
Qi leads to unsmoothness of Blood circulation. This results
in abdominal pain during menstruation, and unsmoothness
of menstruation, distending pain at sternocostal part or
breasts. Also because of the stagnation of Liver Qi, mental
depression results, and if the depression becomes worse, the
patient will experience feelings of dysphoria, and irritability. Because of the irregularity of dispelling and resolving,
the delay and advancement of menstrual period is not fixed.
The dark red texture of the tongue, slight white tongue coating, and tense pulse are all the signs of the stagnation of
Liver Qi.

Treatment Principles: Soothing the Liver and regulating
the circulation of Qi to relieve the depression of the Liver;
restoring the Kidney to enrich Blood.

Prescription: Xin Kaiyu Zhongyu Tang (New Decoction
for Liver-Soothing and Pregnancy) (Prescription based on
the clinical experience of the author)

Bupleurum root (Radix Bupleuri) 9g, Chinese angelica
root (Radix Angelicae Sinensis) 9g, white peony root

(Radix Paeoniae Alba) 9g, Chuangxiong rhezome (Rhizoma Ligustici Chuangxiong) 6g, nutgrass faltsedge rhizoma (Rhizoma Cyperi) 9g, moutan bark (Cortex Moutan Radicis) tree 9g, wolfberry fruit (Fructus Lycii) 15g, dogwood fruit (Fructus Corni) 9g, dodder seed (Semen Cuscutae) 9g, desertliving cistanche (Herba Cistachi) 15g, epimedium (Herba Epimedii) 15g and amethyst (Fluorite) 30g. The above drugs are decocted in water for oral administration, one dose per day, and 6-9 doses successively after completion of the menstrual cycle.

Analysis of the Prescription: Bupleurum root (Radix Bupleuri) can soothe the Liver and relieve the stagnation of Liver Qi. Chinese angelica root (Radix Angelicae Sinensis) and white peony root (Radix Paeoniae Alba) enrich Blood and nourish the Liver, chuangxiong rhezome (Rhizoma Ligustici Chuangxiong) can activate the circulation of Blood and promote the flow of Qi. Nutgrass faltsedge rhizoma (Rhizoma Cyperi) can relieve the depressed Liver, soothe the Liver and regulate the flow of Qi. Moutan bark (Cortex Moutan Radicis) can remove Heat from Blood and activate the circulation of Blood. Wolfberry fruit (Fructus Lycii), dogwood fruit (Fructus Corni), dodder seed (Semen Cuscutae), desertliving cistanche (Herba Cistachi) can nourish the Kidney and the Liver, tonify and benefit Kidney Qi. Epimedium (Herba Epimedii), amethyst (Fluorite) can warm and restore Kidney Yang. The whole prescription relieves the depressed the Liver, soothes the Liver and regulates the flow of Qi, restores the Kidney, nourishes Blood and relieves Qi stagnation, pregnancy may be achieved.

Modifications of the Prescription: For the case with sternocostal distention and fullness, the following drugs are added to the above prescription: Green tangerine peel (Pericarpium Citri Reticulatae) 9g, Sichuan chinaberry (Fructus Meliae Toosendan) 9g, tangerine leaf (Folium Citri Reticulatae) 9g, tangerine seed (Semen Citri Reticulatae) 9g, vaccaria seed (Semen Vaccariae) 15g and sweetgum fruit (Fructus Liquidambaris) 15g. For the case having problem of stagnancy of Qi and Blood, the above prescription is added with safflower (Flos Carthami) 9g, peach kernel (Semen

232

Persicae) 9g, red sage root (Radix Salviae Miltiorrhizae) 30g, Herba Lycopi 9g, motherwort (Herba Leonuri) 30g and common fennel fruit (Fructus Foeniculi) 6g. For the case with clear symptom of Kidney Deficiency, the following drugs are added to the above prescription: Morinda root (Radix Morindae Officinalis) 9g, eucommia bark (Cortex Eucommiae) 9g, dipsacus root (Radix Dipsaci) 15g, curculigo rhizome (Rhizoma Curculiginis) 9g, prepared aconite root (Radix Aconiti) 6g and bark of Chinese cassia tree 6g.

• *Female Sterility due to Blood Stasis*

Main Symptoms and Signs: No pregnancy over a long period of time after marriage, less menstruation with purplish color and with blood clots during the later period of menstruation, abdominal pain and distending and pain with dragging feeling which is intolerant to pressing during menstruation, or usually, pain in lower abdominal, purplish black tongue or with ecchymosis and petechiae along the edge of the tongue with slight white tongue coating, stringy pulse or deep pulse.

Analysis of the Symptoms and Signs: Because Blood Stasis obstructs the Uterine Collaterals, during the later period of menstruation, the amount is less or there are abdominal pain, sensation of distention and fullness, intolerance to pressing. Because Blood Stasis comes out with menstruation, the color of it is purplish black, and there are blood clots. The black tongue with ecchymosis and petechiae, stringy choppy pulse are the symptoms of Blood Stasis.

Treatment Principles: Promoting the circulation of Blood to remove Blood Stasis; warming the channels to help pregnancy.

Prescription: Shaofu Zhuyu Tang (Decoction for Removing Blood Stasis in the Lower Abdomen, from *Corrections on the Errors of Medical Works*, *Yi Lin Gai Cuo*)

Common fennel fruit (Fructus Foeniculi) 6g, dried ginger (Rhizoma Zingiberis) 6g, corydalis tuber (Rhizoma Corydalis) 9g, myrrh (Myrrha) 9g, Chinese angelica root (Radix Angelicae Sinensis) 9g, chuangxiong rhezome (Rhizoma Ligustici Chuangxiong) 6g, cinnamon bark (Cortex Cinnamomi) 6g, red peony root (Radix Paeoniae Rubra) 9g,

233

cat-tail pollen (Pollen Typhae) 9g and trogopterus dung (Faeces Trogopterorum) 9g. The above drugs are decocted in water for oral administration, and 6-9 doses successively after completion of the menstrual cycle.

Analysis of the Prescription: Cinnamon bark (Cortex Cinnamomi), dried ginger (Rhizoma Zingiberis) and common fennel fruit (Fructus Foeniculi) warm the Uterine Collaterals and remove Cold Damp. Chinese angelica root (Radix Angelicae Sinensis) root, chuangxiong rhezome (Rhizoma Ligustici Chuangxiong) and red peony root (Radix Paeoniae Rubra) can nourish Blood, activate Blood circulation and remove Blood Stasis. Corydalis tuber (Rhizoma Corydalis), trogopterus dung (Faeces Trogopterorum), cat-tail pollen (Pollen Typhae) and myrrh (Myrrha) can remove Blood Stasis and pain. The whole prescription warms the Uterine Collaterals and removes Cold, activates the circulation of Blood and removes Blood Stasis and pain.

Modifications of the Prescription: For the case with sensation of cold and pain in lower abdomen, and amenia because of the accumulation of Cold and Blood Stasis, the above prescription is added with argyi leaf (Folium Artemisiae Argyi) 6g, donkey-hide gelatin (Colla Corii Asini) 11g, cyathula root (Radix Cyathulae) 12g, burreed tuber (Rhizoma Sparganii) 9g, zedoary (Rhizoma Zedoariae) 9g, dried hawthorn fruit (Fructus Crataegi) 30g, Herba Siphonoste 9g and chicken's gizzard-skin (Endothelium Corneum Gigeriae Galli) 9g. For the case with uteritis, annexitis, added are the following drugs to the above prescription: Honeysuckle flower (Flos Lonicerae) 24g, (Fructus Forysythiae) 12g, sargentgloryvine (Caulis Sargentodoxae) 30g, patrinia (Herba Patriniae) 30g, dandelion herb (Herba Taraxaci) 18g, diding (Herba Violae) 15g, prepared myrrh (Myrrha) 9g and phellodendron bark (Cortex Phellodendri) 9g. For the case whose oviduct is obstructed or unobstructed but not smooth, added are the following drugs, parched pangolin scales (Squama Manitis), thorns of Chinese honey locus (Spina Gleditsiae) 15g, burreed tuber (Rhizoma Sparganii) 9g, zedoary (Rhizoma Zedoariae) 9g, Japanese sea tangle (Thallus Laminariae) 9g, sargassum (Sargassum) 9g, red sage root (Radix Salviae Miltiorrhizae), peach kernel (Semen Persicae), prunella spike (Spica Prunellae) 9g, vaccaria seed (Semen Vaccariae) 15g, sweetgum fruit (Fructus Liquidambaris) 15g, Sichuan Chinaberry (Fructus Meliae Toosendan) 9g and stemona root (Radix Stemonae) 9g. For the case with Deficiency of Qi and Blood, added are the following drugs: Dangshen (Radix Codonopsis Pilosulae) 18g, astragalus root (Radix Astragali Seu Hedysari) 30g, white atractylodes rhizome (Rhizoma Atractylodis Macrocephalae) 9g, poria (Poria) 9g and prepared licorice (Radix Glycyrrhizae) 6g. For the case with stagnation of Liver Qi and Kidney Deficiency (ovulatory dysfunction), added are the drugs that can soothe the Liver and restore the Kidney (see the previous chapters)

• *Female Sterility due to Phlegm Damp*

Main Symptoms and Signs: No pregnancy over a long period, fat body, delayed or irregular menstruation, much amount of leukorrhea which is sticky, brightly white, dizziness and palpitation, oppression of chest, hyperdynamia, pale tongue with white greasy coating and slippery pulse.

Analysis of the Symptoms and Signs: Fat people usually have problems involving Phlegm, and the accumulation of Phlegm Damp disturbs functional activities of Qi, so Uterine Collaterals are blocked. As a result, the menstruation is delayed or irregular. Water retention due to hypofunction of the Spleen and downward flow of pathogenic Damp result in much amount of viscid leukorrhea. The inner repression of Phlegm Damp, disturbance in ascending and descending, Lucid Yang failing to rise, pale complexion, dizziness, palpitation, oppression of chest and asthenia occur. White greasy tongue coating, slippery pulse are symptoms of accumulation of Phlegm Damp.

Treatment Principles: Eliminating Damp to remove Phlegm; restoring the Kidney to regulate menstruation.

Prescription: Xin Qigong Wan Jiajian (Modified New Pill for Restoring the Function of Uterine, from the author's clinical experience)

Cyperus tuber (Rhizoma Cyperi) 9g, tangerine peel (Pericarpium Citri Reticulatae) 9g, poria (Poria) 9g, Chinese an-

235

gelica root (Radix Angelicae Sinensis) 9g, chuanxiong rhizome (Rhizoma Ligustici Chuanxiong) 6g, prepared pinellia tube (Rhizoma Pinelliae) 9g, grassleaved sweetflag rhizome (Rhizoma Acori Graminei) 9g, pangolin scales (Squama Manitis) 9g, thorn of Chinese honey locus (Spina Gleditsiae) 15g, prepared rehmannia root (Radix Rehmanniae Praeparata) 12g, dodder seed (Semen Cuscutae) 15g, zedoary (Rhizoma Zedoariae) 9g, epimedium (Herba Epimedii) 15g and curculigo rhizome (Rhizoma Curculiginis) 9g. The above drugs are decocted in water for oral administration, one dose per day, and 6-9 doses successively after the completion of the menstrual cycle.

Analysis of the Prescription: Prepared pinellia tube (Rhizoma Pinelliae), poria (Poria), tangerine peel (Pericarpium Citri Reticulatae) can remove Damp and Phlegm. Cyperus tuber (Rhizoma Cyperi), chuanxiong rhizome (Rhizoma Ligustici Chuanxiong) can regulate the flow of Qi to promote Blood circulation. Chinese angelica root (Radix Angelicae Sinensis) can nourish Blood and promote circulation of Blood. Grassleaved sweetflag rhizome (Rhizoma Acori Graminei) can eliminate Damp with aromatics. Pangolin scales (Squama Manitis), thorn of Chinese honey locus (Spina Gleditsiae), zedoary (Rhizoma Zedoariae) can soften hardness and remove Phlegm. Prepared rehmannia root (Radix Rehmanniae Praeparata) and dodder seed (Semen Cuscutae) can nourish and tonify the Liver and the Kidney. Epimedium (Herba Epimedii) and curculigo rhizome (Rhizoma Curculiginis) can warm and restore Kidney Yang. The whole prescription eliminates Damp and removes Phlegm, restores the Kidney and regulates menstruation.

Modifications of the Prescription: For the case with amenorrhea, added are the following drugs to the above prescription: Morinda root (Radix Morindae Officinalis) 9g, antler glue (Colla Cornus Cervi, parched) 9g, red peony root (Radix Paeoniae Rubra) 9g, red sage root (Radix Salviae Miltiorrhizae) 30g, peach kernel (Semen Persicae) 9g, dried hawthorn fruit (Fructus Crataegi) 30g, herba siphonoste 9g, chicken's gizzard-skin (Endothelium Corneum Gigeriae Galli) 9g and common fennel fruit (Fructus Foenicuii) 6g. For

236

the case with dizziness, oppression of chest, hypodynamia which becomes severe, added are the following drugs: Dang-shen (Radix Codonopsis Pilosulae) 18g, astragalus root (Radix Astragali Seu Hedysari) 18g, polygala root (Radix Polygalae) 9g, schisandra fruit (Fructus Schisandrae) 9g, fleece-flower root (Radix Polygoni Multiflori) 15g, wolfber-ry fruit (Fructus Lycii) 15g and bitter orange (Fructus Au-rantii) 9g.

Current Research
1. 215 patients with female sterility due to ovulatory dys-functional were treated with Shiying Yulin Tang (Decoction of Amethyst for Pregnancy). Among them, 141 got preg-nant, with a pregnancy rate of 65.6%. The effect had shown on 31 patients (14.4%). There were effects on 26 patients (12.1%). There were no effects on 17 patients (7.9%). The total effective rate was 92.1%. The prescription was special-ly designed to promote ovulation and restore the functions of corpus luteum. Therefore, besides treating female sterility, this prescription can also be used to treat various cases of de-layed or irregular menstruation, amenorrhea, dysfunctional uterine bleeding due to ovulatory dysfunction. The ingredi-ents of Quartz and Chinese Unicorn Decoction include amethyst (Fluorite) 15-30g, peppertree (Pericarpium Zan-thoxyli) 1.5g, chuanxiong rhizome (Rhizoma Ligustici Chuanxiong) 12-15g, epimedium (Herba Epimedii) 12-18g, dodder seed (Semen Cuscutae) 9g, wolfberry fruit (Fructus Lycii) 9g, cyperus tuber (Rhizoma Cyperi) 9g, Chinese an-gelica root (Radix Angelicae Sinensis) 12-15g, red peony root (Radix Paeoniae Rubra) 9g, white peony root (Radix Paeoniae Alba) 9g, cinnamon bark (Cortex Cinnamomi) 6g and moutan bark (Cortex Moutan Radicis) 9g. The drugs were decocted twice in water for oral use, one dose per day, and to be taken 2 times a day. For the case whose menstrual period was some 40-50 days, whose uterine growth was small, and whose Kidney Deficiency was not severe, the drug was taken according to the original prescription. Start to take the decoction from the 7th day of menstruation over 3 days, stopping for one day (to protect the Spleen and the

Stomach to achieve good appetite). Each month, 6-12 doses of the drug must be taken. Those whose menstrual cycle was 2-3 months long, and whose uterine was 2/3 of the common size, or accompanied by asexuality or whose colpocytological smear examination successively showed a slight influence (unable to reach mediate or high degree of effect), 45g of amethyst (Fluorite) was used with being decocted first; the amount of epimedium (Herba Epimedii) increased to 30g, one dose daily, successively over 3 days with an interval of one days, then stop for one day. Seeing that BBT increased over 3 days, stop taking the drug, and then continue to take the drug from the 7th day of menstruation. The treatment of the accompanying syndromes: For the case with stagnation of Liver Qi and Kidney Deficiency, accompanied by vexation, irritability, distending pain in breast, added were bupleurum root (Radix Bupleuri) 9g, capejasmine (Fructus Gardeniae) 9g; for the case with from Deficiency of Qi and hypodynamia, dangshen (Radix Codonopsis Pilosulae) 15-30g, astragalus root (Radix Astragali Seu Hedysari) 15-30g; for the case feeling the food is tale, amomum fruit (Fructus Amomi) 6g, tangerine peel (Pericarpium Citri Reticulatae) 9g; for the case with edema of face and feet, poria (Poria) 15g, plantain seed (Semen Plantaginis) (wrapped) 9g; for the case whose bilateral ovaries were bigger (including polycystic ovary syndrome), red sage root (Radix Salviae Miltiorrhizae) 30g, peach kernel (Semen Persicae) 9g, or burreed tuber (Rhizoma Sparganii) 9g, zedoary (Rhizoma Zedoariae) 9g; for the case with pain in lower abdomen, common fennel fruit (Fructus Foenicuii) 6g, argyi leaf (Folium Artemisiae Argyi) 6g. Among the patients who used this decoction, the longest period of medical administration was 12 months, and the shortest was one month. The largest number of dose taken was 200 doses, and the smallest number was 6 doses, averaged 14 doses monthly, and 48 doses individually (Li Guangwen, 1990).

The effect of Quartz and Chinese Unicorn Decoction in promoting ovulation and its influence on animal reproductive system: The test results of plasma LH and FSH levels showed that the decoction can markedly raise plasma LH,

FSH contents ($P<0.01$). FSH can stimulate the growth and development of the follicles in the ovary, and with the participation of little luteotropic hormone, it makes the growing follicles excrete estrogen. LH, together with FSH, makes the grown follicles ovulated. And after ovulation, yellow body of ovary is formed which excretes much amount of progestogen and little amount of estrogen. These two points are all consistent with what was observed: The ovary weight notably increased ($P<0.05$), and the contents of plasma dihydrotheelin, progesterone increased remarkably. The increase of dihydrotheelin and progesterone contents naturally promote the growth of the uterine. We also observed that Quartz and Chinese Unicorn Decoction can help the increase of the young rat's uterine weight ($P<0.05$). These hormones and the changes of the reproductive organs are all beneficial to the formation, growth, implantation and even pregnancy.

In isolated uterine experiment, we observed that when the decoction of the prescription was added to the bathing tank, the concentration was 3.69×10^{-2}, it could obviously restrict the uterine contraction caused by lobus posterior hypophyseos; and when the concentration was 7.35×10^2, it could restrict normal uterine contraction. In the isolated oviduct experiment, it could be observed that when the drug concentration reached 7.35×10^{-2}, it could obviously promote rhythmical contraction of the oviduct. Modern pharmaceutical research has proved that cyathula root, white peony root (Radix Paeoniae Alba) and cyperus tuber (Rhizoma Cyperi) can reduce the motion of the isolated uterine, lower the tensile force, and responds against the uterine contraction caused by hypophysin. The decoction of this prescription promotes rhythmical contraction of the oviduct, and is beneficial to the running and ovulation of the follicles in the oviduct. That uterine contraction is reduced is helpful to implantation of the fertilized ovum and pregnancy as well. This is consistent with the measured result of the plasma hormonal content.

In the body, TXB_2 mainly offers strong contraction, and at the same time, it is a strong inducer to promote clotting. 6-K-PGFI$_2$ is a product of metabolism of PGI$_2$ whose function is just opposite to that of TXB$_2$, having a strong function of widening blood vessels and anti-clotting. The result showed that plasma 6-K-PGFI$_2$ content obviously increased ($P < 0.01$), and there was a decline tendency in TXB$_2$ content, but it was not remarkable. This helps to improve the supply of blood to the tissues and organs, and in nourishing the related tissues of gonadal secretion axis. This is related to some ingredients in the prescription: Chuanxiong rhizome (Rhizoma Ligustici Chuanxiong), red sage root (Radix Salviae Miltiorrhizae), and red peony fruit (Radix Paeoniae Rubra) activate the circulation of Blood, remove stagnation, expand blood vessels, improve blood rheological condition. Also, the result is related to the function of its anti-clotting agent.

The experiment of edema hind feet of the animal caused by anti-carrageenin of Quartz and Chinese Unicorn Decoction showed that the effect of anti-inflammation of this prescription was weak, and was obviously weaker than 0.5% DXM Sodium phosphate injection and 0.5% hydrocor tisone ($P < 0.01$), but it was observed that the liquid of this prescription had obvious antagonism against twisting body caused by acetic acid injection ($P < 0.01$). Its pain-removing effect was non-specific. This may be related to the pain-removing effect, and spasmolysis of white peony root (Radix Paeoniae Alba), cyperus tuber (Rhizoma Cyperi).

The acute toxic experiment of this prescription showed that this prescription has little toxicity. 40ml/kg was given to the young rat through enema (equivalent to herbal drug 120g/kg). There was no acute toxic response. According to this, it can be worked out that if a grown-up orally takes 6000ml of this liquid, there will not be acute toxic response. Subacute toxic experiments showed that after this drug was taken successively for 45 days, there are no degeneration, hyperemia, necrosis, edema and inflammatory cellular infiltration in the cells of such organs as the heart, the liver, follicles, uterine, etc. The results of teratogenesis experiment was also negative (Wang Shurong, 1990).

240

2. A clinical report of 257 sterile cases treated according to the basic theories of Treatment Based on Syndrome Differentiation. After the treatment, 257 patients all were cured and became pregnant. Among them, the curative time of 127 patients was shorter than 3 months; that of 76 patients was 4-6 months; that of 37 patients was 7-12 months, and that of 17 patients was longer than one year. The follow-up study of the 257 pregnant patients showed that 17 of them underwent miscarriage, who got pregnant again later and the babies grew well after their births. After the treatment, among 61 pregnant patients, whose oviduct was not unobstructed at first and became unobstructive later, only one of them underwent extrauterine pregnancy, and all the others underwent normal pregnancy. Treatment based on Syndrome Differentiation: ① 71 cases (27.63%) are differentiated as Syndrome of Kidney Deficiency. This type can often be found in patients with endocrine imbalance and hypoplasia of uterus. The treatment should restore the Kidney, warm Yang and regulate menstruation. Yulin Zhu (Chinese Unicorn Pill), Fugui Dihuang Wan (Bolus of Aconite, Cinnamon, and Rehmannia), Wuzi Yanzhong Wan (Bolus of Five Seed Drugs for Pregnancy), Quanlu Wan (Deer Bolus), Guiling Ji (Longevity Powder), etc. were used. The drugs include aconite root (Radix Aconiti), cinnamon bark (Cortex Cinnamomi), rehmannia root (Radix Rehmanniae), white peony root (Radix Paeoniae Alba), dogwood fruit (Fructus Corni), morinda root (Radix Morindae Officinalis), epimedium (Herba Epimedii), fleece-flower root (Radix Polygoni Multiflori), Chinese yam (Rhizoma Dioscoreae), eucommia bark (Cortex Eucommiae), etc. ② 33 cases (12. 84%) are differentiated as Syndrome of Deficiency of both the Spleen and the Kidney. This type is often seen in patients with endocrine imbalance and hypoplasia of uterus. The treatment principle is invigorating the Spleen and restoring the Kidney, tonifying Qi and regulating menstruation. The prescription should be Neibu Wan (Bolus for Internal Tonification) with Shenling Baizhu Wan (Bolus of Dangshen (Radix Codonopsis Pilosulae), Poria (Poria) and White Atractylodes) or with Guipi Wan Jiajian (Modified

241

Spleen-Tonifying Bolus). The drugs used usually are dang-shen (Radix Codonopsis Pilosulae), astragalus root (Radix Astragali Seu Hedysari), white atractylodes rhizome (Rhizoma Atractylodis Macrocephalae), poria (Poria), Chinese yam (Rhizoma Dioscoreae), prepared rehmannia root (Radix Rehmanniae Praeparata), flatstem milkvetch puncturevine, desertliving cistanche (Herba Cistachis), dodder seed (Semen Cuscutae), arborvitae seed, glossy privet fruit (Fructus Ligustri Lucidi), etc. ③ 30 (11.67%) are Syndrome of Deficiency of both the Liver and the Kidney. This type is often seen in patients with irregular menstruation, pelvic inflammation, polycystic ovary syndrome. The principles for the treatment should be nourishing the Liver and restoring the Kidney and regulating the Chong and Ren channels. The prescriptions can be Liuwei Dihuang Wan (Bolus of Six Ingredients Including Rehmannia), Da Bu Yin Wan (Yin-Tonifying Bolus), Tiao Gan Tang (Decoction for Regulating the Liver Functions), etc. The used commonly drugs are dried rehmannia root, prepared rehmannia root (Radix Rehmanniae Praeparata), dogwood fruit (Fructus Corni), moutan bark (Cortex Moutan Radicis), poria (Poria), Chinese yam (Rhizoma Dioscoreae), wind-weed rhizome (Rhizoma Anemarrhenae), tortoise plastron (Plastrum Testudinis), etc. ④ 13 (5.06%) belong Syndrome of Yin Deficiency producing Interior Heat. This type is often seen in patients with irregular menstruation, polycystic ovary syndrome. The principle for the treatment should be nourishing Yin and clearing Heat and regulating menstruation. The prescriptions can be Zhibo Dihuang Wan (Bolus of Anemarrhena, Phellodendron, and Rehmannia), Digupi Yinzi (Powder of Wolfberry bark (Cortex Lycii Radicis), Liangdi Tang (Decoction of Rehmannia). The drugs usually used are wind-weed rhizome (Rhizoma Anemarrhenae), phellodendron bark (Cortex Phellodendri), dried rehmannia root (Radix Rehmanniae Praeparata), dogwood fruit (Fructus Corni), the root bark of the peony tree (Cortex Radix Paeoniae), wolfberry bark (Cortex Lycii Radicis), Chinese yam (Rhizoma Dioscoreae), etc. ⑤ 19 (7.39%) are differentiated as Syndrome of stagnation of Liver Qi. This type is often

242

found in patients having problems of irregular menstruation, endometriosis, polycystic ovary syndrome, obstruction in oviduct. The principle of the treatment should be soothing the Liver to remove stagnation, nourishing blood to regulate menstrua tion. The prescriptions can be Kaiyu Zhongyu Tang (Decoction for Stagnation Removal and Pregnancy), Si Zhi Xiangfu Wan (Bolus of Lance Asiabell Root and A-conite Root), Jisheng Juhe Wan (Life Preserving Bolus of Semen Citri Reticulatae). The common drugs are Chinese angelica root (Radix Angelicae Sinensis), bupleurum root (Radix Bupleuri), cyperus tuber (Rhizoma Cyperi), white atractylodes rhizome (Rhizoma Atractylodis Macrocephalae), moutan bark (Cortex Moutan Radicis), poria (Poria), white peony root (Radix Paeoniae Alba), tangerine leaf (Folium Citri Reticulatae), tangerine seed (Seman Citri Reticulatae), etc. ⑥ 76 patients (29.57%) are Syndrome of Blood Stasis. This type is often found in patients with endometriosis, obstruction of oviduct. The treatment principles of the treatment should be activating the circulation of Blood to remove Blood Stasis and regulating the flow of Qi to alleviate pain. The prescriptions can be Shaofu Zhuyu Tang (Decoction for Removing Blood Stasis in the Lower Abdomen), Dahuang Zhechong Wan (Rhubarb and Betel Nut Bolus), Guizhi Fuling Wan (Cinnamom Twig and Poria (Poria) Bolus), etc. The drugs usually used include Chinese angelica root (Radix Angelicae Sinensis), chuanxiong rhizome (Rhizoma Ligustici Chuanxiong), safflower (Flos Carthami), peach kernel (Semen Persicae), burreed tuber (Rhizoma Sparganii), zedoary (Rhizoma Zedoariae), moutan bark (Cortex Moutan Radicis), red peony root (Radix Paeoniae Rubra), betel nut, etc. ⑦ 8 patients (3.11%) are Syndrome of Phlegm Damp. This type is often found in patients with endocrine unbalance, irregular menstruation, small uterus. The principles of the treatment should be removing Phlegm Damp, invigorating the Spleen and regulating menstruation. The prescriptions can be Qigong Wan (Bolus for Pregnancy), Cangfu Daotan Wan (Bolus of Atractylodes and Aconite for Removing Phlegm), Mengshen Guntan Wan (Bolus of Chlorite— schist for Expelling Phlegm). The drugs

243

used commonly include atractylodes rhizome (Rhizoma A-tractylodis), bighead atractylodes rhizome (Rhizoma A-tractylodis Macrocephalae), tangerine peel (Pericarpium Citri Reticulatae), pinellia tuber (Rhizoma Pinelliae), poria (Poria), arisaema tuber (Rhizoma Arisaematis), bitter orange (Fructus Aurantii), grassleaved sweetflag rhizome (Rhizoma Acori Graminei), curcuma root (Radix Curcumae), chlorite-schist (Lapis Chloriti), etc. ⑧ 7 patients (2. 73%) had problem of accumulation of Cold Damp. This type is often seen in patients with irregular menstruation, poor endocrine function, small uterus. The principles of the treatment should be warming the channels to expel pathogenic Cold, warming the uterus to help pregnancy. The prescriptions can be Wen Jin Tang (Decoction for Warming the Channels), Danggui Sini Tang (Decoction of Chinese Angelica root (Radix Angelicae Sinensis) for Resuscitation), Xianggui Wan (Cyperus and Cinnamon Bolus), Aifu Nuangong Wan (Bolus of Argyi leaf (Folium Artemisiae Argyi) and Aconite for Warming the Uterus), Fuzi Lizhong Tang (Decoction of Aconite for Regulating the Functions of the Middle Jiao), etc. The drugs used commonly are Chinese angelica root (Radix Angelicae Sinensis), aconite root (Radix Aconiti), dangshen (Radix Codonopsis Pilosulae), dried ginger (Rhizoma Zingiberis), cinnamon bark (Cortex Cinnamomi), amethyst (Fluorite), evodia fruit (Fructus Evodiae), cyperus tuber (Rhizoma Cyperi), cnidium fruit (Fructus Cnidii), etc.

The treatment by artificial cyclic therapy in TCM was carried out based on menstrual cycle, and generally, the treatment was conducted by three stages: ① Postmenstruation (i. e., after completion of the menstrual cycle). For example, for the case with Kidney Deficiency, then, warming Yang and restoring the Kidney were needed. For the case with Deficiency of the Liver and the Kidney, then, nourishing and tonifying the Liver and the Kidney were needed. The medical administration period was about 10 days. ② Ovulatory period. On the basis of medical administration during postmenstruation, added were such drugs that warm Yang and activate the circulation of Blood, usually, as epimedium

244

(Herba Epimedii), morinda root (Radix Morindae Officinalis), desertliving cistanche (Herba Cistachi), cuttle-bone (Os Sepiella seu Sepiae), dried madder root (Radix Rubiae), red sage root (Radix Salviae Miltiorrhizae), Herba Lycopi, Alismaceae (Rhizoma Alismatis), etc. For the case with severe Yang Deficiency, added were aconite root (Radix Aconiti), cinnamon bark (Cortex Cinnamomi) in order to activate follicle function, and to promote ovulation. The drug was taken for 5 days. ③ Premenstruation and menstrual period. The treatment of premenstruation was based on postmenstruation medical ad ministration. Added were such drugs that can activate the circulation of Blood and regulate menstruation as Chinese angelica root (Radix Angelicae Sinensis), chuangxiong rhezome (Rhizoma Ligustici Chuangxiong), red sage root (Radix Salviae Miltiorrhizae), red peony root (Radix Paeoniae Rubra), and spatholobus stem (Caulis Spatholobi), etc. During menstrual period, based on the premenstrual treatment, according to individual symptoms and signs, the drugs were modified.

61 patients (23.7%) with oviduct obstruction were statistically collected in this article. To these patients, treatment by drugs of eliminating Blood Stasis was taken as the main factor. The drugs used commonly are burreed tuber (Rhizoma Sparganii), zedoary (Rhizoma Zedoariae), sappan wood (Lignum Sappan), earthworm (Lumbricus), ground beetle (Eupolyphagaseu Steleophaga), leech (Hirudo), centipede (Scolopendra), pangolin scales (Squama Manitis), etc. During the treatment, three combinations should be observed: ① Treatment in combination with Heat-clearing and Toxins-removing. If oviduct obstruction was caused by inflammation, then, besides drugs of eliminating Blood Stasis, Heat-clearing and toxic-removing drugs were added. Usually, used were sargentgloryvine (Caulis Sargentodoxae), patrinia (Herba Patriniae), dandelion herb (Herba Taraxaci), barbat skullcap (Herba Scutellariae Barbatae), phellodendron bark (Cortex Phellodendri), etc. If oviduct obstruction was caused by tuberculosis, scutellaria root (Radix Scutellariae), stemona root (Radix Stemonae), balanophyl lia, leather leaf mahonia (Caulis Mahoniae), etc.

245

② Treatment in combination with hardness-softening and Blood Stasis-removing. Mass-softening drugs can make the connective tissues soft, and adhesive tissues disappear, and oviduct unobstructed. The drugs commonly used for hardness-softening are Sichuan fritillary bulb (Bulbus Fritillariae Cirrhosae), airpotato yam (Rhizoma Dioscoreae Bulbiferae), oyster shell (Concha Ostreae), prunella spike (Spica Prunellae), fritillary bulb (Bulbus Fritillariae), sargassum (Sargassum), sea-tangle (Thallus laminariae seu Eckloniae), etc. ③ Treatment in cimbination with Blood Stasis-removing and Vital Qi-tonifying. Because drugs that remove Blood Stasis can damage Vital Qi, so after these drugs were used for 2 months, the following drugs that tonify Qi and Blood should be added: Dangshen (Radix Codonopsis Pilosulae), astragalus root (Radix Astragali Seu Hedysari), white atractylodes rhizome (Rhizoma Atractylodis Macrocephalae), white hyacinth bean (Semen Dolichoris Album), Chinese yam (Rhizoma Dioscoreae), siberian solomonseal rhizome (Rhizoma Polygonati), etc. (Li Xiangyun, 1987).

3. A clinical observation of Uterus-Nourishing Tablet used to treat 211 patients with functional primary female sterility and irregular menstruation. Of 211 patients, 122 suffered from female sterility, and 89 suffered from irregular menstruation. After the treatment, in the sterile group, 109 patients had ovulation, with an ovulatory rate of 89.3%; 89 got pregnant, with a pregnancy rate of 73%. In the irregular menstruation group, 74 had ovulation, with an ovulatory rate of 83.1%; 54 got recovered, and 23 got improved, with an effective rate of 86.5%. The ingredients of Uterus-Nourishing Tablet include prepared rehmannia root (Radix Rehmanniae), dodder seed (Semen Cuscutae), eucommia bark (Cortex Eucommiae), wolfberry fruit (Fructus Lycii), tortoise-plastron glue (Colla Plastri Testudinis), dangshen (Radix Codonopsis Pilosulae) rhizome, white atractylodes rhizome (Rhizoma Atractylodis Macrocephalae), white peony root (Radix Paeoniae Alba), cyperus tuber (Rhizoma Cyperi), peppertree (Pericarpium Zanthoxyli), etc. Processing method: According to the proportions of each drug in the prescription, the drugs were decocted twice, and the

colature was nebulized, then the drugs were baked and ground into powder and made into tablets with 0.5g of each one. Administration: 3 times a day, and 4-6 tablets each time, and one month making up one course of treatment, and stop taking it during menstruation. Among this 122 patients with primary female sterility, after the treatment, the quickest effect was seen during one course of treatment, and the slowest effect was observed 16 courses of treatment later. The patients who had 3-7 courses of treatment, with an average 5.31 courses of treatment; and to the 89 pregnant patients, they had an averaged 4.49 courses of treatment. No side effects had been found after the treatment.

Uterus-Nourishing Tablet originates from Chinese Unicorn Pill, flavored, from *Complete Works of Zhang Jingyue (Jing Yue Quan Shu)*. In the prescription, prepared rehmannia root (Radix Rehmanniae), dodder seed (Semen Cuscutae), eucommia bark (Cortex Eucommiae), wolfberry fruit (Fructus Lycii), etc. can nourish and tonify the Liver, the Kidney, the Vital Essence, and blood. Tortoise-plastron glue (Colla Plastri Testudinis) is closely related to blood and flesh, can replenish the Vital Essence of the Kidney to activate the Chong and Ren Channels; Dangshen (Radix Codonopsis Pilosulae), white atractylodes rhizome (Rhizoma Atractylodis Macrocephalae), etc. can reinforce the Spleen to benefit Qi. White peony root (Radix Paeoniae Alba) regulates the Liver and benefits Blood. Sichuan peppertree (Pericarpium Zanthoxyli) warms the Du Channel to warm uterus. The drugs used in combination warm the Kidney and strengthen the functions of the Spleen, nourish Blood and regulate menstruation. Kidney Qi is strong, Vital Essence and Blood are profuse, and the Chong and Ren Channels are unobstructed, and menstruation is well regulated.

The experiment study of Uterus-Nourishing Tablet: ① The study of the influence of Uterus-Nourishing Tablet on the uterus weight of the young rat showed that the uterus weight of the administered rats was notably bigger than that of the rats in control group ($P < 0.05$). This suggests that Uterus-Nourishing Tablet has the same functions as estrogen. ② The study of the influence of Uterus-Nourishing Tablet on delayed hypersensitivity of the skin reaction caused by 2, 4-dinitrochlorobenzene showed that Uterus-Nourishing Tablet had remarkable effect in restricting the delayed hypersensitive skin reaction of the rat caused by DNCB, which suggests that Uterus-Nourishing Tablet has distinct effect in restricting cellular immunity. ③ The study of the effect of the drug in the formation of hymolysin antibody caused by SRBC showed that Uterus-Nourishing Tablet can inhibit the formation of the specific antibody caused by SRBC immunity. ④ The spectrophotometry study of the effect of the drug on hemolysis caused by splenocyte showed that Uterus-Nourishing Tablet 5g/kg notably inhibits the formation of hemolysin. ⑤ The study of the effect of the drug on macrophagocytes phagocytic function in reticuloendothelial system (RES) showed that Uterus-Nourishing Tablet restrains their phagocytic function. ⑥ The study of the effect of the drug on rat antitiredness test. The study of the effect of the drug on the young rat given prednisone showed that after being given Uterus-Nourishing Tablet, the swimming time was longer than that of the ones given prednisone and salt liquid ($P<0.05$). The effect of the drug in the young rat given thyroxin tablet showed that after being given Uterus-Nourishing Tablet, the swimming time of the young rat was obviously prolonged ($P>0.02$) (Yang Wenlai, et al, 1990).

4. The treatment experimental analysis of 110 with female sterility. After gynecological examination, 59 patients were found to have organic diseases, including oophoritic cyst, polycystic ovary syndrome, endometriosis, hysteromyoma, uterus malformation and obstructed oviduct, etc. 59 patients were found to have no organic diseases, including the patients with ovulatory dysfunction, incomplete functions of yellow body of ovary, abnormal immune function, etc. One menstrual cycle was considered to be one course of treatment. The period from administration to pregnancy was at least one course of treatment, and the longest was 24 courses of treatment. Those having organic diseases needed averagedly 6.75 courses of treatment, (Among this, those with complete oviduct obstruction needed 8.38 courses of treatment). 8.38 courses of treatment were the averaged course of treatment of the patients with Kidney Deficiency. The pa-

tients with stagnation of Liver Qi needed averagedly 5. 65 courses of treatment, and the patients with Blood Stasis needed averagedly 7. 41 courses of treatment. Methods of treatment: Nourishing the Kidney. Prescription No. I for Pregnancy and Prescription No. II for Pregnancy were the essential prescriptions (See the detail at the end of this chapter). Starting the treatment when one menstrual period was over, the patients took 7 doses of Prescription No. I for Pregnancy, during the middle stage (ovulatory period), 8 doses of Prescription No. II for Pregnancy will be given. During menstruation, the patients were treated according to symptoms and signs: For the case with Deficiency of Kidney Yin, added were the following drugs to the above two prescriptions: Ophiopogon root (Radix Ophiopogonis), tortoise plastron (Plastrum Testudinis) and wolfberry fruit (Fructus Lycii), etc. ; for the case with Deficiency of Kidney Yang, such drugs as one sees fit as cinnamon bark (Cortex Cinnamomi), aconite root (Radix Aconiti), Wuji Baifeng Wan (White Phoenix Bolus of Black-bone Chicken), and Heche Dazao Wan (Bolus of Placenta for Nourishment), etc. For the case having problem of stagnation of Liver Qi, the first method discussed above can be used and according to illness condition, the drugs that warm Yang were reduced, and added were bupleurum root (Radix Bupleuri), white peony root (Radix Paeoniae Alba), cyperus tuber (Rhizoma Cyperi), Sichuan Chinaberry (Fructus Meliae Toosendan), Xiaoyao Wan (Ease Pill), Sizhi Xiangfu Wan (Bolus of Lance Asiabell and Cyperus tuber (Rhizoma Cyperi), which soothe the Liver and regulate the flow of Qi. For the case with accumulation of Phlegm Damp, Cangsha Daotan Wan Jiajian (Modified Phlegm-Removing Bolus of Atractylodes and Seabuckthorn) can be applied; or the above method could be used, but taking away Siberian solomonseal rhizome (Rhizoma Polygonati), prepared rehmannia root (Radix Rehmanniae) greasy and sticky in nature, and added were grassleaved sweetflag rhizome (Rhizoma Acori Graminei), white mustard seed (Semen Sinapis Albae), prepared arisaema tuber (Rhizoma Arisaematis), prepared pinellia tuber (Rhizoma Pinelliae), atractylodes rhizome (Rhizoma Atractylodis Macrocephalae), white atractylodes rhizome (Rhizoma Atractylodis Macrocephalae), sargassum (Sargassum), prunella spike (Spica Prunellae) and Zhimi Fuling Wan (Regulating Bolus of Poria (Poria) to dry Damp and remove Phlegm. For the case of accumulation of Cold Damp, the above method could be used except the following drugs such as Dried rehmannia root (Radix Rehmanniae), glossy privet fruit (Fructus Ligustri Lucidi), etc., and added were atractylodes rhizome (Rhizoma Atractylodis Macrocepha lae), argyi leaf (Folium Artemisiae Argyi), evodia fruit (Fructus Evodiae), Aifu Nuangong Wan (Uterus-Warming Bolus of Argyi leaf (Folium Artemisiae Argyi) and Aconite root (Radix Aconiti). For the case with slight accumulation of Damp Heat, the previous method could be used and the following drugs were taken away: Prepared rehmannia root (Radix Rehmanniae), siberian solomonseal rhizome (Rhizoma Polygonati), added were such drugs that can clear Heat and remove Damp as patrinia (Herba Patriniae), sargentgloryvine (Caulis Sargentodoxae), dayflower (Herba Commelinae); and for the case with accumulation of Damp Heat used was the prescription of removing Damp Heat in the Lower Jiao to cool Blood and eliminate Blood Stasis. After the patients became better, or the symptoms disappeared, Prescription No. I for Pregnancy and Prescription No. II for Pregnancy were used with modification. For the case with stagnation of menstrual blood, three prescriptions were specially designed: Prescription No. I for Endometriosis, Prescription No. II for Endometriosis, and Prescription No. III for Endometriosis. This is because that when menstrual blood stagnates, it turns to blood clots, which causes problems to the patients. This belongs to endometriosis in western medicine. Prescription No. I was used for the cases with dysmenorrhea, and Prescription No. II was used to the ones with profuse menstruation, and one of the two was selected according to different Syndromes, and 7 doses were taken 3 days before menstruation according to Syndromes Defferentiation, and 10 doses of No. III were taken successively to eliminate Blood Stasis and to remove blood clots. After the patient got slightly recovered, according to the

250

needs, selected was one of Prescription No. I for Pregnancy and Prescription No. II for Pregnancy to nourish the Kidney and regulate the functions of the Kidney. For the case with tuberculosis in inner reproductive system, after the completion of menstrual cycle, 10 doses of Kanglao Wan (Anti-tuberculosis Bolus) were taken, and then the patient was diagnosed and treated by according to Syndrome Differentiation. If the patients were found to have restrained and critical pain usually in the lower abdomen with polychromatic yellow and ill smell, and to have problem of thickened adnexa, or of obstructed oviduct or incomplete obstructed oviduct, or of hydrops after tubal patent test, prescription for clearing and activating the collaterals (See the appendix later) can be used with other various prescriptions to ease Uterine Collaterals; however, the prescriptions should not be used during the later stage of menstruation. Of 110 cases recorded in the article, 59 patients (53.64%) were found to suffer from various organic diseases in the reproductive system to the varying degree. This is objective counterevidence to some people who hold that TCM can only treat functional female sterility. However, it is indeed difficult to treat the patients with female sterility with organic diseases. The curative duation was in average two courses of treatment longer than those with no organic diseases. For the case with oviduct obstruction, the curative duation was even longer.

Attached Prescriptions are shown as follows:

① Prescription No. I for Pregnancy: Yunnan poria (Poria) 12g, dried rehmannia root (Radix Rehmanniae) 9g, prepared rehmannia root (Radix Rehmanniae) 9g, Huai achyranthes root (Radix Achyranthis Bidentatae) 9g, sweetgum fruit (Fructus Liquidambaris) 9g, stir-baked tortoise-shell (Concha Testudinis) 9g, cloves (Flos Caryophylli) 2.5g, epimedium (Herba Epimedii) 12g, photinia leaf (Folium Photiniae) 9g, prepared siberian solomonseal rhizome (Rhizoma Polygonati) 12g and cinnamom twig (Ramulus Cinnamomi) 2.5g.

② Prescription No. II for Pregnancy: Yunnan poria (Poria) 12g, dried rehmannia root (Radix Rehmanniae) 9g, prepared rehmannia root (Radix Rehmanniae) 9g, photinia leaf

(Folium Photiniae) 9g, amethyst (Fluorite) 12g, prepared glossy privet (Fructus Ligustri Lucidi) 9g, cibot rhizome (Rhizoma Cibotii) 12g, desertliving cistanche (Herba Cistachi) 9g, curculigo rhizome (Rhizoma Curculiginis) 9g, deglued antler powder (Cornu Cervi Degelation) 9g and epimedium (Herba Epimedii) 12g.

③ Prescription for Clearing Heat and Drying Damp: Yunnan poria (Poria) 12g, cinnamon twig (Ramulus Cinnamomi) 2.5g, bupleurum root (Radix Bupleuri) top 4.5g, red peony root (Radix Paeoniae Rubra) 9g, patrinia (Herba Patriniae) 20g, moutan bark (Cortex Moutan Radicis) 9g, dayflower (Herba Commelinae) 20g, Sichuan Chinaberry (Fructus Meliae Toosendan) 9g, sargentgloryvine (Caulis Sargentodoxae) 15g, corydalis tuber (Rhizoma Corydalis) 9g and Huai achyranthes root (Radix Achyranthis Bidentatae) 9g.

④ Prescription No. I for Endometriosis: Baked Chinese angelica root (Radix Angelicae Sinensis) 9g, red sage root (Radix Salviae Miltiorrhizae) 12g, chuangxiong rhezome (Rhizoma Ligustici Chuangxiong) 4.5g, cyathula root (Radix Cyathulae) 9g, prepared cyperus tuber (Rhizoma Cyperi) 9g, corydalis tuber (Rhizoma Corydalis) 9g, red peony root (Radix Paeoniae Rubra) 9g, dragon's blood (Resina Draconis) 3g, prepared myrrh (Myrrha) 6g, sappan wood (Lignum Sappan) 9g and Shixiao San (Wonderful Powder for Relieving Blood Stagnation) (wrapped).

⑤ Prescription No. II for Endometriosis: Stirred Chinese angelica root (Radix Angelicae Sinensis) 9g, red sage root (Radix Salviae Miltiorrhizae) 6g, red peony root (Radix Paeoniae Rubra) 9g, white peony root (Radix Paeoniae Alba) 9g, dried cat-tail pollen (Pollen Typhae) 30g (wrapped), ophicalcite (Ophicalcitum) 15g, dragon's blood (Resina Draconis) 3g, notoginseng (Radix Ginseng) powder 1.5g (infused), Huai achyranthes root (Radix Achyranthis Bidentatae) 9g, prepared cyperus tuber (Rhizoma Cyperi) 9g, Zhenling Dan (Pill for Tranquilizing the Mind and Relieving Palpitation) 12g (wrapped).

⑥ Prescription No. III for Endometriosis: Fried Chinese angelica root (Radix Angelicae Sinensis) 9g, red sage root

252

(Radix Salviae Miltiorrhizae) 12g, prepared cyperus tuber (Rhizoma Cyperi) 9g, mashed peach kernel (Semen Persicae) 9g, cyathula root (Radix Cyathulae) 9g, cinnamom twig (Ramulus Cinnamomi) 2.5g, dried lacquer (Rhus Verniciflua Strokes) 4.5g, dragon's blood (Resina Draconis) 3g, zedoary (Rhizoma Zedoariae) 12g, thorn of Chinese honey locus (Spina Gleditsiae) 12g, vaccaria seed (Semen Vaccariae) 9g, stir-baked tortoise-shell (Concha Testudinis) 9g, Chinese honey locust spine (spina Gleditsiae) 12g and ground beetle (Eupolyphage Sinensis 9g.

⑦ Prescription for Anti-tuberculosis: Red sage root (Radix Salviae Miltiorrhizae) 12g, stemona root (Radix Stemonae) 12g, vaccaria seed (Semen Vaccariae) 9g, shanhailuo (Rhizoma Codonopsis Lanceolata) 15g, houttuynia (Herba Houttuyniae) 12g, mahonia stem (Caulis Mahoniae) 15g, prunella spike (Spica Prunellae) 12g, thorn of Chinese honey locus (Spina Gleditsiae) 12g, achyranthes root (Radix Achyranthis Bidentatae) 9g, big dried rehmannia root (Radix Rehmanniae) 9g and sweetgum fruit (Fructus Liquidambaris) 9g.

⑧ Prescription for Clearing Obstruction from and Invigorating the Collaterals: Thorn of Chinese honey locus (Spina Gleditsiae) 15g, vaccaria seed (Semen Vaccariae) 9g, Chinese rose (Flos Rosae Chinensis) 4.5g, earthworm (Lumbricus) 6g, Diding (Herba Violae) 6g and slices of dalbergia wood (Lignum Dalbergiae Odoriferae) 4.5g (Cai Xiaosun, 1985).

5. An observation of 95 patients with various ovulatory dysfunctions treated with Cu Pailuan Tang (Decoction for Promoting Ovulation). The report says that better results had been obtained through the use of Cu Pailuan Tang (Decoction for Promoting Ovulation) consisting of Kidney-restoring prescription and prescription for promoting the circulation of Blood and strengthening the functions of the Kidney. The drugs of the prescriptions were modified according to different Syndromes. Of 95 patients, 35 suffered from polycystic ovary syndrome, 19 suffered from anovulatory dysfunctional uterine bleeding, 23 suffered from secondary amenorrhea, 3 had problem of oligo-ovulation, 4 had prob-

lem of anovulatory amenorrhea, and 11 suffered from insufficient function of the yellow-body of ovary. The prescription consisted of Prescription for Restoring the Kidney and Prescription for Activating Blood Flow and Invigorating the Kidney. Prescription for Restoring the Kidney which is comprised of prepared rehmannia root (Radix Rehmanniae), fleece-flower root (Radix Polygoni Multiflori), dodder seed (Semen Cuscutae), desertliving cistanche (Herba Cistachi), curculigo rhizome (Rhizoma Curculiginis), epimedium (Herba Epimedii), glossy privet fruit (Fructus Ligustri Lucidi), eclipta (Herba Ecliptae), wolfberry fruit (Fructus Lycii), Chinese angelica root (Radix Angelicae Sinensis), dipsacus root (Radix Dipsaci), 9g respectively; Chinese yam (Rhizoma Dioscoreae) 15g and donkey-hide (Corium Asini) 12g. After the completion of menstrual cycle, the drugs are taken for 7-10 days, one dose daily. The patient was then observed for 2-3 weeks, after which, continued to take the drug according to the method explained previously. Prescription for Activating Blood Flow and Invigorating the Kidney including Bupleurum root (Radix Bupleuri), red peony root (Radix Paeoniae Rubra), white peony root (Radix Paeoniae Alba), alismaceae (Rhizoma Alismatis), motherwort (Herba Leonuri), Herba Siphonoste, dried cat-tail pollen (Pollen Typhae), achyranthes root (Radix Achyranthis Bidentatae), dodder seed (Semen Cuscutae), wolfberry fruit (Fructus Lycii), curculigo rhizome (Rhizoma Curculiginis), epimedium (Herba Epimedii), 9g respectively; spatholobus stem (Caulis Spatholobi), glossy privet fruit (Fructus Ligustri Lucidi), raspberry (Fructus Rubi), 15g respectively. For the case having no regular menstrual cycle, three doses were taken with an interval of 7 days, and 9 doses monthly. For the case having menstruation, three doses were taken during menstruation, and another three doses on 11th to 13th day after the completion of menstrual cycle, and six doses per month. The effect of the treatment was evaluated according to menstrual cycle. There are 133 cycles in which the prescription for restoring the Kidney was solely used. Those getting pregnant needed eight cycles, and those having gained effects needed 51 cycles, and one cycle brought effect. The effective rate was 44.3%. There are 61 cycles in which prescription for promoting the circulation of Blood and restoring the Kidney; those becoming pregnant took 8 cycles; those having gained effect needed 33 cycles. One cycle brought effect. The effective rate was 67.2%. It can be seen that the latter prescription is superior to the former with obvious differences ($P < 0.01$) (Zhao Songquan, 1985).

Chapter Six
Treatment of
Common Diseases

Endometriosis

Endometriosis is one of the main causes of sterility. Statistically, 25-50% of infertile patients suffer from endometriosis. Because the ectopic endometrium is affected periodically by ovary hormones, and thus periodical changes result to it with manifestations of degeneration, necrosis, bleeding, thus typical ectopic focus is formed. The ectopic endometrium pathologic change can cause tubal obstruction. Great amount of prostaglandin (PG) is produced in tuberal part of the focus, which makes the contents of $PGF_{2\alpha}$ and PGE_2 in abdominal cavity increase. This directly affects the normal peristalsis, and the normal running state of the ova is affected. The great amount of prostaglandin also causes uterine abnormal contraction and incomplete ovary function. Endometriosis can lead to the increase of serum prolactin which inhibits pituitary gonadotropic hormones, and thus the function of ovary is affected, which leads to functional ovulatory obstruction or LUFS, to the increase of the C_3-proactivator convertase concentration and C_4-proactivator convertase concentration of the ectopic focus, to the increase of blood Igm, and to the increase of macrophages in abdominal fluids, which phagocytize spermia. All these overall and local immune responses can lead to sterility.

Etiology and Pathogenesis
TCM holds that the disease is caused by extreme of the seven emotions, indulgence of sexual activity or injury from

operations, thus causing stagnation of Blood and Qitagnation, and Blood Stasis appears long time later. This can also be caused by Wind, Cold and Damp retained in the Chong and Ren Channels, Uterine Collaterals, thus resulting in stagnation of menstruation; or caused by accumulation of Damp Heat accumulating in the body, entering the Chong and Ren Channels, and obstructing the circulation of Blood and Qi; or during menstruation, after pregnancy, the patient is infected with pathogenic Damp Heat which accumulates in the Chong and Ren Channels or in Uterine Collaterals together with stagnant Heat, pseudo-blood appears, leading to Blood Stasis occurring in the abdomen.

Main Points of Diagnosis
• *Clinical Diagnosis*
① Progressive dysmenorrhea; ② Discomfort in lower abdomen and lumbosacral portion during menstruation, and the feeling exacerbates progressively; ③ Periodical rectal irritating symptom which exacerbates progressively; ④ Tender nodes in posterior fornix, uterine sacral ligament or uterine isthmus area; ⑤ Adnexa adherent lumps together with capsule nodes and patent oviduct; ⑥ Before and after the completion of menstrual cycle, the lumps of adnexa obviously change in size (No anti-inflammation drugs are used). With any point among ①, ② and ③ and one of the points among ④, ⑤ and ⑥ existing at the same time, it can be confirmed that the patient suffers from endometriosis.

• *Pathologic Diagnosis*
The following proofs should be obtained after incisional biopsy: ① Body of gland of endometrium; ② Interstitial matter of endometrium; ③ Internal bleeding of the tissues, and confirmed diagnosis can be obtained if red cells, ferric xanthematin, and growth of local connective tissues are observed. (The above standards for diagnosis of the disease were established on the Second Academic Conference of the Committee of Gynecology and Obstetrics of TCM and Western Medicine in Combination, October, 1986, Kunming.)

257

Treatment Based on Syndrome Differentiation

• *Blood Stasis due to Stagnation of Qi*

Main Symptoms and Signs: No pregnancy long after marriage, distending or stabbing pain in lower abdomen before or during menstruation, which spreads to lumbosacral area or perineum, the dragging feeling of anus, or distending pain in chest, limbs and breast, or scanty menstruation, unpatent flow of menstruation, purple in color and containing blood clots, the pain being reduced if blood clots come out, purple tongue with ecchymosis and petechiae with white tongue coating, tense and slippery pulse, the uterine being slightly larger and comparatively fixed revealed through gynecological examination, tender nodes in posterior fornix and uterine sacral ligament, or adherent lumps in adnexa, and the lumps changing in size before or after the completion of menstrual cycle.

Analysis of the Symptoms and Signs: Blood Stasis obstructs at Uterine Collaterals; thus, there is no pregnancy long after marriage. The depression of Qi and Blood Stasis at the Chong and Ren Channels result in obstruction in Blood and Qi flow. This is why before or after menstruation, there is distending pain of tenderness in lower abdomen. The pain spreads to lumbosacral and perineum area accompanying by dragging feeling of anus. Less menstruation or non-patent flow of menstruation will occur. Because the Liver is poorly regulated, there is distending pain in the chest, limbs and breasts. Because of the accumulation of Blood Stasis, the color is dark violet accompanied by blood clots. After blood clots come out, the accumulation of Blood Stasis is reduced, and the flow of Blood and Qi can continue temporally; therefore, the pain is alleviated. The conditions of the tongue and the pulse indicate stagnation of Qi and Blood Stasis. Because Blood Stasis accumulates, blood clots appear; thus, masses in lower abdomen are formed. That is why in the uterine, posterior fornix, and sacral ligament, there are tender nodes or adnexa adherent masses. If Blood Stasis and nodes are not removed, they either will recur in the next menstrual period, or continue to worsen progressively.

258

Treatment Principles: Promoting the circulation of Blood to remove Blood Stasis; removing nodes to dissolve lumps.

Prescription: Xiaoyi Tang (Decoction for Eliminating Endometriosis) (Prescription based on clinical experience of the author)

Burreed tuber (Rhizoma Sparganii) 9g, zedoary (Rhizoma Zedoariae) 9g, stir-baked pangolin scales (Squama Manitis) 9g, prepared frankincense (Olibanum) 9g, prepared myrrh (Myrrha) 9g, red peony root (Radix Paeoniae Rubra) 9g, red sage root (Radix Salviae Miltiorrhizae) 30g, peach kernel (Semen Persicae) 9g, prepared cyperus tuber (Rhizoma Cyperi) 9g, corydalis tuber (Rhizoma Corydalis) 9g, chuangxiong rhezome (Rhizoma Ligustici Chuangxiong) 9g, motherwort (Herba Leonuri) 30g, dried cat-tail pollen (Pollen Typhae) 9g, parched trogopterus dung (Faeces Trogopterorum) 9g and dragon's blood (Resina Draconis) 3g (to be taken in boiled water). The drugs are decocted in water for oral administration, one dose per day, and taking continuously over 1-3 months.

Analysis of the Prescription: Burreed tuber (Rhizoma Sparganii), zedoary (Rhizoma Zedoariae) remove Blood Stasis and resolve lumps. Prepared pangolin scales (Squama Manitis), prepared frankincense (Olibanum), prepared myrrh (Myrrha), dried cat-tail pollen (Pollen Typhae), parched trogopterus dung (Faeces Trogopterorum) remove obstruction in the channels, remove Blood Stasis and pain. Red peony root (Radix Paeoniae Rubra), red sage root (Radix Salviae Miltiorrhizae) peach kernel (Semen Persicae), chuangxiong rhezome (Rhizoma Ligustici Chuangxiong), corydalis tuber (Rhizoma Corydalis), motherwort (Herba Leonuri) can promote the circulation of Blood and remove stasis, regulate the flow of Qi and alleviate pain. Dragon's blood (Resina Draconis) can remove Blood Stasis and pain. The whole prescription promotes the circulation of Blood to remove Blood Stasis, softens hardness to resolve lumps.

• *Blood Stasis due to Cold*

Main Symptoms and Signs: No pregnancy long after marriage; pain in lower abdomen with cold sensation before or

259

after the completion of menstrual cycle which spreads to lumbosacral bone, perineum and anus, and which is reduced by warmth; infrequent menstruation with dark color accompanied by blood clots; aversion to cold and cold limbs, slightly pale tongue coating with ecchymosis and petechiae, deep and thready pulse; tender nodes in the areas of posterior fornix, uterine sacral ligament revealed through gynecological examinations.

Analysis of the Symptoms and Signs: Blood Stasis and Cold accumulate in the Uterine Channel, thus sperm obtaining is impossible. This leads to non-pregnancy long after marriage. The pathogenic Cold stays in the Chong and Ren Channels, thus menstrual flow can not be smooth. This is the reason of pain with dragging and discomfortable feeling in anus and the lower abdomen, lumbosacral area and perineum. After warmth, Blood Stasis and Cold are reduced slightly, pain can be alleviated. Blood is stagnated due to Cold, thus scanty dark menstruation with blood clots will occur. Because of insufficient Kidney Yang, cold limbs occurs, too. The deep thready pulse is an indication of Blood Stasis due to Cold. Because of Cold and Blood Stasis, pseudo-blood gets stagnated and thus blood clots are formed. This is why tender nodes can be found in the areas of posterior fornix, uterine sacral ligament.

Treatment Principles: Warming the channels to remove Blood Stasis; removing nodes to resolve lumps.

Prescription: Wenyi Tang (Decoction for Warming Endometriosis) (Prescription based on the clinical experience of the author)

Prepared aconite root (Radix Aconiti) 6g, cinnamom twig (Ramulus Cinnamomi) 9g, common fennel fruit (Fructus Foeniculi) 6g, burreed tuber (Rhizoma Sparganii) 9g, zedoary (Rhizoma Zedoariae) 9g, parched pangolin scales (Squama Manitis) 9g, red peony root (Radix Paeoniae Rubra) 9g, red sage root (Radix Salviae Miltiorrhizae) 30g, peach kernel (Semen Persicae) 9g, Chinese angelica root (Radix Angelicae Sinensis) 9g, chuangxiong rhezome (Rhizoma Ligustici Chuangxiong) 9g, prepared cyperus tuber (Rhizoma Cyperi) 9g, corydalis tuber (Rhizoma Corydalis)

260

9g, dahurian angelica root (Radix Angelicae Sinensis) 9g and dragon's blood (Resina Draconis) 3g (to be taken with boiled water). The above drugs are decocted in water for oral administration, one dose per day, and taking continuously over 1-3 months.

Analysis of the Prescription: Aconite root (Radix Aconiti) warms the Kidney and helps Yang, removes Cold and alleviate pain. Cinnamom twig (Ramulus Cinnamomi) warms and removes obstruction in the channels and collaterals. Common fennel fruit (Fructus Foeniculi) removes Cold, regulates the flow of Qi and alleviates pain. Chinese angelica root (Radix Angelicae Sinensis), pungent in taste and warm in nature, nourishes Blood and promotes the circulation of Blood. Burreed tuber (Rhizoma Sparganii), zedoary (Rhizoma Zedoariae), pangolin scales (Squama Manitis), red peony root (Radix Paeoniae Rubra), red sage root (Radix Salviae Miltiorrhizae), peach kernel (Semen Persicae), chuangxiong rhezome (Rhizoma Ligustici Chuangxiong), prepared cyperus tuber (Rhizoma Cyperi), corydalis tuber (Rhizoma Corydalis), dragon's blood (Resina Draconis) can remove Blood Stasis and resolve lumps, regulate the flow of Qi and alleviate pain. Dahurian angelica root (Radix Angelicae Sinensis) can relieve inflammation and alleviate pain. The whole prescription warms the channels and collaterals, removes Blood Stasis and resolves lumps.

• *Downward Flow of Damp Heat*

Main Symptoms and Signs: No pregnancy long after marriage, occasional pain in lower abdomen, which exacerbates before or during menstruation, high fever with a feeling of burning and tenderness, or the pain spreading to lumbosacral area, perineum, and anus, profuse dark red sticky menstruation with blood clots, rising and falling low fever, yellowish sticky whites, scanty dark urine, occasional dry stool, red tongue with ecchymosis and petechiae on the tip of the tongue with yellowish greasy tongue coating, thready and rapid pulse, slightly larger uterine with tenderness revealed through gynecological examinations, adnexa being thickened, and tender; or lumps that can be felt, tender nodes in posterior fornix uterine sacral ligament.

261

Analysis of the Symptoms and Signs: The combined Damp, Heat and Blood block in the Chong and Ren Channels and the uterus, which makes it impossible to obtain spermia, which results in non-pregnancy long after marriage. The downward flow of Damp Heat causes pain in lower abdomen with tenderness and burning sensation, or the pain spreads to lumbosacral area, perineum, and anus. Before and during menstruation, Heat at the Chong Channel exacerbates and leads to pain in lower abdomen. The stagnated Heat interferes with Blood and forces it to flow downward. This is the reason of increased menstruation with dark red color, and blood clots. The menstruation is sticky. The lingering Damp Heat causes the rising and falling of low fever. Downflow of Damp Heat in the Lower Jiao causes yellowish, thick and sticky leukorrhea, scanty dark urine and dry stool. The conditions of the tongue and pulse reflect Syndromes of Damp Heat and Blood Stasis. The accumulation of Blood Stasis and Excess Heat combined causes masses in abdomen. This is the reason of increased adnexa and the reason of tender nodes in the posterior fornix, uterine sacral ligament.

Treatment Principles: Clearing Heat to remove Blood Stasis; dissolving the nodes to resolve masses.

Prescription: Qingyi Tang (Decoction For Clearing Away Endometriosis) (Prescription based on clinical experience of the author)

Sargentgloryvine (Caulis Sargentodoxae) 15g, (Fructus Forysythiae) 12g, phellodendron bark (Cortex Phellodendri) 9g, prunella spike (Spica Prunellae) 9g, parched pangolin scales (Squama Manitis) 9g, fresh-water turtle shell (Carapax Trionycis) 30g, Japanese sea tangle (Thallus Laminariae) 9g, sargassum (Sargassum) 9g, moutan bark (Cortex Moutan Radicis) 9g, red peony root (Radix Paeoniae Rubra) 9g, red sage root (Radix Salviae Miltiorrhizae) 30g, peach kernel (Semen Persicae) 9g, corydalis tuber (Rhizoma Corydalis) 9g, prepared cyperus tuber (Rhizoma Cyperi) 9g and dragon's blood (Resina Draconis) 3g (to be taken with boiled water). The above drugs are decocted in water for oral administration, one dose per day, and taking successively over 1-3 months.

Analysis of the Prescription: Sargentgloryvine (Caulis Sargentodoxae), (Fructus Forysythiae), phellodendron bark (Cortex Phellodendri), prunella spike (Spica Prunellae) clear Heat and remove Toxins and resolve masses. Parched pangolin scales (Squama Manitis), fresh-water turtle-shell remove obstruction in the channels and dissolve nodes. Japanese sea tangle (Thallus Laminariae), seaweed clear Heat and remove Phlegm, soften hardness and dissolve nodes. Root bark of peony tree, red sage root (Radix Salviae Miltiorrhizae), red peony root (Radix Paeoniae Rubra), peach kernel (Semen Persicae), corydalis tuber (Rhizoma Corydalis), prepared cyperus tuber (Rhizoma Cyperi), dragon's blood (Resina Draconis) promote the circulation of Blood to remove Blood Stasis, regulate the flow of Qi and alleviate pain. The whole prescription clears Heat and removes Blood Stasis, dissolves nodes and resolves lumps.

Besides the endometriosis discussed above, a few of the patients may be accompanying by Kidney Deficiency, insufficiency of Qi and Blood, or accumulation of Phlegm. Supplementary drugs for restoring the Kidney and regulating menstruation, reinforcing Qi and nourishing Blood, or removing Phlegm and softening lumps must also be added respectively. Whatever the case it is, during the later stage of the treatment, drugs for restoring the Kidney should be added. Only after the circulation of Blood is promoted and the Kidney is tonified, will it be much more effective to promote ovulation; therefore, pregnancy may occur.

Current Research

1. 40 patients with endometriosis were treated mainly with promoting the circulation of Blood and removing Blood Stasis. Method of Treatment: ① 16 patients (40%) were treated according to the principle of promoting the circulation of Blood to remove Blood Stasis, warming the channels to remove obstruction in the collaterals. Prescription: Taohong Siwu Tang (Pink Decoction of Four Ingredients), together with Fu Gui Dihuang Wan Jiajian (Modified Bolus of Aconite, Cinnamon, and Rehmannia) including Aconite root (Radix Aconiti), cinnamom twig (Ramulus Cinnamomi),

263

peach kernel (Semen Persicae), safflower (Flos Carthami), Chinese angelica root (Radix Angelicae Sinensis), prepared rehmannia root (Radix Rehmanniae), red peony root (Radix Paeoniae Rubra), dragon's blood (Resina Draconis), red sage root (Radix Salviae Miltiorrhizae), chuangxiong rhezome (Rhizoma Ligustici Chuangxiong), Chinese yam (Rhizoma Dioscoreae), alismaceae (Rhizoma Alismatis), moutan bark (Cortex Moutan Radicis) and poria (Poria). For the case also with dragging feeling in lower abdomen, dangshen (Radix Codonopsis Pilosulae), white atractylodes rhizome (Rhizoma Atractylodis Macrocephalae), astragalus root (Radix Astragali Seu Hedysari) and cimicifuga rhizome (Rhizoma Cimicifugae) are added; for the case with exacerbated pain, corydalis tuber (Rhizoma Corydalis), dahurian angelica root (Radix Angelicae Sinensis) and Sichuan Chinaberry (Fructus Meliae Toosendan); for the case whose BBT increase was not good, amethyst (Fluorite), epimedium (Herba Epimedii) and desertliving cistanche (Herba Cistachi) are added. ② 6 patients (15%) were treated according to the principle of promoting the circulation of Blood to remove Blood Stasis, clearing Heat to dissolve lumps. Prescription: Qing Re Tiao Xue Tang (Decoction for Clearing Away Heat and Regulating Blood Flow) including Chinese angelica root (Radix Angelicae Sinensis), chuangxiong rhezome (Rhizoma Ligustici Chuangxiong), white peony root (Radix Paeoniae Alba), dried rehmannia root (Radix Rehmanniae), goldthread root (Rhizoma Coptidis), sargentgloryvine (Caulis Sargentodoxae), septemlobum, cyperus tuber (Rhizoma Cyperi), peach kernel (Semen Persicae), safflower (Flos Carthami), zedoary (Rhizoma Zedoariae), dragon's blood (Resina Draconis), corydalis tuber (Rhizoma Corydalis), moutan bark (Cortex Moutan Radicis) and prunella spike (Spica Prunellae). For the case with low fever, wolfberry bark (Cortex Lycii Radicis) and sweetworm wood (Herba Artemisiae) are added; for the case with depressed mind and irritability, pittosporm root (Radix Pittospori) and Sichuan Chinaberry (Fructus Meliae Toosendan) are added; for the case with masses in abdomen and lumps, eupolyphage sinensis and burreed tuber (Rhizoma

264

Sparganii) are added; for the case with preceded menstruation, scutellaria root (Radix Scutellariae) and phellodendron bark (Cortex Phellodendri) are added. ③ 10 patients (25%) were treated according to the principle of regulating the flow of Qi and promoting the circulation of Blood, removing Blood Stasis, and resolving lumps. Prescription: Jun Jun Jian (Decoction of Drastic Purgatives for Eliminating Blood Stasis and Masses) (Prescription based on clinical experience of the author) including Burreed tuber (Rhizoma Sparganii), zedoary (Rhizoma Zedoariae), pangolin scales (Squama Manitis), sweetgum fruit (Fructus Liquidambaris), eupolyphage sinensis, prunella spike (Spica Prunellae), cyperus tuber (Rhizoma Cyperi), clematis root, baked frankincense (Olibanum), prepared myrrh (Myrrha), red sage root (Radix Salviae Miltiorrhizae), red peony root (Radix Paeoniae Rubra), cinnamon twig (Ramulus Cinnamomi). After operation, if intestinal adhesion was resulted in, added were white peony root (Radix Paeoniae Alba) and licorice (Radix Glycyrrhizae). For the case with obstruction in oviduct, Chinese sage and dried oyster shell (Concha Ostreae) are added; for the case with distending breasts, whole trichosanthes and tangerine seed (Semen Citri Reticulatae) are added; for the case with non-patent menstruation, motherwort (Herba Leonuri) and Shixiao San (Wonderful Powder for relieving Blood Stagnation) are added. ④ 6 patients (15%) were treated by promoting the circulation of Blood to remove Blood Stasis, restoring the Kidney to regulate menstruation. Prescription: Chong Ren Jian (Decoction for Activating the Chong and Ren Channels) together with Shaofu Zhuyu Tang Jiajian (Modified Decoction for Removing Blood Stasis in the Lower Abdomen) including Chinese angelica root (Radix Angelicae Sinensis), chuangxiong rhezome (Rhizoma Ligustici Chuangxiong), cyperus tuber (Rhizoma Cyperi), common fennel fruit (Fructus Foeniculi), tortoise plastron (Plastrum Testudinis), antler powder (to be taken with boiled water), dangshen (Radix Codonopsis Pilosulae), dried rehmannia root (Radix Rehmanniae), dodder seed (Semen Cuscutae), epimedium (Herba Epimedii), red sage root (Radix Salviae

Miltiorrhizae), red peony root (Radix Paeoniae Rubra) and corydalis tuber (Rhizoma Corydalis). For the case also with profuse menstruation, added was donkey-hide gelatin (Colla Corii Asini). For the case with soreness of lumbar area and knees, eucommia bark (Cortex Eucommiae) and parasitism are added; for the case with slow BBT increase, desertliving cistanche (Herba Cistachi) is added. ⑤ 1 patient (2.5%) was treated by promoting the circulation of Blood to remove Blood Stasis, removing Phlegm and softening hardness. Prescription: Shen Tan Wan (Bolus for Removing Phlegm and Blood Stasis in the Kidney) including Chinese angelica root (Radix Angelicae Sinensis), prepared rehmannia root (Radix Rehmanniae), Chinese yam (Rhizoma Dioscoreae), epimedium (Herba Epimedii), desertliving cistanche (Herba Cistachi), thorn of Chinese honey locus (Spina Gleditsiae), blue chlorite-schist (Lapis Chloriti), airpotato yam (Rhizoma Dioscoreae Bulbiferae), arisaema tuber (Rhizoma Arisaematis), sprunella spike (Spica Prunellae), fritillary bulb (Bulbus Fritillariae) and dogwood fruit (Fructus Corni). For the case with preceded menstruation, dried rehmannia root (Radix Rehmanniae) and wolfberry bark (Cortex Lycii Radicis) are added; for the case with abdominal pain, corydalis tuber (Rhizoma Corydalis) and common fennel fruit (Fructus Foeniculi) are added. Mass resolving required to use earthworm (Lumbricus), zedoary (Rhizoma Zedoariae). ⑥ 1 patient (2.5%), was treated by promoting the circulation of Blood to remove Blood Stasis, removing water to relieve tuberculosis. Prescription: Jiawei Qin Bai Dan (Modified Bolus of Scutellaria and Stemona) including Scutellaria root (Radix Scutellariae), stemona root (Radix Stemonae), red sage root (Radix Salviae Miltiorrhizae), lepidium seed (Semen Lepidii seu Descurainiae), plantain seed (Semen Plantaginis), umbellate pore fungus (Haematitum), poria (Poria), prunella spike (Spica Prunellae), genkwa, dried oyster shell (Concha Ostreae) and Xiao Jin Dan (Little Gold Pill). For the case also with slow BBT increase, added were amethyst (Fluorite), epimedium (Herba Epimedii); for the case with constipation, cynomorium, dried rehmannia root (Radix Rehmanniae); for the case with preceded menstruation, dried rehmannia root (Radix Rehmanniae), sweetworm wood (Herba Artemisiae); for the case with abdominal pain, corydalis tuber (Rhizoma Corydalis), Sichuan Chinaberry (Fructus Meliae Toosendan). Therapeutic effects: All the patients were cured and got pregnant (Li Xiangyun, 1989-1990).

2. A clinical summary and experimental study of 40 patients with endometriosis holds that Blood Stasis accompanying by Kidney Deficiency was the basic pathogenesis, but Blood Stasis was the main aspect. Therefore, promoting the circulation of Blood to remove Blood Stasis, and warming the Kidney to nourish Blood should be applied. Clinically, the patients were divided into two types: Type of Dysmenorrhea (31 cases) and Type of Amenorrhea (9 cases). The main drugs for Type of Dysmenorrhea include red sage root (Radix Salviae Miltiorrhizae), red peony root (Radix Paeoniae Rubra), epimedium (Herba Epimedii) and zedoary (Rhizoma Zedoariae); for the case with soreness of waist, added were eucommia bark (Cortex Eucommiae) and dodder seed (Semen Cuscutae); for the case with Blood Deficiency, added was Siwu Tang (Decoction of Four Ingredients); for the case with Qi Deficiency, Si Junzi Tang (Decoction of Four Noble Drugs); for the case with profuse menstruation, added were cat-tail pollen (Pollen Typhae) and Zhenling Dan (Pill for Tranquilizing the Mind and Relieving Palpitation); for the case with obstructed oviduct or unpatent oviduct, pangolin scales (Squama Manitis) and sweetgum fruit (Fructus Liquidambaris). The commonly used drugs are Dangshen (Radix Codonopsis Pilosulae) rhizome, astragalus root (Radix Astragali Seu Hedysari), prepared rehmannia root (Radix Rehmanniae), red sage root (Radix Salviae Miltiorrhizae), sprunella spike (Spica Prunellae), etc. The drugs were taken one week before menstruation, and zedoary (Rhizoma Zedoariae), ophicalcitum (Ophicalcitum), bos taurus domesticus Gemelin being taken away. For the case with severe pain, added was Shixiao San (Wonderful Powder for Relieving Blood Stagnation), etc.

Therapeutic effects: 24 patients got pregnant with a pregnancy rate of 60%. Modern pharmacological effect of drugs

267

promoting blood flow and warming the Kidney shows that drugs promoting the circulation of Blood to remove Blood Stasis can improve uterine microcirculation, promote absorption of blood clots, stimulate the hematopoietic function of bone marrow of red blood cells and platelet, achieve depolymerization, and promote reproduction of the cells, inhibit carcinoma growth, reinforce the function of phagocytes, relieve inflammation and pain, and prevent adhesion. Drugs warming the Kidney, like epimedium (Herba Epimedii), regulate female's hormones, and BBT (Dai Deying, 1988).

3. Treatment comparison of 50 patients with endometriosis and female sterility. After peritoneoscopy, 50 patients were found to have endometriosis together with sterility. After operation, they were treated with materia medica, and Tablet for Woman. In the group treated with materia medica, Red sage root (Radix Salviae Miltiorrhizae), red peony root (Radix Paeoniae Rubra), stir-baked cat-tail pollen (Pollen Typhae), trogopterus dung (Faeces Trogopterorum), Chinese angelica root (Radix Angelicae Sinensis), prepared cyperus tuber (Rhizoma Cyperi) and corydalis tuber (Rhizoma Corydalis) are used with dosage of 10g respectively, Burreed tuber (Rhizoma Sparganii) and zedoary (Rhizoma Zedoariae) 6-10g respectively. For the case of Qi Deficiency, added were dangshen (Radix Codonopsis Pilosulae), astragalus root (Radix Astragali Seu Hedysari) 10-15g respectively. After the completion of menstrual cycle, the drugs were taken after being decocted, one dose daily, and for 15-20 days. Three months made a course of treatment. Most of the 32 patients (64%) in this group took the drugs for 2-3 courses of treatment, and the longest period was four courses of treatment. In the group treated with Tablet for Woman, Tablet for Woman is prescribed, 2.5mg, 1-2 times daily, and the medicine was taken from the fifth day of menstruation for 20-22 days. One course of treatment consisted of 3 months. Generally, the 14 patients in this group took the medicine for 1-2 courses of treatment. The longest curative period was 3 courses of treatment. In the group with temporization, no any medicine was administered to 4 pa-

tients. As a result, in the group treated with materia medica, 14 among 32 patients got pregnant. In the group treated with Tablet for Woman, 1 among 14 became pregnant; and 2 among 4 patients in the group treated with temporization became pregnant. After statistical processing of the three groups, it was found $P<0.05$. This indicates that pregnancy rate is related to treating methods. The total pregnancy rate of TCM Group was 43.5%, but that of Tablet for Woman Group was only 7.1%. This indicates that Tablet for Woman can only relieve the symptoms and make the focus disappear. So this method should not be applied (Fan Huaguang, 1987).

4. An observation of animal experiment of endometriosis prevented by promoting the circulation of Blood to remove Blood Stasis. In order to observe the cure effect of endometriosis treated with the prescription of promoting the circulation of Blood to remove Blood Stasis, by applying animal experiment, the author observed the general and histological cure effect of the medicine to transplanted endometrium to offer scientific proof for TCM treating endometriosis. A control group (No medicine was given) was set up for observation. Materials and methods: 16 white never- pregnant female, weighting 3kg, rabbits from New Zealand were chosen. To benefit the growth of endometrium and the surviving of ectopic intima, 3-6 days before laparotomy was applied. each received 30μg/kg/day of estradiol benzoate by way of intramuscular injection. The rabbits were divided into two groups, each group with 8 ones. The first group was TCM Group. Three days before operation, they were given TCM drugs, one dose daily until 25 days after operation. Then ventrotomy was applied, and the material was dissected for test. Prescription: Astragalus root (Radix Astragali Seu Hedysari) 30g, chuangxiong rhezome (Rhizoma Ligustici Chuangxiong) 15g, peach kernel (Semen Persicae) 15g, zedoary (Rhizoma Zedoariae) 15g, safflower (Flos Carthami) 15g and pseudostellaria (Radix Pseudostellariae) 30g. The drugs were decocted in longer time, and decoction was taken in 3 days, and one time daily. Animal Mold of Ectopic Endometrium was made in the following way. The operation

was carried out under the anesthesia of pentobarbital (30mg/kg intravenous injection). The uterus on the left was dissected, and the cut part was sutured. The dissected uterus was dissected open into four pieces, and they were transplanted on the peritoneum of the uterine rectum fossa, mesentery of the oviduct on the left, right oviduct mesentery, and on the left 2cm away from the dissected part. The method was applied to the above two groups. The rabbits in the control group did not receive TCM drugs. After mold making, the rabbits of the two groups received intramuscular injection of $30\mu g/kg$ of estradiol benzoate in 4 days. 25 days later, celiotomy was applied again. Result: Including general examination and pharmacological etiology examination. The first group (Medicated Group): The transplanted intimas were all alive, and appear to be fibroid lumps or multilocular small vesiculae in which there is yellow or white serous fluid. Etiological examination showed that the ectopic transplanted uterine intima appears to be in withered state whose surface turns to be in low cubic state or to be appanate, some having no glands, and interstitial fluid is scanty. It has a tendency of fibrosis. The second group (control group): General examination showed that the condition of ectopic transplanted intima was similar to that of the first group. Etiological examination showed that the growth of ectopic transplanted intima gland and interstitial fluid was fine, and glandular epithelium and surface epithelium appeared to be in high column state, some of the glands appeared to be papilliform which pushes into glandular cavity, and the interstitial fluid turned to be fusiformly dense.

All the transplanted intimas in this study were alive. General examination and etiological examination showed that the drugs that promote the circulation of Blood to remove Blood Stasis had some effect in preventing and treating endometriosis. Among the six drugs of the prescription, two tonify Qi and the remained four relieve stagnation of Qi and promote the circulation of Blood. By reviewing through the prescriptions of all the dynasties, we found all the prescriptions that promote the circulation of Blood and remove Blood Stasis and the prescriptions that promote the circula-

270

tion of Blood and regulate the flow of Qi were added with drugs tonifying Qi largely because after the break-out of Blood Stasis, there is obstruction in the channels and collaterals, which leads to Deficiency of Qi and Blood; therefore, Qi tonifying and Yang reinforcing are needed so that the circulation of Blood can remove the accumulation of Blood Stasis. The patients with endometriosis mostly have problem of Deficiency due to lingering diseases, so Yang-supporting and pathogens-removing are needed so that the goal of treatment is achieved. Modern medical study of astragalus has shown that astragalus contains 8 main ingredients, among which F_3 has strong immune reinforcing effect, but F_2 can inhibit immunity. So two-dimensional regulation is achieved (Su Yanhua, 1989-1990).

5. Preliminary observation of endometriosis treated with drugs promoting the circulation of Blood and removing Blood Stasis and uterine artery hemodynamic change. The author used pulse ultrasonic doppler blood-flow detector to measure the artery hemodynamic indices of the uterus of the two sides of the 22 patients with endometriosis before and after the treatment by drugs of promoting the circulation of Blood and removing Blood Stasis. The other 10 healthy women formed a control group. Bupleurum root (Radix Bupleuri), red peony root (Radix Paeoniae Rubra), moutan bark (Cortex Moutan Radicis), red sage root (Radix Salviae Miltiorrhizae), corydalis tuber (Rhizoma Corydalis), Sichuan chinaberry (Fructus Meliae Toosendan), dried cattail pollen (Pollen Typhae), trogopterus dung (Faeces Trogopterorum), leech (Hirudo), peach kernel (Semen Persicae), aucklandia root (Radix Aucklandiae), cyperus tuber (Rhizoma Cyperi), dried oyster shell (Concha Ostreae), sargentgloryvine (Caulis Sargentodoxae), patrinia (Herba Patriniae), sprunella spike (Spica Prunellae). For the case with Yang Deficiency, curculigo rhizome (Rhizoma Curculiginis) and epimedium (Herba Epimedii) were added; for cases of Yin Deficiency, dried rehmannia root (Radix Rehmanniae), ophiopogon root (Radix Ophiopogonis). The drugs were taken one dose daily. Each dose was decocted 2 times and taken cool. Drugs for enema: Purple gromwell

271

root (Radix Arnebiae seu Lithospermi), moutan bark (Cortex Moutan Radicis), red sage root (Radix Salviae Miltiorrhiz ae), corydalis tuber (Rhizoma Corydalis), sargentgloryvine (Caulis Sargentodoxae), patrinia (Herba Patriniae), Herba Hedyotis and phellodendron bark (Cortex Phellodendri). Every night before sleep, 100ml of the strongly decocted fluid was used for anus retention-enema. The drug was used throughout the menstruation (including menstrual period). Averagedly, all the patients took 73 doses of the medicine, and 54 doses for enema and and the averaged course of treatment was 2. 4 months. Result of treatment: Symptoms and Signs were reduced and improved to the varying degree. Among all the patients, 6 got pregnant, with a pregnancy rate of 27. 7%. The indices of uterine artery hemodynamics showed that after the treatment, the amount of the uterine artery the circulation of Blood. The pregnancy rate in 22 patients with endometriosis was obviously lowered.

The 22 patients in the treated group received the drugs promoting the circulation and Blood to remove Blood Stasis, and clearing Heat and removing Toxins, and received the drugs soothing the Liver and regulating the flow of Qi, and removing stagnation of Qi and masses in abdomen. The patients took the drugs orally and in enema and were treated both locally and overally. The averaged course of treatment was 2. 4 months. The illness condition of 21 patients with dysmenorrhea were improved, and retroflexion fixed uterus of three patients could move, and the bilateral chocolate cyst of 16 patients reduced in size (That of four patients disappeared). Six were pregnant. The cure effect in treating adhesion of the peripheral tissues caused by the focus of endometriosis and the medicine could be taken for a long time without side effects. TCM calls endometriosis "xue xia," (meaning blood clots) and holds that it is caused by "obstruction of Blood Vessles," and "Blood Stasis and Qi Stagnation." Modern medicine holds that the local focus of endometriosis exfoliate and bleed periodically, and blood accumulates in the tissue space. This causes hyperplasia of the peripheral fibroid tissue, thus lumps in different sizes form,

called endometrial stromal sarcoma. According to contemporary pharmacological study of promoting the circulation of Blood to remove Blood Stasis, red sage root (Radix Salviae Miltiorrhizae), red peony root (Radix Paeoniae Rubra), leech (Hirudo), moutan bark (Cortex Moutan Radicis) in the prescription can enlarge peripheral blood vessels and coronary artery. Trogopterus dung (Faeces Trogopterorum), moutan bark (Cortex Moutan Radicis), aucklandia root (Radix Aucklandiae), red sage root (Radix Salviae Miltiorrhizae), red peony root (Radix Paeoniae Rubra) have the effect of fibrinolysis. Sargentgloryvine (Caulis Sargentodoxae), patrinia (Herba Patriniae) and sprunella spike (Spica Prunellae) can clear Heat and remove inflammatory lumps. As a result, Blood Stasis and enema in the local focus disappeared, and peripheral fibroid tissues were dissected and disappeared and infectional response gradually disappeared, too. The pressure around the uterine artery was lowered, and blood and oxygen supply to the body of the uterus and adnexa was improved. This is why the amount and the rate of blood in the uterine artery gradually were restored. In the prescription, red sage root (Radix Salviae Miltiorrhizae), moutan bark (Cortex Moutan Radicis), cattail pollen (Pollen Typhae), trogopterus dung (Faeces Trogopterorum), corydalis tuber (Rhizoma Corydalis), peach kernel (Semen Persicae), etc. were proved through animal experiment to be able to lower the tension of local focus of the endometriosis, and to help wither or reduce the focus volume. The measured indices of the uterine artery hemodynamics can reflect the main source of blood supply. Compared with the condition before treatment and after treatment, the volume and the averaged velocity of the circulation of Blood of the 22 patients obviously increased and were quickened. This indicates that the infectional inflammatory response around the focus of endometriosis. This is caused by self-protection system with compensatory regulation to local blood circulation. After treatment, the volume of the circulation of Blood of the uterine artery was reduced, and the averaged velocity of the circulation of Blood was slowed. This may be related to the reduced local focus, im-

273

proved infectional, and local oxygen supply. This also indicates that this method of treatment can enlarge Blood Vessels, improve microcirculation, relieve blood from the strong, adhesive, and accumulating condition and dissolve fibrin. The above-mentioned effects in combination can regulate the physiochemical property of blood and regulate hemodynamic functions (Zhu Wenxin, et al, 1989-1990).

Polycystic Ovary Syndrome (PCOS)

PCOS refers to that the abnormal relation of hormone secretory volume among hypothalamus, hypophysis and ovary result in scanty menstruation, or amenorrhea, or irregular uterine bleeding, or polytrichosis, obesity, sterility, enlarged bilateral ovary and polycystic diseases, etc.

There is no special account about this disease in TCM, but it can be found here and there in the accounts about irregular menstruation or female sterility.

Etiology and Pathogenesis

Though there has been much research on the anovulatory mechanism of PCOS, the reason of anovulation is still unknown.

Modern research holds that it is related to the following factors: ① Adrenal dysfunction results in abnormal relation among hypothalamus-hypophysis-ovary axis and abnormal hormone secretion. ② Because of the break-down of cyclic center of hypothalamus, the positive and negative feedback of estrogen to hypothalamus is abnormal; that is, the lowered dihydrotheelin can not reach its proper lowest level. As a result, FSH release volume can not stimulate the follicles to grow; or estradiol level can not reach the high level before ovulation, so it can not lead to LH peak. Therefore, ovulation is impossible. ③ Because of the lack of some enzymes or of the disturbance of ovary enzyme system, androstenedione and testosterone are unable to synthesize estrone and dihydrotheelin. ④ Various factors affect the pulse release of gonadotropin-releasing hormone; therefore, normal release of gonadotropic hormone is affected. Thus, ovulation is impossible.

TCM holds that the disease has relation with the following items of pathogenesis: ① Exhaustion due to marrying too early, Yang Deficiency due to vegetarian diet, Deficiency of the Chong and Ren Channels due to insufficiency of Kidney Qi—all of this leads to Deficiency of Essence and Blood, thus the Uterine Collaterals can not be nourished. ② Obesity together with vegetarian diet, or with rich fatty diet, accumulation of Phlegm Damp, disturbance of visceral function—all of this leads to obstruction of the Uterine Collaterals, or Phlegm obstructing in capsule, and Essence can not be stored; therefore, pregnancy is impossible. ③ Depression of mind, stagnation of Liver Qi which leads to disturbance between dispelling and excretion, and derangement of Qi and Blood and the disorder between the Chong and Ren Channels. With the depressed emotions and worsened stagnation, the function of the uterus is affected, leading to sterility. ④ After menstruation or child-bearing, some blood still remains which forms Blood Stasis which obstructs in the Interior. Because Blood Stasis obstructs in the uterus which can not receive the nourishment of new blood; therefore, to obtain sperm for pregnancy is impossible.

Main Points of Diagnosis

Manifestations: Scanty menstruation, amenorrhea, sterility, some with dysfunctional uterine bleeding, and manifestations of polytrichia, obesity or facial acne; pneumoperitoneo graphy and pelvic pneumography, peritoneoscopy or B-ultrasonic scanning examination show that the bilateral follicles are 1/4 larger than the normal uterus. In the follicles, there are polycystic follicles. Hyperplasia of thecacells. No yellow body of ovary is seen. The ratio of LH/FSH is greater than 3.

Treatment Based on Syndrome Differentiation

• *Kidney Deficiency Accompanying by Phlegm Syndrome*
   Main Symptoms and Signs: No pregnancy over a long period of time after marriage, scanty menstruation or amenia,

soreness of the waist and lassitude of legs, tiredness, obesity with more hairs, distressed chest, nausea, or thin and loose stool, thick pale tongue with thin greasy tongue coating, thready and slippery pulse.

Analysis of the Symptoms and Signs: Kidney Deficiency leading to insufficiency of Essence and Blood, and the uterus can not be nourished. Together with Phlegm obstruction to functional activities of Qi, and to the uterus, to obtain sperm for pregnancy is impossible. Therefore, there is no pregnancy long after marriage. The Chong and Ren Channels fail to be nourished leading to Kidney Deficiency, or Phlegm obstructing the functional activities, the obstructed Uterus can lead to scanty menstruation or amenorrhea. Deficiency of Kidney Yang results in decline of Fire from the Gate of Life. That is the reason of soreness and flaccidity of lumbar area and legs, listlessness and aversion to cold. Deficiency of Kidney Yang results in Deficiency of the Spleen and Vital Qi and results in poor digestion, and Phlegm appears because of the accumulation of the fluid. This is the reason of obesity and polytrichia, choking sensation in chest and nausea. Deficiency of Spleen Yang and Kidney Yang results in loose and thin stool. Other symptoms and signs suggest Kidney Deficiency and accumulation of Phlegm.

Treatment Principles: Restoring the Kidney and removing Phlegm.

Prescription: Bu Shen Hua Tan Tang (Decoction for Restoring the Kidney and Removing Phlegm) (Prescription based on clinical experience of the author)

Prepared rehmannia root (Radix Rehmanniae) 12g, dodder seed (Semen Cuscutae) 9g, psoralea fruit (Fructus Psoraleae) 9g, epimedium (Herba Epimedii) 15g, dogwood fruit (Fructus Corni), eucommia bark (Cortex Eucommiae) 9g, parched pangolin scales (Squama Manitis) 12g, thorn of Chinese honey locus (Spina Gleditsiae) 15g, Japanese sea tangle (Thallus Laminariae) 9g, seaweed (Sargassum) 9g, sprunella spike (Spica Prunellae) 9g, red peony root (Radix Paeoniae Rubra) 9g and red sage root (Radix Salviae Miltiorrhizae) 30g. The above drugs are decocted strongly with water for oral administration, one dose daily, and taking

276

successively over 1-3 months.

Analysis of the Prescription: The first six drugs nourish and tonify the Liver and the Kidney, warm and reinforce Kidney Yang. The next five drugs soften hardness and remove Phlegm. The last two drugs promote the circulation of the circulation of Blood to remove Blood Stasis to help restore the Kidney and remove Phlegm.

• *Stagnation of Liver Qi Producing Liver Fire*

Main Symptoms and Signs: No pregnancy long after marriage, scanty menstruation, amenorrhea, or irregular bleeding, strong body with thick hair on the head, facial acne, distending pain and full feeling in the chest ribs, dry mouth and hanger for cold drinks, constipation, thin and yellow tongue coating, tense and rapid pulse.

Analysis of the Symptoms and Signs: The disorder of Liver Qi, the prolonged stagnation of Liver Qi worsens so that the uterus is heated, which leads to non-pregnancy long after marriage. The stagnation of Liver Qi causes unsmooth circulation of Blood so scanty menstruation, amenorrhea, or irregular bleeding, distention and pain in breasts, chest and hypochondrium occur. The stagnation of Liver Qi accompanying by Spleen Deficiency cause abnormal growth of hair and facial acne. Stagnation of Liver Qi producing Liver Fire causes dry mouth, desire for cold drinks and constipation. The remaining signs suggest stagnation of Liver Qi.

Treatment Principles: Clearing Heat from the Liver to relieve Fire.

Prescription: Qing Gan Xie Huo Tang (Decoction for Clearing Away Heat of the Liver to Relieve Fire) (Prescription based on the clinical experience of the author)

Gentian root (Radix Gentianae) 9g, capejasmine seed (Fructus Gardeniae) 9g, scutellaria root (Radix Scutellariae) 9g, bupleurum root (Radix Bupleuri) 9g, plantain herba (Herba Plantaginis) 15g, dried rehmannia root (Radix Rehmanniae) 12g, rhizome of wind-weed (Rhizoma Anemarrhenae) 9g, trichosanthes root (Radix Trichosanthes) 9g, trichosanthes fruit (Fructus Trichosanthes) 12g, motherwort (Herba Leonuri) 30g, wolfberry fruit (Fructus Lycii) 15g, dodder seed (Semen Cuscutae) 9g, Japanese sea tangle

277

(Thallus Laminariae) 9g and seaweed (Sargassum) 9g. The drugs are decocted in water for oral administration, one dose per day, and continuously over 1-3 months.

Analysis of the Prescription: Gentian root (Radix Gentianae) relieves Fire from the Liver and the Gallbladder. Scutellaria root (Radix Scutellariae), capejasmine seed (Fructus Gardeniae), bitter in taste and cold in nature, clear Heat. Bupleurum root (Radix Bupleuri) removes Blood Stasis by soothing the Liver. Plantain herba (Herba Plantaginis) induces diuresis to remove pathogenic Heat, so that Heat is removed through urination. Dried rehmannia root (Radix Rehmanniae) nourishes Yin and cools Blood. Rhizome of wind-weed (Rhizoma Anemarrhenae) clears Heat, nourishes Yin and moistens Dryness. Trichosanthes root (Radix Trichosanthes) clears Heat and promotes salivation. Trichosanthes fruit (Fructus Trichosant hes) clears Heat and removes Phlegm, promotes circulation of Qi and removes depressed chest, loosening the bowel to relieve constipation. Motherwort (Herba Leonuri) promotes the circulation of Blood and removes Phlegm, induces diuresis to remove Toxins. Wolfberry fruit (Fructus Lycii) and dodder seed (Semen Cuscutae) invigorate the Kidney to benefit Essence, nourish Yin and Blood. Japanese sea tangle (Thallus Laminariae) and seaweed (Sargassum) clear Heat, and remove Phlegm, soften hardness to induce diuresis. The whole prescription purges Liver Fire, resolve the hard lumps and removes Phlegm together with reinforcing the Kidney to promote the circulation of Blood.

• *Blood Stasis Accompanying by Kidney Deficiency*

Main Symptoms and Signs: No pregnancy long after marriage, scanty menstruation, or amenorrhea, or profuse slight dark menstruation with blood clots, aversion to cold, soreness of waist and faint legs, dizziness, tinnitus, dark red tongue with ecchymosis and petechiae along its edge, deep thready pulse or deep slippery pulse.

Analysis of the Symptoms and Signs: Kidney Deficiency leads to Deficiency and impairment of the Chong and Ren Channels. As a result, insufficiency of Essence and Blood occurs. What's more, Blood Stasis, accumulating in the

278

uterus, obstructs in the Interior, thus obtaining sperm for pregnancy is impossible. This is the reason of non-pregnancy long after marriage. Blood Stasis due to Kidney Deficiency leads to scanty menstruation, amenorrhea or profuse slight dark menstruation with blood clots. Deficiency of Kidney Yang leads to aversion to cold, soreness and flaccidity of lumbar area and legs, dizziness and tinnitus. Other symptoms and signs reflect Blood Stasis accompanying by Kidney Deficiency.

Treatment Principles: Restoring the Kidney and removing Blood Stasis.

Prescription: Bu Shen Qu Yu Tang (Decoction for Restoring the Kidney and Removing Blood Stasis) (Prescription based on clinical experience of the author)

Prepared rehmannia root (Radix Rehmanniae) 12g, dogwood fruit (Fructus Corni) 9g, morinda root (Radix Morindae Officinalis) 9g, dodder seed (Semen Cuscutae) 12g, desertliving cistanche (Herba Cistachi) 12g, epimedium (Herba Epimedii) 15g, burreed tuber (Rhizoma Sparganii) 9g, zedoary (Rhizoma Zedoariae) 9g, Chinese angelica root (Radix Angelicae Sinensis) 9g, chuangxiong rhezome (Rhizoma Ligustici Chuangxiong) 9g, peach kernel (Semen Persicae) 9g, safflower (Flos Carthami) 9g, red sage root (Radix Salviae Miltiorrhizae) 30g and motherwort (Herba Leonuri) 30g. The drugs are decocted in water for oral administration, one dose daily, and successively over 1-3 months.

Analysis of the Prescription: In the prescription, the first six drugs nourish and invigorate the Liver and the Kidney, warm and restore Kidney Yang. All the other drugs promote the circulation of Blood to remove Blood Stasis.

This disease is mainly divided into above three types. Clinically, most of the cases are found to be both Deficiency accompanying by Excess, particularly Syndrome of Kidney Deficiency accompanying by Phlegm Syndrome; what's more, the dominance of Kidney Deficiency, and dominance of Phlegm in individual cases, so the treatment should be correspondingly emphasized on tonifying weakness and removing Phlegm. Whatever the case is, after the treatment, activating the circulation of Blood and invigorating the Kidney should be done.

Current Research

1. 133 cases with PCOS treated with method of invigorating the Kidney and removing Phlegm. According to treatment based on Syndrome Differentiation, the disease was divided into three types: Phlegm Syndrome, Phlegm accompanying by Kidney Deficiency Syndrome and Kidney Deficiency Syndrome. For Phlegm Syndrome, Phlegm removal and lumps resolving are considered, supplemented with drugs that restore the Kidney such as Sprunella spike (Spica Prunellae) 12g, Japanese sea tangle (Thallus Laminariae), pangolin scales (Squama Manitis) 12g, thorn of Chinese honey locus (Spina Gleditsiae) 12g, pleione rhizome (Rhizoma Pleionis) 12g, fritillary bulb (Bulbus Fritillariae) 12g, arisaema with bile (Arisaem cum Bile) 6g, red peony root (Radix Paeoniae Rubra) 9g, dodder seed (Semen Cuscutae) 12g and epimedium (Herba Epimedii) 12g. For Kidney Deficiency accompanying by Phlegm Syndrome, drugs restoring the Kidney and drugs removing Phlegm and resolving lumps were used in combination such as Prepared rehmannia root (Radix Rehmanniae) 9g, dodder seed (Semen Cuscutae) 12g, raspberry (Fructus Rubi) 12g, epimedium (Herba Epimedii) 12g, curculigo rhizome (Rhizoma Curculiginis) 9g, sprunella spike (Spica Prunellae) 12g, pangolin scales (Squama Manitis) 12g, thorn of Chinese locus 12g, fritillary bulb (Bulbus Frittillariae) 12g, Japanese sea tangle (Thallus Laminariae) 12g. For the case intolerant to cold, aconite root (Radix Aconiti) 9g, cinnamon bark (Cortex Cinnamomi) 3g were added; for the case with loose stool, Chinese yam (Rhizoma Dioscoreae) 12g and fenugreek seed (Semen Trigonellae) 12g. For Syndrome of Kidney Deficiency, Kidney-restoring drugs are used mainly, supplemented with the drugs removing Phlegm and resolving lumps such as Prepared rehmannia root (Radix Rehmanniae) 12g, deglued antler powder (Cornu Cervi Degelation) 12g, dodder seed (Semen Cuscutae) 12g, raspberry (Fructus Rubi) 12g, fenugreek seed (Semen Trigonellae) 12g, epimedium (Herba

280

Epimedii) 12g, aconite root (Radix Aconiti) 9g, cinnamon bark (Cortex Cinnamomi) 3g, fritillary bulb (Bulbus Frittillariae) 9g and pangolin scales (Squama Manitis) 12g. After the finish of menstruation, the drugs were taken until basal BBT went up. For consolidating the cure effect, Taro Bolus and set TCM medicines removing Phlegm and restoring the Kidney were added. Therapeutic effects: Biphasic curve of BBT was considered to be standard of judging ovulation, 110 cases (82.7%) got this result. Those having menarche received ovulatory assay, and among 999 menstrual cycles, ovulation took place in 407 (40%) menstrual cycles. Among the married 76 cases, 36 got pregnant except for two cases having problem of obstructed oviduct. It was believed that that Kidney-restoring drugs can cure PCOS may be through regulating hypothalamus-hypophysis-ovary, then the goal of treatment was achieved. While using the drugs restoring the Kidney, added were such Phlegm-removing and hardness-softening drugs as sprunella spike (Spica Prunellae), fritillary bulb (Bulbus Frittllariae), pangolin scales (Squama Manitis), thorn of Chinese honey locus (Spina Gleditsiae) and arisaema tuber (Rhizoma Arisaematis), thus, problem of more hair will be improved, and cure effect will be improved, too. This suggests that those drugs may have the effects on regulating ovary enzyme system and on ovary capsule (Sun Yueli, 1981).

2. An analysis of 70 cases with PCOS treated based on Syndrome Differentiation. For Syndrome of Liver Fire, purging Liver Fire was applied. The prescriptions are Longdan Xie Gan Tang (Decoction of Gentian for Purging Liver Fire), Danggui Long Hui Wan (Bolus of Chinese Angelica root (Radix Angelicae Sinensis), Gentian root (Radix Gentianae), and Aloes), or Zhibo Bawei Wan (Pill of Eight Ingredients Including Anemarrhena and Phellodendron). For Syndrome of Deficiency of both Qi and Blood, benefiting Qi and nourishing Blood was used. Gui Pi Tang Jiajian (Modified Spleen-Tonifying Decoction) was applied. For Syndrome of Deficiency of Spleen Yang and Kidney Yang, invigorating and benefiting the Spleen and the Kidney was applied. The prescriptions used was Fugui Bawei Wan (Bolus

of Eight Ingredients Including Aconite and Cinnamon), Roucongrong Pian (Tablet of Desertliving Cistanche (Herba Cistachi), or Liu Zi Tang Jiajian (Modified Decoction of Six Seed Drugs) including astragalus root (Radix Astragali Seu Hedysari) 15g, bighead atractylodes rhizome (Rhizoma Atractylodis Macrocepha lae) 9g, aconite root (Radix Aconiti) 9g, cinnamom twig (Ramulus Cinnamomi), wolfberry fruit (Fructus Lycii) 9g, glossy privet fruit (Fructus Ligustri Lucidi) 9g, dodder seed (Semen Cuscutae) 9g, raspberry (Fructus Rubi) 9g, vaccaria seed (Semen Vaccariae) 9g and motherwort fruit (Semen Leonuri) 9g. For the case with Phlegm Syndrome, drugs softening hard lumps and removing Phlegm are used such as Pangolin scales (Squama Manitis) 12g, thorn of Chinese honey locus (Spina Gleditsiae) 12g, Japanese sea tangle (Thallus Laminariae) 9g, earthworm (Lumbricus) 9g, red sage root (Radix Salviae Miltiorrhizae) 12g, zedoary (Rhizoma Zedoariae) 9g, cyperus tuber (Rhizoma Cyperi) 9g, white mustard seed (Semen Sinapis Albae) 9g and lepidium seed (Semen Lepidii seu Descurainiae) 9g. For the case with fewer symptoms and no obvious changes in tongue and pulse but amenorrhea as the main symptom, because of varying drugs used, and varying methods of treatment were categorized into "Type of the Others." Standards of Cure Effect are divided into four degrees. Category I: On the whole, menstruation was normal. Biphasic BBT appeared over 3 times (Difference of Temperature 0. 3-0. 45 degree centigrades, increasing for over 9 days). Periodical changes took place to vaginal exfoliated cells, pregnancy may occur. Category II: On the whole, menstruation was normal. Biphasic BBT happened for many times or there are obvious changes to vaginal exfoliated cells. Category III: Menstruation was improved, but there were no obvious changes to BBT and vaginal exfoliated cells. Category IV: After treatment, there were no obvious changes to BBT, menstruation, exfoliated cells. Therapeutic effects: Three months accounted for one course of treatment. 30 cases underwent one course of treatment. 24 experienced two courses of treatment. Ten underwent three courses of treatment, and 46 experienced four courses of treatment. 36 cases (51.4%), obtained effect of Category I, among whom 14 married patients got pregnant. 18 cases (25.7%) obtained effect of Category II. 10 cases (14.3%), obtained effect of Category III, and 6 cases (8.6%) obtained effect of Category IV. Considering the cure effect of the five types of the diseases according to Syndrome Differentiation, the cure effect of each type was by the large the same, and had no obvious differences. The author held that it is not enough to differentiate the diseases only. It should be combined with Syndrome Differentiation. The treatment could be conducted according to the causes (Shi Lingyi, etc., 1984).

3. 19 cases with PCOS treated with materia medica. Pneumoperitoneography and pelvic pneumography or double contrast radiography had confirmed that the bilateral ovary of the patients was over 1/4 larger than the uterus. The treatment based on Syndrome Differentiation is discussed as follows. ① For the case with Kidney Deficiency and accumulation of Phlegm, restoring the Kidney to remove Phlegm are the principles. Drugs include Chinese angelica root (Radix Angelicae Sinensis), Chinese yam (Rhizoma Dioscoreae), eucommia bark (Cortex Eucommiae), dogwood fruit (Fructus Corni), dodder seed (Semen Cuscutae), amethyst (Fluorite), epimedium (Herba Epimedii), morinda root (Radix Morindae Officinalis), pleione rhizome (Rhizoma Pleionis), thorn of Chinese honey locus (Spina Gleditsiae), sprunella spike (Spica Prunellae), fritillary bulb (Bulbus frittillariae), etc. ② For the case with Yin Deficiency and Interior Heat, the principles are nourishing Yin and clearing Heat. The drugs are trichosanthes fruit (Fructus Trichosanthes), dendronbium (Herba Dendrobii), goldthread root (Rhizoma Coptidis), trichosanthes, Chinese pink herb (Herba Dianthi), ophiopogon root (Radix Ophiopogonis), tortoise plastron (Plastrum Testudinis), dried rehmannia root (Radix Rehmanniae), achyranthes root (Radix Achyranthis Bidentatae), plantain seed (Semen Plantaginis), motherwort (Herba Leonuri) and rhizome of wind-weed (Rhizoma Anemarrhenae). ③ For the case of Blood Stasis accompanying by Kidney Deficiency, the principle is restoring the Kid-

283

ney to remove Blood Stasis. The commonly used drugs are Chinese angelica root (Radix Angelicae Sinensis), prepared rehmannia root (Radix Rehmanniae), dogwood fruit (Fructus Corni), epimedium (Herba Epimedii), desertliving cistanche (Herba Cistachi), cynomorium (Herba Cynomorii), fenugreek seed (Semen Trigonellae), Herba Lycopi, burreed tuber (Rhizoma Sparganii), zedoary (Rhizoma Zedoariae), sprunella spike (Spica Prunellae), cyperus tuber (Rhizoma Cyperi), corydalis tuber (Rhizoma Corydalis) and red sage root (Radix Salviae Miltiorrhizae). ④ For the case of Fire Syndrome which is due to stagnation of Liver Qi, the principle for treatment is purging Liver Fire. Longdan Xie Gan Tang (Modified Decoction of Gentian for Purging the Liver Fire) is used. Therapeutic effects: There were effects on 16 patients, among whom 14 got pregnant (Li Xiangyun, 1989).

4. Observation of ovary morphological change of adult rats with from PCOS treated with drugs restoring the Kidney. To observe the change of the endocrine axis from the point of morphology after treatment of restoring the Kidney, testosterone propionate was injected to make PCOS mold in male rats for observation of Kidney-restoring treatment. The drugs including Aconite root (Radix Aconiti) 12g, cinnamon bark (Cortex Cinnamomi) 3g, psoralea fruit (Fructus Psoraleae) 12g, epimedium (Herba Epimedii) 12g, dodder seed (Semen Cuscutae) 12g and siberian solomonseal rhizome (Rhizoma Polygonati) 15g. The water-soluble part was extracted out and was made into dry extracts 324mg/ml, equal to dried herb 3g. The drug was administered 20 times the dose per person, and an animal weighting 100g was given 1ml. The adult white rat with PCOS were also given watersoluble preparation of TCM drugs restoring the Kidney. It was found that interstitial gland obviously increased, which appeared as big balls. This suggests that the drug has certain effect to the ovary. Interstitial glands result from the fact that thecacells become fat when secondary follicles degenerate. The interstitial glands can synthesize steroid hormone. Under microelectrometry, in the rats of testosterone propionate, after perfusion of the TCM fluid restoring the Kid-

284

ney, lipid droplets in cytoplasm of ovary interstitial glands obviously decreased. The decrease of lipid droplets suggests that the synthesis ability of steroid hormone is raised, and the raised ability suggests that drugs restoring the Kidney have some effect on ovary hormone metabolism (Wei Meijuan, 1990).

Luteinized Unruptured Follicle Syndrome (LUFS)

LUFS refers to the syndrome which is marked by regular menstrual cycle but with unruptured follicles and even no ovulation in the middle of menstruation. This is one of the important causes of female sterility.

The research has proved that LH peak value of LUFS is obviously lower than that in normal menstrual period. Therefore, a series of changes caused by normally higher LH peak value before and during ovulation takes place; and the maturity, rupture of the follicles, and ovulation are obstructed. Research also has proved that because LH level is not high enough, the increase of cAMP is affected; therefore, the activity of plasminogen activator in the ovary is lowered, which affects fibrinolysis and self-digestion of folliclular wall. Therefore, coagulation of liquor folliculi occurs. Not only does abdominal fluid of LUFS decrease, but also the levels of internal estradiol and pregnendione are obviously lower than those of the normal people. In the past, the reason that clomiphine could treat the cases with high "ovulatory rate," low pregnancy rate is probably because the peak value induced by clomiphine is not higher; as a result, LUFS results. Dmowski (1980) reported that the patients with endometriosis and dysfunction of corpus luteum complicated with LUFS took up 16-79%. There are no remarkable differences between the degree of seriousness of endometriosis and LUFS incidence. He also put forward that that the above two diseases cause LUFS is probably because of ovary adhesion. Hamilten (1985) called it mechanically unruptured follicle syndrome.

There are no records and special account about this disease in TCM documents. I think the main pathogenic factors of mechanism are exhaustion due to too early marriage, or weakness due to vegetarian diet, Deficiency of Kidney Qi, Deficiency and impairment of the Chong and Ren Channels, and follicles are unable to be ovulated; or remained blood during menstruation or after birth-giving turns to be Blood Stasis long time later, which accumulates and obstructs in the uterus, the collaterals of the uterus. Therefore, follicles are unable to to be ovulated.

Main Points of Diagnosis
This disease is often misdiagnosed as female sterility due to unknown causes, endometriosis, pelvic inflammation, dysfunction of corpus luteum, etc. Various monitoring examinations of ovulatory function are normal; however, after BBT increases for 2-4 days, no stigma can be observed under abdominoscope. Ovary biopsy pharmacological examination under abdominoscope is much more significant to confirm diagnosis, so is serial B-ultrasonic examination of monitoring of growth and development of follicles of ovary. That is, the examinations are conducted 4-5 days before ovulation until 3-4 days after BBT increases, one time per day. Normally, there are B-ultrasonic signs of ovulation: Before ovulation, the averaged diameter of the follicles is 21 ± 0.5mm; after ovulation, the dominant follicles become smaller or their border becomes vague with folds. There are minute rarefactive light-spots on the area, and 1-2 days later, these light-spots form an area of dense light-spots indicating the formation of corpus luteum. And the whole ovary becomes low echo area, and there may be dropsy in the retrorectal excavation area. After examining the patients with LUFS with B-ultrasonic, no ovulatory signs stated above can be seen; what's more, after LH peak, follicles continue to enlarge with the diameter being over 35mm averagedly. No area of dense light spots and hydrops appear. It is convenient and undamageable to use B-ultrasonic scanning examination; furthermore, it can be used for successive observation. Therefore, it is an important means in diagnosing the disease.

286

Treatment Based on Syndrome Differentiation

Main Symptoms and Signs: No pregnancy long after marriage, normal or abnormal menstrual cycle and amount of menstruation, with its color being light dark, or with blood clots, or pain with dragging feeling in lower abdomen during menstruation, aversion to cold, cold arms and legs, soreness and flaccidity of lumbar area and knees, dizziness and tinnitus, light dark tongue with ecchymosis and petechiae along its margin, deep and slippery pulse.

Analysis of the Symptoms and Signs: Deficiency and impairment of the Chong and Ren Channels due to Kidney Deficiency, insufficiency of Essence and Blood together with Blood Stasis in the channels and collaterals of the Uterus, the impossibility of follicle ovulation to combine with spermia—all of these lead to non-pregnancy long after marriage. Deficiency and impairment of the Chong and Ren Channels, the less severe condition of Blood Stasis make it possible to regulate menstruation temporally, but if Deficiency and impairment become very severe, then, irregular menstruation results. Insufficiency of Kidney Qi results in aversion to cold and cold limbs, soreness and flaccidity of lumbar area s and knees, dizziness and tinnitus. Tongue and pulse indicate Blood Stasis accompanying by Kidney Deficiency.

Treatment Principles: Restoring the Kidney and removing Blood Stasis; activating the collaterals and reducing blood clots.

Prescription: Bushen Quyu Tang Jiajian (Modified Decoction for Restoring the Kidney and Removing Blood Stasis)

Prepared rehmannia root (Radix Rehmanniae) 12g, dogwood fruit (Fructus Corni) 9g, morinda root (Radix Morindae Officinalis) 9g, dodder seed (Semen Cuscutae) 9g, epimedium (Herba Epimedii) 15g, amethyst (Fluorite) 30g (Decocted first), burreed tuber (Rhizoma Sparganii) 9g, zedoary (Rhizoma Zedoariae) 9g, parched pangolin scales (Squama Manitis) 12g, Japanese sea tangle (Thallus Laminariae) 9g, sea weed (Sargassum) 9g, peach kernel (Semen Persicae) 9g, safflower (Flos Carthami) 9g, red sage root (Radix Salviae Miltiorrhizae) 30g and prepared myrrh (Myrrha) 9g. The above drugs are decocted in water

287

for oral administration, one dose per day, and successively over 1-3 months.

Analysis of the Prescription: The first six drugs nourish the Liver and restore the Kidney, warm and promote Kidney Yang. Burreed tuber (Rhizoma Sparganii) and zedoary (Rhizoma Zedoariae) remove Blood Stasis and resolve hard lumps. Parched pangolin scales (Squama Manitis), Japanese sea tangle (Thallus Laminariae) and sea weed remove obstruction from collaterals and dissolve hardness. Peach kernel (Semen Persicae), safflower (Flos Carthami), red sage root (Radix Salviae Miltiorrhizae) and prepared myrrh (Myrrha) promote the circulation of Blood to remove Blood Stasis.

The drugs that restore the Kidney and promote the circulation of Blood can regulate the normal secretory function of hypothalamus-hypophysis-ovary axis, and the drugs removing Blood Stasis, activating the collaterals and resolving hardness are used to promote the ovulation of the mature ova after the foliclular wall is broken. Better curative effect can be obtained to those patients who have no obvious symptoms and signs.

Current Research

1. LUFS is one of the important reasons of female sterility due to unknown causes. This disease may also refer to the patients who suffer from ovulatory dysfunction and is still unable to get pregnant even if inducing ovulation is successful. Besides manifestations of the related diseases, the patients have no other symptoms and signs. In examinations, regular menstrual cycle and biphasic BBT can be found. Before menstruation, endometrium through diagnostic curettage show secretory period change. After the increase of BBT, estrogenemia, pregnendione can be in normal range. 2-4 days after the increase of BBT, no stigmas in ovary under abdominoscope are found. To sum up, a confirmed diagnosis about this disease can be made, on one hand, on the basis of overall analysis of the above conditions; and, on the other hand, on the basis of successive observation for 2-3 menstrual periods. At present, the following methods are

288

adopted for confirmed diagnosis: ① Abdominoscopy: The method is applied at the best time, usually at 12-48 hours after ovulation suggested by BBT and B-ultrasonic examinations. If there is no stigma or corpus luteum in the ovary after the increase of BBT for 2-4 days, then, on the whole, the diagnosis of LUFS can be confirmed. Under abdominoscope, ovary biopsy pharmacological examination is more important in making a confirmed diagnosis. ② Monitoring of Growth and Development: For the convenience of evaluating the growth and development of ovary follicles, B-ultrasonic examination should be conducted during menstrual period, i. e., 4 days before predicted ovulation until 3 days after blood LH peak, one time per day, but one time every 2-3 days during the other days. Normally, before ovulation, follicular diameter is 21. 2 ± 0. 53mm. After ovulation, the dominant follicles become smaller or their border becomes vague with plicae. 1-2 days later, an area of dense light spots appears, indicating the formation of corpus luteum. The whole ovary becomes low echo area, and hydrops can be seen in the retrorectal excavation area. B-ultrasonic scanning examination of LUFS patients shows none of the above symptoms and signs of ovulation before LH peak. There is no difference in follicular growing curve between LUFS patient and the normal one. After LH peak, follicles continue to become large with an averaged diameter of 33. 5mm. No area of dense light spots and hydrops are observed. B-ultrasonic scanning examination has such advantages as simplicity, ease, no injury, successive observation and follow-up study. ③ Abdominal Fluid Examination: 2-4 days after BBT increases, abdominal fluid is aspirated through abdominoscope or posterior fornix for observation. If abdominal fluid coagulates quickly, and estradiol and pregnendione contents in it are remarkably lower than normal values, then LUFS confirmed diagnosis can be made. ④ Endocrine Examination: After measurement, blood LH peak value, FSH value are lower than those of the normal ones or BBT is slowly lowered in returning to normal condition. This is for reference (Gui Suiqi, 1987).

2. In the case with female sterility due to unknown causes,

ultrasonic scanning is applied to estimate LUFS. The scanning is carried out with real-time fan-shaped probe with a working frequency of 3.5MHz. If at first scanning confirms that the averaged diameter of the follicles is shorter than 17mm, then it is carried out again 48 hours later. If the diameter is longer or equal to 17mm, scanning is conducted the next day. The cycle can be determined through BBT and next menstruation. The scanning is conducted until follicular rupture appears or BBT increases for 4 days during luteal phase. The diagnosis of rupture of follicles is determined through ruptured follicle together with reduced volume, inner echo, and increased hydrops in retrorectal excavation area. The average diameter of each follicle is calculated out of the averaged value of longitudinal, transverse and anteroposterior meridiani. Of 30 patients in this study, ultrasonic scanning confirmed that the averaged follicular diameter before follicular rupture was 22.1mm, and 3 days before rupture, the averaged increasing rate was 2.35mm. The incidence of LUFS among the infertile patients was 6-79% after abdominoscopy; but, 47% of the women having reproductive ability were found to have no ovulatory spots 2-4 days before predicted ovulatory date after abdominoscopy. This may be related to the quick restoration of epithelium of ovulatory spots. Recent reports declared that in patients with female sterility due to unknown causes, 57% of the patients suffered from LUFS, among whom, part of the patients were found to have ovulatory spots observed under abdominoscope. Because ovulatory spots can not be found through ultrasonic scanning, the incidence of LUFS is overpredicted. Generally, if unruptured follicles happen during two successive menstrual periods, it can be confirmedly diagnosed that the patient suffers from LUFS (Daly, et al, 1985).

3. Evaluation of ultrasonic examination and abdominoscopy in the diagnosis of LUFS

For further examination, B-ultrasonic examination and abdominoscopy were conducted to 23 sterile patients with normal menstruation, biphasic BBT, except for obstruction in oviduct. They underwent abdominoscopy in 2-4 days when

290

BBT increased. Among them, 10 had ovulation, and were found to have stigma and blood stain on the surface of one side of ovary under abdominoscope. The result is consistent with the result of B-ultrasonic monitoring. There were ovulatory signs. 13 patients were found to have LUFS, and no stigma and blood stain were found on the surface of the ovary under abdominoscope. What was found only was ova with diameters about 15-20mm. The "B-ultrasound" monitoring suggested no signs of ovulation. It was also found that five LUFS patients were complicated with light endometriosis, and one with middle-degree endometriosis. The report held that abdominoscopy is significant in confirming LUFS, but it is best to apply the method in 2-4 days after BBT increases, combined with serial B-ultrasonography, the diagnostic correctness can be improved. Abdominoscopy is only applied in one menstrual cycle, and repeated application of it is not suggested; however, ultrasonography is better in confirming ovulation. What's more, it is simple, easy and undamageable. A definite conclusion of the observation and evaluation of the growth and development of the follicles, of whether ovulation happens and curative effect can be got through monitoring of the same menstruation or several menstrual cycles; therefore, it has greater clinical value (Gui Suiqi, et al, 1990).

Hyperprolactinemia

Hyperprolactinemia is caused by pathologic changes of hypothalamus-hypophysis, manifested as lactorrhea, hyposexual function, which leads to anovulation and sterility. The cases of this kind take up 13-33% of the total cases whose female sterility is due to endocrine factors. Hyperlactinemia, no matter what etiological factors, can all cause anovulation or amenorrhea. 3% of primary amenorrhea and 30-33% of secondary amenorrhea are caused by hyperlac tinemia, especially, the incidence rate of hyperlactinemia in the cases with amenorrhea complicated with lactation is even higher (80% of them have hyperlactinemia). To any hyperlactine-

291

mia patients, pituitary adenoma and micropituitary adenoma should be excluded. If female sterility is complicated with irregular menstruation or lactorrhea, or both, the incidence of hyperlactinemia increases.

There are no specialized accounts about this disease in TCM. It can be found in the accounts about menstrual disorders and female sterility.

Etiology and Pathogenesis
• *Deficiency of Kidney and Liver Yin*

Deficiency of the congenital Essence together with the unprosperous Kidney Qi and insufficient Vital Qi and Liver Blood leads to poor nourishment to the Chong and Ren Channels; therefore, there is nothing to be turned into menstruation; or tiredness due to sexual indulgence, abortion, or the Kidney affected because of lingering diseases leads to excessive consumption of Kidney Essence, scanty and insufficiency of Liver Blood, Deficiency of Essence and Blood, insufficiency and impairment of the Chong and Ren Channels. So there is no Blood in the uterus. As a result, scanty menstruation, amenorrhea, the increase of lactin in blood result. At last, female sterility occurs.

• *Stagnation of Heat in the Liver Channel*

Mental depression or impairment of the Liver due to anger leads to the Liver's failure to govern the normal flow of Qi, derangement of Qi and Blood, menoxenia due to dysfunction of the Chong Channel; or long term stagnation of Liver Qi leads to Heat which burns the Uterus, scanty menstruation, the increase of lactin in Blood and female sterility are induced.

Main Points of Diagnosis
Aphoria, scanty menstruation, amenorrhea, or with lactorrhea; serum prolactin (PRL) > 23ng/ml (This can be a standard for diagnosis); enlargement of sella turcica which may be observed from radiograph, defect which can be seen from visual field examination; pituitary adenoma and micropituitary adenoma may be found after CT examination.

Treatment Based on Syndrome Differentiation

● *Deficiency of Liver and Kidney Yin*

Main Symptoms and Signs: Aphoria over a long period of time after marriage, PRL > 23ng/ml, scanty menstruation or amenorrhea, distending pain in breasts, lactorrhea, dysphoria with feverish sensation in chest, palms and soles, headache, dream-disturbed sleep, soreness and weakness of waist and knees, pale and red tongue with thin coating, deep feeble pulse, or thready choppy pulse.

Analysis of the Symptoms and Signs: The excessive consumption of the Liver and the Kidney leads to Deficiency of Essence and Blood; therefore, Deficiency and impairment of the Chong and Ren Channels result. This is the reason of scanty menstruation or amenorrhea, the increase of PRL in serum; and at last, female sterility occurs. Because of Deficiency of Liver Blood and Kidney Essence, the Liver Collaterals can not get nourishment. This is the reason of distending breasts and occasional lactorrhea. Other symptoms and signs indicate Deficiency of Liver and Kidney Yin.

Treatment Principles: Nourishing the Liver and restoring the Kidney.

Prescription: Gui Shen Wan Jiajian (Modified Bolus for Invigorating the Spleen-Yin)

Prepared rehmannia root (Radix Rehmanniae) 12g, dogwood fruit (Fructus Corni) 9g, wolfberry fruit (Fructus Lycii) 15g, mulberry (Fructus Mori) 15g, dodder seed (Semen Cuscutae) 9g, eucommia bark (Cortex Eucommiae) 9g, Chinese yam (Rhizoma Dioscoreae) 15g, poria (Poria) 9g, Chinese angelica root (Radix Angelicae Sinensis) 9g, white peony root (Radix Paeoniae Alba) 9g, epimedium (Herba Epimedii) 15g, moutan bark (Cortex Moutan Radicis) 9g, red sage root (Radix Salviae Miltiorrhizae) 30g and motherwort (Herba Leonuri) 30g. All the above drugs are decocted in water for oral administration, one dose daily, and continuously over 1-3 months.

Analysis of the Prescription: The first four drugs in the prescription nourish and invigorate the Liver and the Kidney. Dodder seed (Semen Cuscutae) and eucommia bark (Cortex Eucommiae) tonify and replenish Kidney Qi. Chi-

293

nese yam (Rhizoma Dioscoreae) and poria (Poria) reinforce the Spleen and regulate Qi in the Middle Jiao. Chinese angelica root (Radix Angelicae Sinensis) and white peony root (Radix Paeoniae Alba) decrease Yin exhaustion with astringent and replenish Blood. Epimedium (Herba Epimedii) warms and restores Kidney Yang. Moutan bark (Cortex Moutan Radicis), red sage root (Radix Salviae Miltiorrhizae), motherwort (Herba Leonuri) clear Heat and cool Blood, promote the circulation of Blood to remove Blood Stasis.

• *Liver Heat due to Stagnation of Liver Qi*

Main Symptoms and Signs: *No pregnancy over a long period of time after marriage, serum PRL >23ng/ml, uncertainty of the delay and precedence of menstruation, scanty menstruation or amenorrhea, distending pain of breasts before menstruation, lactorrhea, dysphoria, feverish sensation in both palms and soles, dry mouth and constipation, red tongue with thin yellowish coating, stringy rapid and thready pulse.*

Analysis of the Symptoms and Signs: Mental depression leads to the Liver's failure to govern the flow of Qi. As a result, derangement of Qi and Blood, menoxenia due to dysfunction of the Chong Channel happens. This is the reason of uncertainty of the delay and precedence of menstruation. The lingering stagnation of Liver Qi leads to Heat transmission which burns the Uterus; as a result, there is no Blood for menstruation. This is the reason of scanty menstruation, amenorrhea and the increase of serum PRL. As a result, it leads to female sterility. The stagnation of Liver Qi and transmission due to the lingering stagnation of Liver Qi force the milk to overflow or squeeze out. Irritability and feverish sensation in both palms and soles, dry mouth and constipation. Tongue and pulse conditions indicate Liver Heat produced by stagnation of Liver Qi.

Treatment Principles: Removing Heat from the Liver and regulating the flow of Liver Qi.

Prescription: Dan Zhi Xiaoyao San Jianjian (Modified Ease Powder Supplemented with Moutan bark and Capejasmine Fruit)

294

Moutan bark (Cortex Moutan Radicis) 9g, capejasmine fruit (Fructus Gardeniae) 9g, scutellaria root (Radix Scutellariae), bupleurum root (Radix Bupleuri) 9g, Chinese angelica root (Radix Angelicae Sinensis) 9g, white peony root (Radix Paeoniae Alba) 9g, poria (Poria) 9g, white atractylodes rhizome (Rhizoma Atractylodis Macrocephalae) 9g, cyperus tuber (Rhizoma Cyperi) 9g, chuangxiong rhezome (Rhizoma Ligustici Chuangxiong) 9g, motherwort (Herba Leonuri) 30g, glossy privet fruit (Fructus Ligustri Lucidi) 12g, eclipta (Herba Ecliptae) 12g and germinated barley (Fructus Hordei Germinatus) 30g. The above drugs are decocted in water for oral administration, one dose daily and continuously over 1-3 months.

Analysis of the Prescription : Moutan bark (Cortex Moutan Radicis), capejasmine fruit (Fructus Gardeniae), scutellaria root (Radix Scutellariae) remove irritability, induce diuresis, clear Heat and cool Blood. Bupleurum root (Radix Bupleuri) soothe the Liver and regulate the flow of Qi. Chinese angelica root (Radix Angelicae Sinensis) and white peony root (Radix Paeoniae Alba) nourish Blood and tonify the Liver. The three drugs combined together invigorate the Liver itself and assist the function of the Liver. Poria (Poria) and white atractylodes rhizome (Rhizoma Atractylodis Macrocephalae) tonify the Middle Jiao and regulate the Spleen. Cyperus tuber (Rhizoma Cyperi), chuangxiong rhezome (Rhizoma Ligustici Chuangxiong) and motherwort (Herba Leonuri) soothe the Liver and regulate the flow of Qi, promote the circulation of Blood to remove Blood Stasis. Glossy privet fruit (Fructus Ligustri Lucidi), eclipta (Herba Ecliptae) reinforce and nourish the Liver and the Kidney. Germinated barley (Fructus Hordei Germinatus) removes distending pain of the breasts and stops milk secretion.

Current Research

1. According to case history and laboratory examinations, after the treatment based on Syndrome Differentiation in combination with differentiation of diseases, of 76 cases, except for two cases who were confirmedly diagnosed to suffer

from from hypophysis carcinoma, 49 (66.2%) normally got pregnant. PRL of 23 cases returned to normal state, and that of five cases decreased to 50ng/ml. The total effective rate was 93.2%.

Nourishing and Restoring the Liver and the Kidney: It was applied to the cases with amenorrhea, lactation, ovulatory disorder, scanty menstruation, dysfunction of part of corpus luteum. Liuwei Dihuang Wan Jiajian (Modified Decoction of Six Ingredients Including Rehmannia) is used including Prepared rehmannia root (Radix Rehmanniae), Chinese yam (Rhizoma Dioscoreae), poria (Poria), moutan bark (Cortex Moutan Radicis), dogwood fruit (Fructus Corni), epimedium (Herba Epimedii), curculigo rhizome (Rhizoma Curculiginis), dodder seed (Semen Cuscutae), wolfberry fruit (Fructus Lycii) and glossy privet fruit (Fructus Ligustri Lucidi).

Clearing Away Heat from the Liver and Removing Stagnation: It was applied to the cases with dysfunction of corpus luteum. Dan Zhi Xiaoyao San Jiajian (Modified Ease Powder Added with Moutan Bark and Capejasmine Fruit) is used including Bupleurum root (Radix Bupleuri), scutellaria root (Radix Scutellariae), pinellia tuber (Rhizoma Pinelliae), moutan bark (Cortex Moutan Radicis), capejasmine fruit (Fructus Gardeniae), Chinese angelica root (Radix Angelicae Sinensis), chuangxiong rhezome (Rhizoma Ligustici Chuangxiong), peony root (Radix Paeoniae), eclipta (Herba Ecliptae), glossy privet fruit (Fructus Ligustri Lucidi). During menstruation, Taohong Siwu Tang (Pink Decoction of Four Ingredients) was used together with motherwort (Herba Leonuri). The author held that 20-30% of the endocrine female sterility cases are caused by hyperlactinemia. Therefore, in the gynecological cases with endocrine diseases, routine PRL determination is helpful in obtaining correct diagnosis and finding reasons of female sterility. Clinical curative effects and results from laboratory show that method of clearing Heat from the Liver and removing stagnation can regulate the functions of hypothalamus-hyophysis-ovary sexual gland axis so that therapeutic effects are improved (Niu Dehui, 1990).

296

2. It holds that hyperlactinemia is one of most commonly seen in hypothalamus-hyophysis disorders. The increase of serum lactin caused by any reasons is accompanied with sexual dysfunction or female sterility. The common Syndrome types are stagnation of Liver Qi, stagnation of Heat in the Liver Collaterals. The following prescriptions are commonly used including Dan Zhi Xaoyao San (Ease Powder Supplemented with Moutan Bark and Capejasmine Fruit), Longdan Xigan Tang (Decoction of Gentian for Purging Liver Fire), Zhibo Dihuang Tang (Decoction of Anemarrhena, Phellodendron and Rehmannia) and Zengyie Tang (Decoction for Increasing Fluid) combined with such drugs that activate the circulation of Blood and remove obstruction from collaterals as chuangxiong rhezome (Rhizoma Ligustici Chuangxiong), Chinese angelica root (Radix Angelicae Sinensis), red peony root (Radix Paeoniae Rubra), red sage root (Radix Salviae Miltiorrhizae), peach kernel (Semen Persicae), vaccaria seed (Semen Vaccariae), sweetgum fruit (Fructus Liquidambaris), etc. to clear Heat and activate the Liver Channel, nourish Yin and purge Liver Fire, promote the circulation of Blood and remove Blood Stasis, and regulate the flow of Qi and relieve Qi stagnation. For the case complicated with unpatent oviduct, added were such drugs that remove Heat Phlegm, soften and resolve hardness as Japanese sea tangle (Thallus Laminariae), sea weed (Sargassum), sprunella spike (Spica Prunellae), burreed tuber (Rhizoma Sparganii), etc. For the case complicated with immune female sterility, anti-immunity materia medica were added. Through lactin inhibiting factor PIF secreted from hypothalamus, the above prescriptions and drugs influence dopaminergic neurons to decrease lactin level in Blood, or directly act at the cells secreting lactin of hyophysis, and stimulate dopaminergic receptor. What's more, they may make the enlarged hypophysis return to normal state. Through blood rheology, microcirculation determination, and the weight of hypophysis, ovary and the uterus, determination of FSH, LH, E_2, P, PRL, PGE_2, $PGF_{2\alpha}$, TXB_2 and the determination of follicle count, pregnancy indices, animal experimental research support the results of clinical research (Jin Weixin,

297

1989-1990).

3. 19 cases with hyperlactinemia treated with TCM and western medicine combined. Determination showed that PRL was 470-4,000mIu/L, and no cancer was found in sella turcica radiographs of the 19 patients. Microglandular cancer was found through CT examination of two of them, and the remaining cases having no obvious symptoms of cancer belonging to Adson's syndrome (idiopathic amenorrhea-lactorrhea syndrome). Among them, 13 with amenorrhea, and 5 with scanty menstruation, and 1 without any symptoms and signs. 11 were given bromocriptine together, doses were different from 2.5mg×14 to 2.5mg×180, etc.

Treatment based on Syndrome Differentiation is discussed as follows: ① Heat-Transmission due to Stagnation of Liver Qi: Prescription: Dan Zhi Xiao Yao San (Ease Powder Supplemented with Moutan Bark and Capejasmine Fruit) including Moutan bark (Cortex Moutan Radicis) 10g, stir-baked capejasmine fruit (Fructus Gardeniae) 10g, white atractylodes rhizome (Rhizoma Atractylodis Macrocephalae), bupleurum root (Radix Bupleuri) 10g, Chinese angelica root (Radix Angelicae Sinensis) 10g, red peony root (Radix Paeoniae Rubra) 10g, white peony root (Radix Paeoniae Alba) 10g, poria (Poria) 10g, cyperus tuber (Rhizoma Cyperi) 10g, Sichuan Chinaberry (Fructus Meliae Toosendan) 10g, curcuma root (Radix Curcumae), fruit of Crataegus (Fructus Crataegi) 10g respectively, motherwort (Herba Leonuri) 15g, Herba Lycopi 10g and trichosanthes fruit (Fructus Trichosanthes) 12g. For the case with breasts lumps, vaccaria seed (Semen Vaccariae) is added. ② Impairment of the Kidney and Deficiency of Blood: Prescription: Bushen Gujing Tang Er Hao (Decoction No. II for Restoring the Kidney and Promoting Menstruation) together with Cu Huangti Tang (Decoction for Promoting the Development of Corpus Luteum) including Astragalus root (Radix Astragali Seu Hedysari) pseudostellaria root (Radix Pseudostellariae), prepared rehmannia root (Radix Rehmanniae), chuangxiong rhezome (Rhizoma Ligustici Chuangxiong), Chinese angelica root (Radix Angelicae Sinensis), white peony root (Radix Paeoniae Alba), dodder seed (Semen Cuscutae), wolfberry

298

fruit (Fructus Lycii), raspberry (Fructus Rubi), mulberry (Fructus Mori), desertliving cistanche (Herba Cistachi), antler glue (Colla Cornus Cervi), motherwort (Herba Leonuri), Herba Lycopi. Drugs of the other prescriptions include bupleurum root (Radix Bupleuri), Chinese angelica root (Radix Angelicae Sinensis), white peony root (Radix Paeoniae Alba), chuangxiong rhezome (Rhizoma Ligustici Chuangxiong), Sichuan Chinaberry (Fructus Meliae Toosendan), cyperus tuber (Rhizoma Cyperi), lindera root (Radix Linderae), sweetgum fruit (Fructus Liquidambaris), dodder seed (Semen Cuscutae), epimedium (Herba Epimedii), wolfberry fruit (Fructus Lycii), antler glue (Colla Cornus Cervi), motherwort (Herba Leonuri) and herba lycopi. ③ Impaired Liver and Yang Deficiency: Prescription: Flavored Decoction for Restoring the Kidney and Invigorating the Channels No. I including Baked astragalus root (Radix Astragali Seu Hedysari), dangshen (Radix Codonopsis Pilosulae), Chinese angelica root (Radix Angelicae Sinensis), chuangxiong rhezome (Rhizoma Ligustici Chuangxiong), prepared rehmannia root (Radix Rehmanniae), white peony root (Radix Paeoniae Alba), dodder seed (Semen Cuscutae), wolfberry fruit (Fructus Lycii), morinda root (Radix Morindae Officinalis), curculigo rhizome (Rhizoma Curculiginis), epimedium (Herba Epimedii), antler glue (Colla Cornus Cervi), motherwort (Herba Leonuri), Herba lycopi, cinnamon bark (Cortex Cinnamomi) and safflower (Flos Carthami). Prescription for Soaking Feet: Cinnamon bark (Cortex Cinnamomi), tail of Chinese angelica root (Radix Angelicae Sinensis), cyathula root (Radix Cyathulae), clematis root (Radix Clematidis), safflower (Flos Carthami), common fennel fruit (Fructus Foeniculi), morinda root (Radix Morindae Officinalis) and chuangxiong rhezome (Rhizoma Ligustici Chuangxiong).

Therapeutic effects: 6 became pregnant after the treatment (Zhou Wenyu, 1989-1990).

Immunological Sterility

Immunological sterility refers to sterility due to immunological factors. 20% of the sterile couple suffer from sterility due to unknown causes. With the progress of genesioimmunological research, it is believed that most cases of the sterility are caused by immunological factors. Because of female's inflammation of genital duct, local exudate increases, the immune correlated cells enter genital duct; and at the same time, the change of mucosal osmosis of the genital duct enhances the absorption of spermia antibody; and as natural adjuvants, the infective agents like bacteria and viruses, etc. strengthen immune response of the human body to antibodies. Therefore, antisperm antibody appears in the local area of the genital duct and in the serum, which affects the activity of the spermia, and interferes with fertilization. Therefore, sterility occurs. Or the human body is invaded by an antigen which cross-reacts with pellucid zone, or the degeneration of pellucid zone caused by infective agents stimulates the body to produce anti-pellucid zone, interferes with combination of spermia and pellucid zone, and blocks fertilizing process. As a result, sterility occurs. This is called zona pellucida immunology.

Etiology and Pathogenesis

In TCM, there is no record of immune sterility which is most often found in the records of irregular menstruation and female sterility.

• *Excessive Consumption of Kidney Yin*

The excessive consumption of Kidney Yin leads to insufficiency of Essence and Blood and the Chong and Ren Channels, and to poor nourishment of Uterine Collaterals. As a result, female sterility occurs. Or hyperactivity of Fire due to Yin Deficiency leads to Heat accumulation in the Chong Channel and to the burning of the Uterus. As a result, sterility occurs.

• *Blood Stasis due to Cold*

300

The remaining blood during menstruation and in fetal abortion, infected with pathogenic Cold, Blood Stasis due to accumulation of Cold, obstruction of Uterine Collaterals—all of this leads to female sterility.

Main Points of Diagnosis
1. Other causes of sterility of both female and male are excluded through clinical and various examinations.
2. Positive antisperm antibody of serum or cervical mucus; or positive antiovazona antibody.
3. Two hours before ovulation and after sexual activity, fewer than five spermia that can sthenically go forward in cervical mucus are found under high power perimeter.
4. Before ovulation, under the test mirror of contact test of spermia and cervical mucus, the spermia on the contacting surface of cervical mucus are seen to be trembling, inactive, or acting slowly.

To sum up, to a couple with sterility due to unknown causes, male's spermia are normal after routine examination, and many times of Huhner's test show negative, and in the serum or cervical mucus, there are antispermia antibodies, or the antibodies of antiovazona pellucida show positive, then immune sterility can be diagnosed confirmedly.

Treatment Based on Syndrome Differentiation
 • *Excessive Consumption of Kidney Yin*
Main Symptoms and Signs: No pregnancy long after marriage, immune test being positive, preceded scanty menstruation, dark red and sticky, with no blood clots; or regular menstruation, thin body, weakness and soreness of lumbar area and knees, dizziness and palpitations, dysphoria with feverish sensation in chest, palms and soles, dry mouth and throat, red tongue with thin coating, thready and rapid pulse.

Analysis of the Symptoms and Signs: Excessive consumption of Kidney Yin leads to accumulation of Heat in the Chong Channel, dysfunction of sexual gland axis and hypophysis-adrenal cortex system. This results in immune test being positive and no pregnancy long after marriage. Defi-

301

ciency of Kidney Yin results in Interior Heat which interferes with the Chong Channel and forces Blood to advance. As a result, menstruation is preceded. Deficiency of water and hyperactivity of Fire leads to scanty, dark and sticky menstruation. Insufficiency of Essence and Blood leads to poor nourishment of the limbs, which results in emaciation. The Kidney is located in lumbar area. The insufficiency of Kidney Essence leads to weakness and soreness of the lumbar area and knees. Insufficiency of Blood and Yin results in poor nourishment of the Heart and the Liver. Then dizziness and palpitations result. Yin and Blood Deficiency leads to rising of the Monarch Fire (Heart Fire) which results in dysphoria with feverish sensation in chest, palms and soles, dry mouth and throat. Other symptoms and signs suggest hyperactivity of Fire due to Yin Deficiency.

Treatment Principles: Restoring the Kidney to enrich Essence; helping pregnancy by anti-immunity.

Prescription: Kang Mianyi Yihao (Prescription No. I for Anti-immunity) (Prescription based on clinical experience of the author)

Dried rehmannia root (Radix Rehmanniae) 12g, dogwood fruit (Fructus Corni) 9g, ophiopogon root (Radix Ophiopogonis) 9g, white peony root (Radix Paeoniae Alba) 9g, eclipta (Herba Ecliptae) 12g, tortoise plastron (Plastrum Testudinis) 30g, fresh-water turtle-shell (Carapax Trionycis) 30g, moutan bark (Cortex Moutan Radicis) 9g, red sage root (Radix Salviae Miltiorrhizae) 30g, astragalus root (Radix Astragali Seu Hedysari) 30g, prepared siberian solomonseal rhizome (Rhizoma Polygonati) 15g, scutellaria root (Radix Scutellariae) 9g, panicled swallowwort root (Radix Cynanchi Paniculati) 9g and dried licorice (Radix Glycyrrhizae) 9g. All the above drugs are decocted in water for oral administration, one dose daily, and successively over 1-3 months.

Analysis of the Prescription: The first 5 drugs clear Heat and promote the production of body fluids, nourish and tonify the Liver and the Kidney. Moutan bark (Cortex Moutan Radicis), red sage root (Radix Salviae Miltiorrhizae) remove Blood Stasis and promote the circulation of Blood. Astragalus root (Radix Astragali Seu Hedysari) tonifies Qi of the Middle Jiao to prevent drugs bitter in taste and cold in nature from damaging the Spleen and Stomach. Prepared siberian solomonseal rhizome (Rhizoma Polygonati) nourishes Yin and nourishes Blood. Scutellaria root (Radix Scutellariae) clears Heat and purges Fire. Panicled swallowwort root (Radix Cynanchi Paniculati) expels Wind and removes Toxins. Dried licorice (Radix Glycyrrhizae) clears Heat and removes Toxins, and coordinates the actions of various ingredients in the prescription.

Research has shown such drugs that nourish Yin and cool Blood as dried rehmannia root (Radix Rehmanniae), ophiopogon root (Radix Ophiopogonis), white peony root (Radix Paeoniae Alba), moutan bark (Cortex Moutan Radicis), eclipta (Herba Ecliptae), tortoise plastron (Plastrum Testudinis) and fresh-water turtle shell can inhibit hyperimmunity, counteract against allergic pathological changes, reduce or remove the side effects caused by treatment of immunosuppressants. What's more, tortoise plastron (Plastrum Testudinis), fresh-water turtle shell can help increase phagocytic activity of reticuloendothelial system. Dogwood fruit (Fructus Corni), white peony root (Radix Paeoniae Alba), dried rehmannia root (Radix Rehmanniae), ophiopogon root (Radix Ophiopogonis), eclipta (Herba Ecliptae), fresh-water turtle shell not only strengthen immunity but also restrain immunity. Moutan bark (Cortex Moutan Radicis) and red sage root (Radix Salviae Miltiorrhizae) promote the circulation of Blood to remove Blood Stasis, relieve inflammation, decrease permeability of capillary, reduce exudate from inflammation, strengthen absorption and restrict cellular immunity and humor immunity. Astragalus root (Radix Astragali Seu Hedysari) and prepared siberian solomonseal rhizome (Rhizoma Polygonati) can improve non-specific immunological functions. For example, it can increase lymphocyte transformation rate and phagocytic activity of reticuloendothelial system. Astragalus root (Radix Astragali Seu Hedysari) also can increase the content of plasma cAMP, enhance body fluids immunity and increase immunoglobulin (Ig) content, possess the function of dual-directional regula-

303

tion of immunity activity. Scutellaria root (Radix Scutellariae) clears Heat and removes Toxins, and not only has the function of dual-directional regulation of immunity activity, but also can increase lymphocyte transformation rate and improves phagocytic activity of white blood cells (WBC). Panicled swallowwort root (Radix Cynanchi Paniculati) has comprehensive anti-immune function. Dried licorice (Radix Glycyrrhizae) has hormonal function which is similar to that of deoxycorticosterone. Therefore, it is considered as immunosuppressant used for anti-allergy and removing inflammation.

• *Blood Stasis due to Accumulation of Cold*

Main Symptoms and Signs: No pregnancy long after marriage, immune test being positive, scanty and dark menstruation during the latter stage of menstruation, usually pain in lower abdomen which becomes severe by coldness and which is relieved by warmth, purplish dark tongue or with ecchymosis and petechia along the border, tense thready or deep thready pulse.

Analysis of the Symptoms and Signs: Blood Stasis obstructs at Uterine Collaterals and stops at the Uterus with pathogenic Cold. Therefore, dysfunction of the body's sexual glandular axis and hypophysis-adrenocortical system. It results in immune test being positive, and non-pregnancy occurs. Cold accumulates and obstructs in the Uterus and Uterine Collaterals; as a result, menstruation is scanty at the latter stage of menstruation. Blood clots come out with menstruation; therefore, menstrual color is dark purplish with blood clots. If Blood Stasis is not severe, menstruation can be normal, pathogenic Cold stays and combines with Blood, which leads to pain in lower abdomen and the pain gets more severe by coldness and is relieved by warmth. The conditions of tongue and pulse indicate Blood Stasis.

Treatment Principles: Promoting the circulation of Blood to remove Blood Stasis; helping pregnancy by anti-immunity.

Prescription: Kang Mianyi Erhao (Prescription No. II for Anti-immunity) (Prescription from clinical experience of the author)

Chinese angelica root (Radix Angelicae Sinensis) 9g, white peony root (Radix Paeoniae Alba) 9g, chuangxiong rhezome (Rhizoma Ligustici Chuangxiong) 9g, peach kernel (Semen Persicae) 9g, safflower (Flos Carthami) 9g, corydalis tuber (Rhizoma Corydalis) 9g, red sage root (Radix Salviae Miltiorrhizae) 30g, motherwort (Herba Leonuri) 18g, cinnamon bark (Cortex Cinnamomi) 6g, epimedium (Herba Epimedii) 15g, dodder seed (Semen Cuscutae) 9g, astragalus root (Radix Astragali Seu Hedysari) 30g, panicled swallowwort root (Radix Cynanchi Paniculati) 9g and dried licorice (Radix Glycyrrhizae) 9g. All the above drugs are decocted in water for oral administration, one dose daily, and successively over 1-3 months.

Analysis of the Prescription: The first eight drugs promote the circulation of Blood and remove Blood Stasis, promote the flow of Qi and alleviate pain. Cinnamon bark (Cortex Cinnamomi), epimedium (Herba Epimedii) and dodder seed (Semen Cuscutae) warm and restore Kidney Yang. Astragalus root (Radix Astragali Seu Hedysari) tonifies Qi of the Middle Jiao. Panicled swallowwort root (Radix Cynanchi Paniculati) dispels Wind and removes Toxins, and coordinates the actions of various ingredients in the prescription.

Modern research has shown that Chinese angelica root (Radix Angelicae Sinensis), white peony root (Radix Paeoniae Alba), chuangxiong rhezome (Rhizoma Ligustici Chuangxiong), peach kernel (Semen Persicae), safflower (Flos Carthami), corydalis tuber (Rhizoma Corydalis), red sage root (Radix Salviae Miltiorrhizae), motherwort (Herba Leonuri) have anti-inflammation function to several experimental inflammations of different types, decrease permeability of capillary and reduce exudate from inflammation, strengthen absorption and improve blood rheological property. What's more, safflower (Flos Carthami), chuangxiong rhezome (Rhizoma Ligustici Chuangxiong) and white peony root (Radix Paeoniae Alba) can increase lymphocyte transformation rate, strengthen cellular immunity. Cinnamon bark (Cortex Cinnamomi), epimedium (Herba Epimedii) and dodder seed (Semen Cuscutae) enhance formation or the preceded formation of antibody. Chinese angelica root (Radix Angelicae Sinensis), astragalus root (Radix Astragali Seu Hedysari) possess dual-directional regulating function of immunity. Panicled swallowwort root (Radix Cynanchi Paniculati), dried licorice (Radix Glycyrrhizae) have hormonal function.

Current Research

1. Preliminary observation of related immunological study of TCM drugs. According to their acting behavior and locations of action, drugs were divided into immunostimulant, immunosuppressant, immunomodulator and antiallergic transmitter. Clinically, according to organism immunity in different states, corresponding treatment was conducted. For the case with immune hypofunction, immunostimulants, some acting mainly for cellular immunity, and some chiefly for humor immunity, are applied. For the cases of immune hyperfunction, immunosuppressants are applied. For the case with immune hypofunction, some were caused by insufficiency of T helper lymphocyte (TH); some are caused by hyperfunction of suppressor T lymphocyte; some need block allergic reaction process to relieve pathological damage from the process, for example, the release of allergic inhibiting transmitter; some need to improve tissue damage from allergic reaction process or counteracted against the toxic effect of it. For example, the use of drugs of hormones. To sum up, the nature and location of abnormal immune reaction of the individual patient should be found out, and the corresponding treatment is applied so immune function can be restored and the patient recovers from the disease.

Immunostimulants

Generally, materia medica that strengthen the body resistance and/or restore normal functioning of the body to consolidate the constitution are considered to have immunoenhancement function for the components they stimulate are different. Some stimulate mainly reticuloendothelial system, some mainly cellular immunity, and some mainly humor immunity.

306

Reticuloendothelial System: It is an important constituent in organism protection function and much important in protection against the pathogenic factors like infection, toxicity, radioactive injury, carcinoma and the formation of specific immune reaction, and also involves in metabolism of such substances like fat, protein, steroid, and is closely related to aging process. Generally, in a large degree, the function of reticuloendothelial system reflects the organism's non-specific immunologic function, and is an important indicator of organism's general resistance. In recent years, there have been many reports in literature on the effects of materia medica on reticuloendothelial system. Drugs that have received much observation are Qi-tonifying drugs, Yin Nourishing drugs, drugs that remove Blood Stasis and promote Blood circulation, drugs that clear Heat and remove Toxins and acupuncture as well. Such Qi-tonifying drugs as Chinese angelica root (Radix Angelicae Sinensis), astragalus root (Radix Astragali Seu Hedysari), dangshen (Radix Codonopsis Pilosulae), white atractylodes rhizome (Rhizoma Atractylodis Macrocephalae), licorice (Radix Glycyrrhizae), lucid ganoderma (Gaboderma Lucidium), Chinese yam (Rhizoma Dioscoreae), siberian solomonseal rhizome (Rhizoma Polygonati), etc. are proved to strengthen phagocytic function. The experimental research of Beijing Clinical Medicine Laboratory has found that San Jia Yang Yin Tang (Decoc tion of Three Shell Drugs for Nourishing Yin) which is comprised of tortoise plastron (Plastrum Testudinis), turtle-shell (Carapax Trionycis), oyster shell (Concha Ostreae), dangshen (Radix Codonopsis Pilosulae), red sage root (Radix Salviae Miltiorrhizae) and white peony root (Radix Paeoniae Alba) can obviously enhance phagocytic power of reticuloendothelial system, and it also held that this may be helpful in explaining the concept of nourishing Yin. Such drugs that remove Blood Stasis and promote the circulation of Blood as red sage root (Radix Salviae Miltiorrhizae), red peony root (Radix Paeoniae Rubra), peach kernel (Semen Persicae), burreed tuber (Rhizoma Sparganii), zedoary (Rhizoma Zedoariae), chuangxiong rhezome (Rhizoma Ligustici Chuangxiong), etc. are proved after animal experiment to excite great numbers of macrophages released from reticuloendothe lial system, increase the activity of serum opsonin, enhance phagocytosis and bacterial digestion, and sheep red blood cell (SRBC) digestion of the white cells. What's more, common drugs removing Blood Stasis to promote the circulation of blood all can influence the velocity of the circulation of Blood. If velocity of the circulation of blood is quickened, blood circulation is improved, then phagocytic function is enhanced. This is also a factor of the drugs, promoting the circulation of blood to remove Blood Stasis, increase phagocytic activity of reticuloendothelial system. Such drugs that clear Heat and remove Toxins as honeysuckle flower (Flos Lonicerae), green chiretta (Herba Andrographitis), houttuynia (Herba Houttuyniae), subprostrate sophora root (Radix Sophorae Subprodtratae), wild chrysanthemum flower (Flos Chrysanthemi Indici), oldenlandia (Herba Hedyotis Diffusae) and coptis root (Rhizoma Coptidis), etc. all can enhance phagocytic function of reticuloendothelial system. Clinically, the reasons that drugs clearing Heat and removing Toxins show their effects on curing the infective diseases are, on one hand, because the drugs are proved to be able to kill directly and restrict bacterial through drug sensitive test in vitro; and, on the other hand, that they can enhance the function of immune reaction may be an important factor.

Humor Immunity: Materia medica that can stimulate body fluids immunity include mainly drugs that replenish Qi to invigorate the Spleen and drugs that reinforce the Kidney to support Yang. Astragalus root (Radix Astragali Seu Hedysari), a Qi-replenishing drug, can strengthen the body's power of producing interferon, increase the titer of IF, accelerate the formation of 19S antibody. Pharmacological research has proved that astragalus can not only strengthen humor immunity, increase Ig content, and the titer of plasma thromboplastin, but also improve nourishment to cells, advance protein synthesis and metabolism, enlarge peripheral blood vessels, promote the circulation of Blood. All of this is beneficial to strengthen body resistance against disease.

Cellular Immunity: It is one of the main protective functions of the human body. Generally, it is believed that excessive consumption of Vital Qi in TCM is related to modern medicine's hypoimmunity of the antibody, especially with poor cellular immunocompetence. Drugs that are proved to increase T cells specific value include dangshen (Radix Codonopsis Pilosulae), astragalus root (Radix Astragali Seu Hedysari), Chinese angelica root (Radix Angelicae Sinensis), siberian solomonseal root (Rhizoma Polygonati), white atractylodes rhizome (Rhizoma Atractylodis Macrocephalae), pilose antler (Cornu Cervi Pantotrichum), lucid ganoderma (Gaboderma Lucidium), Chinese yam (Rhizoma Dioscoreae), rehmannia root (Radix Rehmanniae), eclipta (Herba Ecliptae), schisandra fruit (Fructus Schisandrae), dodder seed (Semen Cuscutae), etc. Drugs that accelerate lymphacytic transformation rate include loranthus mulberry mistletoe (Ramulus Loranthi), eclipta (Herba Ecliptae), diding (Herba Violae), buffalo horn (Cornu Rhinocerotis), ephedra (Herba Ephedrae), coptis root (Rhizoma Coptidis), scutellaria root (Radix Scutellariae), schisandra fruit (Fructus Schisandrae), white peony root (Radix Paeoniae Alba), and Liuwei Dihuang Wan (Bolus of Six Ingredients Including Remannia), etc.

Immunosuppressants

They refer to the drugs that inhibit immune reaction. Clinical observation and experimental research have proved that drugs that promote the circulation of Blood and remove Blood Stasis have some inhibiting function to humor immunity and cellular immunity. Clinically, Chinese angelica root (Radix Angelicae Sinensis), white peony root (Radix Paeoniae Alba), chuangxiong rhezome (Rhizoma Ligustici Chuangxiong), motherwort (Herba Leonuri), aucklandia root (Radix Aucklandiae), etc., have better effect in treating immune diseases. Through hemolytic phaque technique, saline agglutination test or serum immunoglobulin content determination, Chinese angelica root (Radix Angelicae Sinensis), peach kernel (Semen Persicae), gentian root (Radix Gentianae), date (Fructus Ziziphi Jujubae), etc. were found to have immunologic inhibiting function. Spatholobus stem (Caulis Spatholobi), safflower (Flos

309

Carthami), red sage root (Radix Salviae Miltiorrhizae), etc. can strengthen absorptive and removal function to sedimented antigen-antibody complex. Motherwort (Herba Leonuri), pangolin scales (Squama Manitis), leech (Hirudo), gradfly can restrain pathologic damage caused by immune reaction of antigen and antibody. Red sage root (Radix Salviae Miltiorrhiz ae), notoginseng (Radix Ginseng), curcuma root (Radix Curcumae) can remove the extra antigens in blood stream to prevent the formation of immunocomplex. Chuangxiong rhezome (Rhizoma Ligustici Chuangxiong), red peony root (Radix Paeoniae Rubra), dalbergia wood (Lignum Dalbergiae Odoriferae), red sage root (Radix Salviae Miltiorrhizae) can improve rheological property of blood. From the above clinical and experimental data, it is believed that the function of removing Blood Stasis and producing healthy energy of these drugs is very much similar to homeostasis of immune reaction. They can be used for the treatment of immune diseases, especially autoimmune diseases. The mechanism is that the drugs can improve and restore the homeostasis of the body's immune system. Such drugs that nourish Yin and cool Blood as rehmannia root (Radix Rehmanniae), moutan bark (Cortex Moutan Radicis), peony root (Radix Paeoniae), glossy privet fruit (Fructus Ligustri Lucidi), eclipta (Herba Ecliptae), glehnia root (Radix Glehniae), ophiopogon root (Radix Ophiopogonis), scrophularia root (Radix Scrophulariae), lucid asparagus (Radix Asparagi), etc. can inhibit hyperimmunologic function, counteract against allergic pathologic changes, reduce or relieve the side effects caused by treatment of immunosuppressants. Licorice (Radix Glycyrrhizae) can also obviously counteract against allergic reaction and have the immunologic inhibiting function. There have also been reports that the drugs clearing Heat and removing Toxins can inhibit immune reaction.

Anti-allergic Transmitters

Pathologic inflammatory changes of allergic reaction are caused by allergic transmitters or biologically active lymphacytic factors, for instance, histamine, 5-hydroxytryptamine (5-TH), bradykinin and slow reacting sub-

310

stance, etc. These active transmitters can cause smooth muscle spasm, the increase of capillary permeability, the oozing of inflammatory cells, necrosis and hyperplasia of tissues, etc.; therefore, inflammatory reaction and pathologic damage result, and various allergic diseases appear. According to clinical and experiment research on materia medica in recent years, such drugs that dispel Wind to remove Damp Cold as large-leaf gentian root (Radix Gentianae), ledebouriella root (Radix Ledebouriellae), tetrandra root (Radix Stephaniae Tetrandrae), earthworm (Lumbricus), portulaca (Herba Portulacae), sweetgum fruit (Fructus Liquidambaris), tribulus fruit Fructus Tribuli), flavescent sophora root (Radix Sophorae Flavescentis), etc. have the effects of anti-allergy, removing inflammation, inhibiting the release of allergic transmitters and regulating permeability of Blood Vessels. Baicalin and baicalein both have the effects of anti-allergy, anti-histamine, and anti-angiotensin. The drugs that remove Blood Stasis by promoting the circulation of Blood like moutan bark (Cortex Moutan Radicis), red peony root (Radix Paeoniae Rubra), Chinese angelica root (Radix Angelicae Sinensis), peach kernel (Semen Persicae), safflower (Flos Carthami), corydalis tuber (Rhizoma Corydalis) have anti-inflammatory effect on several experimental inflammations of different types, and lower the permeability of capillary, reduce inflammatory exudate and strengthen absorption. The water-soluble component part of cyathula root (Radix Cyathulae) can also inhibit the release of allergic transmitters.

Hormones Pharmaceutics

Hormones, showing their effects on immune reaction in different areas, can not only inhibit immune reaction, but also relieve or reduce pathological damage from allergic reaction. Many herbal drugs have hormonal function, and more and more drugs come into being that can stimulate hypothalamus-adrenocortical system whose function will be strengthened. The active principle of common licorice (Radix Glycyrrhizae) is glycyrrhetinic acid whose chemical structure is similar to that of adrenocortical hormones. Therefore, it has an effect similar to that of deoxycorti-

311

costerone. Personal experience proves that drugs that restore the Kidney to reinforce Yang can excite the functions of hypothalamus-adr enocortical system, relieve the side effects of hormones, or assist withdrawal hormones, and reduce dependence on hormones to prevent the state of illness from reoccurrence. Some drugs that replenish Qi and reinforce the Spleen like Yi Gong San (Powder with Marvelous Effect), are also proved to have hormonal functions.

2. TCM and Western Medicine Combined in the Treatment of Immune Female Sterility. 85 couples, serum antisperm antibody being positive, the results of other examinations being normal, with sterility, were given small dose of prednisone 5mg, 2 times a day, and one of the each couple with positive sperm antibody together was treated according to Syndrome Differentiation with such materia medica that promote the circulation of Blood to remove Blood Stasis, and relieve stagnation of Qi to induce diuresis as burreed tuber (Rhizoma Sparganii), zedoary (Rhizoma Zedoariae), pangolin scales (Squama Manitis), thorn of Chinese honey locus (Spina Gleditsiae), etc. Three months accounted for one course of treatment. If antibodies of the both were positive, then they were treated at the same time; what's more, condom should be used. For the case with inflammation, antibiotics were added. For the case with high spermia viscosity, big dose of vitamin C was given. Among 85 cases with positive antibodies, 35 were pregnant with a successful rate of 47% which was markedly higher than that abroad gained only through treatment by cortical hormones (Sun Ce, et al, 1986).

3. "Immune Factors of Female Sterility". It held that 20-40% of the infertile cases are caused by immune factors. Therefore, immunological factors hold an important position in female sterility. Long term sterility of the married couples whose reproductive organs are not found to have organic or dysfunctional diseases is called "non-reason sterility." For this kind of cases, immune sterility should be considered at first. Clinically, some of the patients were found to carry special antisperm antibodies. The antibodies of this kind can cause spermia to agglutinate. The spermia can not move for-

ward or immobilize; therefore, it is hard for them to go across cervical mucus which leads to sterility. The cases with antibodies that brake spermia take up 8. 95% of the whole female sterility cases, but normal men, pregnant women and non-married women were not found to have positive antibodies. Antibodies exist in serum or reproductive duct of both men and women. The antibodies in serum mainly are IgG, IgM and the ones in reproductive duct mainly are IgA and IgG. Some people found that in blood circulation of some infertile women, there are antibodies. They can cause spermia to agglutinate. No antibodies are found in cervical fluid. The reasons that women carry antisperm antibodies generally are that the immune reaction takes place when sperm antigens contact vagina and the uterus during sexual intercourse. But some of the infertile women having no history of sexual activity carry antisperm antibodies. The reason for that is in some tissues of them, there are homologous antigen substances which automatically produce antispermia antibodies. Some other people think that the infected reproductive duct can produce local immune reaction. The antibodies produced from it usually appear in the secretions of cervical canal, uterine cavity, and vagina. That in mucus of cervical canal, there is complement essential for antibodies causing spermia to brake, and the titer of antisperm antibodies in cervical canal is generally higher than that of blood illustrate that the local areas of cervical canal can also produce antisperm antibodies. At present, methods for immune sterility examination include sperm-cervical mucus penetration test, sperm-cervical mucus contact test, sperm agglutination test (SAT), sperm immobilization test (SIT), FLISA, etc. For the case with positive antisperm antibodies, there have been no satisfactory effects. The following methods can be applied: ① Condom Treatment. Condom is used continuously for half a year, even one year. The titer of antibodies is measured periodically. The pregnancy rate is 40-60%. After the use of condom, antisperm antibodies produced in local areas of reproductive duct can be reduced. If condom has been used continuously for 12 months, but antibody titer dose not decrease, it is needed to stop using condom. ② Ar-

313

tificial Fertilization in Cervical Canal. There has been research on artificial fertilization after cervical mucus is removed from the cervical canal. The subjects selected were those whose Huhner's test was abnormal, and whose cervical mucus prevented spermia from going upward in woman's reproductive duct. After being treated with this method, the pregnancy rate of 32 couples reached 44%. ③ Artificial Fertilization in the Uterus. It is referred to the case that there are antibodies in woman's cervical mucus and there are autoantibodies in man. The improved Biggers', Whitten's, and Wlttlngham's solutions were used to douche husband's seminal fluid, and high density sperm suspension without seminal serous fluid was obtained for artificial fertilization in the uterus. This is often successful in treating the couple with immune sterility. ④ Treating infection of reproductive organs (Wu Shuxi, 1987).

Appendix

TO Treat Female's Sterility due to Ovulatory Dysfunction with Sweet Basil

Sweet basil was recorded early in *Materia Medica Written in the Year of Jiahu* (*Jia Hu Ben Cao*), and *Compendium of Materia Medica* (*Ben Cao Gang Mu*), "Because its fragrance is pure, and the ancient people used it for resolving Damp and promoting digestion, it is popularly called Western Queen Vegetable. It is healthily beneficial if eaten." So *Dietary Guidelines* (*Yin Shan Zheng Yao*) says, "Eaten with other vegetables, it tastes pungent and fragrant and can dispel fish-stench smell."

Contemporarily, there has been much research about the volatile oil of sweet basil, both nationally and internationally, most of which is for extract from it as perfume. There has had no research about sweet basil as a herb for treating female sterility.

The Appearance of Sweet Basil

This drug is the dry stalk, branch of sweet basil with leaves fallen. There are brown glandular points on the back of the leaf. The drug is yellowish green. The stalk is in square form with white lanugo hair. When the stalk is broken, it is still linked with fibers, and its center is the white pulp. The petals are in umbrella inflorescence. The host sepal is membranous with fawny color, divided into five parts. It smells fragrant with a refrigerant effect. Its small nut is dark brown, which becomes sticky and slippery, enlarged in size with white mucosa if put into water (Wang Changyong, 1987).

315

Analysis of Chemical Composition

There are 5 species with 3 variants of sweet basil family. What was studied in this research is Ocimum Basilicum L. During protophase of blossoming and the height of blossoming, The volatile oil content contained in it varies greatly, and the compositions of the oil are noticeably different. Because the contents of the two masses ability to be moved: Foeniculoum and linalool are different. The contents of them in the height of blossoming are higher than those in the protophase of blossoming, it is advised to use clinically the drug collected in the height of blossoming when the foeniculoum and linalool of it have estrogen activity and the effect of removing inflammation and analgesia according to both national and international studies. So, these two ingredients are chosen as the active principles to treat female sterility due to ovulatory dysfunction and dysmenorrhea (Wang Zhaolun, et al, 1987).

After measuring the trace elements of sweet basil collected in different times and its different parts by means of atomic absorption spectrophotometer flame photometry, graphite furnace, and fluorospectrophotometry, the results show that there are rich trace elements during the height of sweet basil blossoming (iron 293. 6ppm, manganese 51. 7ppm, zinc 30. 5ppm, copper 12. 6ppm) and also selenium. Compared with such drugs for promoting Blood circulation and removing Blood Stasis as red sage root (Radix Salviae Miltiorrhizae), corydalis tuber (Rhizoma Coptidis), siberian solomonseal rhizome and fresh-water turtle shell, Liuwei Dihuang Wan (Bolus of Six Drugs Including Rehmannia), except that the content of iron of siberian solomonseal rhizome is higher than that of sweet basil (522. 0ppm), the contents of all other elements in sweet basil are higher during the height of sweet basil blossoming. The result of this experiment suggests that the reason why sweet basil can treat female sterility resulting from ovulatory dysfunction not only is because of the estrogen activity contained in it, but also related to the rich trace elements of it (Wang Zhaolun, et al, 1990).

The volatile oil of protophase blossoming and the height of blossoming of Ocimum Basilicum L. of sweet basil is extracted by means of steaming distillation method and analog industrial chemical analysis. The volatile oil of sweet basil of protophase blossoming is 0. 66%, which is noticeably higher than that of sweet basil in the height of blossoming (0.48%). After measuring the compositions of the volatile oil by means of gas chromatograph-mass spectrometer-computer, the result show that the volatile oil of sweet basil in protophase blossoming and in the height of blossoming contains cinnamic acid methyl ester, linalool, foeniculoum, ocimenum and borneol. Different compositions are found in two collection times. For example, there is R-myrcene in the protophase blossoming. The contents of foeniculoum and linalool of the two phases are measured by using work tracing analysis. The result shows that the content of the two matters in the height of blossoming are obviously higher than those of the protophase blossoming. This experiment suggests that collection time should be considered if the drug is used clinically. This experiment shows, too, that the sweet basil oil extracted with analog industrial method is noticeably lower than that extracted with ordinary extraction method, but foeniculoum in the volatile oil is obviously higher than that of the volatile oil extracted with ordinary extraction method. This is for the reference of the production plants to improve extraction technology (Wang Zhaolun, et al, 1990).

Clinical Study
• *Study of Sweet Basil Treating Female Ovulatory Dysfunction*

100 cases were treated with the drug, and 76 cases had complete data and follow-up study. All the cases were married for one year but no pregnancy occurs. All the men received routine seminal fluid analysis, and all the women underwent gynecological examination, while oviduct was tested to see whether it was unobstructed or not, including other examinations except all those functional ovulatory obstacle female sterility factors. Every patient both before and after treatment underwent routine basal body temperature (BBT) measurement in order to observe the clinical curative effects.

317

Indications and Course of Treatment: Ten packages for each menstrual period, start to take the drug, 3 days before menstruation, one night one package (27g/per package), and all together five packages. After the menstruation, take another five packages. Three menstrual periods make one course of treatment. The drug is to be decocted in water for 2 times, for oral administration. Take the decoction before going to bed with little red sugar added, and little sweating will result.

Analysis of Curative Effect: After one course of treatment, 70 cases proved to respond effectively to the treatment, among whom 18 got pregnant. 6 failed to respond to the treatment. The total curative rate was 92.1%. The pregnancy rate was 23.68% and ineffective rate was 7.9%. If considering that 19 had problem of abnormal seminal fluid, 2 with oviduct obstruction, 1 with myoma, muscle gland disease, the pregnancy rate after correction was 35.3%. 1 case underwent natural abortion with an abortion rate was 5.88%.

Research of Mechanism: Sweet basil was taken 3 days before menstruation, then successively for 5 days, and it was the time when estrogen and progesterone were reduced to their lowest levels. Their negative feedback effect toward gonadotropic hormone disappeared. The levels of FSH and LH began to raise. It was a time when the new folliculi of the menstrual period began to develop. When sweet basil was used at the early stage of folliculi, though the levels of FSH and LH increased, the increase was not big enough. At this time, the estrogen secretion from the oviduct was slow and steady, and the active feedback effect of the estrogen was not obvious. Before about 7-8 days, the secretion of estrogen turned from slowness to rapidness and reached its peak. The estrogen of usual oviduct was E_2, 95% of E_2 and sexual hormones combined with SHBG, then with albumin, only 2-5% of E_2 were in free state, and had biological activity.

For intensifying the effect of the drug, 2-3 days after finish of menstruation, (i. e., about 7-8 days before ovulation), sweet basil should be used 5 days more continuously. This intensified the active feedback effect of E_2, and promoted FSH and LH to rise to their peaks rapidly. 24 hours after LH peak, mature folliculi were ovulated. The noticeable cure effect of sweet basil showed that the estrogen sterol extracted from it is a estrogen compound with biological activity and in free state, and so according to hormone level and receptor, it also illustrated that sweet basil can not only promote the growth and development of folliculi, but also the formation of yellow body of ovary (Jin Weixin, et al, 1987).

• *Clinical Observation of the Use of Sweet Basil Capsules in Treating Female Sterility due to Ovulatory Dysfunction*

Clinical Data : 140 cases of patients were observed, among whom, 91 cases were treated with sweet basil capsules (Experimental Group). 49 were treated with clomiphene (control group). Before medical treatment, all the cases underwent gynecological routine examinations, test of unobstruction of oviduct. Before and after medical treatment, all the cases also received examinations of routine basal body temperature, some of whom underwent crystallization test of cervical mucus, endometrium biopsy, radio-immunity examination of blood hormones, the successive measurement of folliculi growth with B-ultrasonic examination. The spouses of the patients underwent routine seminal laboratory analysis. All the 140 cases were married over two years, and were diagnosed to suffer from ovulatory dysfunction after BBT examination. 9 received a combined treatment of clomiphene and/or diethyl stilbestrol, chorionic gonadotropin, 13 were given materia medica, and 34 were given western medicines and materia medica as well.

Therapeutic methods : The experimental group took orally sweet basil capsule on the fifth day of menstruation, three capsules each time, and 2 times a day, and for 5 days. Three menstrual periods accounted for one course of treatment. Sweet basil capsules are produced by Shandong Yantai Traditional Chinese Medicines Pharmaceutical Plant. Each capsule of sweet basil contains 0.25g of water soluble extraction and fat-soluble extraction.

The control group took orally clomiphene capsules on the

319

fifth day of menstrual cycle, one capsule (50mg) a day, and for 5 days. In the second, and the third menstrual cycle, the patients took two capsules a day over 5 days. Three menstrual cycles accounted for one course of treatment.

Therapeutic effects: The changes of BBT was regarded as the indication of curative effect. Before treatment, the BBT of those patients was monophasic, or not typical diphasic, or though diphasic but with poor function of yellow body of ovary. After the treatment, they got pregnant or their BBT changed to be diphasic type, and the function of corpus luteum was improved or excellent. All those whose BBT remained the same were considered to fail. The experimental group took orally sweet basil capsules. For one course of treatment, 83 gained effect, and 8 failed to respond to the treatment. The total effective rate was 91.2%. After the treatment, 23 got pregnant with a pregnancy rate of 25.3%. Considering that the seminal fluid of the spouses of 8 cases was not normal, 1 patient had problem of obstruction of oviduct, the corrected pregnancy rate was 28.1%. After pregnancy, two experienced natural abortion with an abortion rate of 8.7%. After the control group took clomiphene for one course of treatment, 39 gained effects and 10 failed to respond to the treatment. The effective rate was 79.6%. After the treatment, 10 got pregnant with a pregnancy rate of 20.4%. 1 underwent natural abortion, with an abortion rate of 10%.

Personal Experience of Treatment: To use sweet basil capsules to treat female sterility resulting from ovulatory dysfunction, its effect can be seen after one course of treatment. If the effect is not good enough, another course of treatment is needed. If the patient's menstruation is delayed, every menstruation after forty to fifty days, then, prolonging drug-taking time is necessary, i.e., to take the drug on the fifth day of menarche and continuously for seven or more days. In clinical application, there has not had any side or toxic effect found. Animal acute experiments and long-term toxic tests have shown that the drug is safe and reliable.

Animal experiments have confirmed that after sweet basil

320

extract or sweet basil oil is given, the number of ova in the oviduct of the two sides of rats and the content of pregnendione in plasma are obviously higher than those of the control group. The animal pregnancy rate is also noticeably higher than that of the control group. It was found in animal ovulatory test that after being given sweet basil extract or sweet basil oil, the big folliculi and the weight of uterus of rabbit were obviously higher than those of the contrast. Its blood E_2 content was also higher than that of the control group. The chemical extract shows that sweet basil contains E_2, E_3, foeniculoum, and linalool, etc. According to some documental reports, foeniculoum and linalool have estrogen activity and can relieve inflammation and get rid of pain. The estrogen contained in sweet basil through receptor and feedback mechanism promotes the growth of folliculi in ovary and the secretion of pituitary gonadotropic hormone FSH and LH, therefore, promotes ovulation and the restoration of the function of the yellow body of ovary. This has been confirmed in animal experiments.

At present, female sterility due to ovulatory dysfunction is treated with western medicine clomiphene. According to the reports abroad, ovulatory rate because of the use of clomiphene is 70-80%, and the pregnancy rate is 20-30%. What has been reported at home is similar to that abroad. The total effective rate of using sweet basil is 91.2%, and the pregnancy rate is 28.1%, and abortion rate is 8.7%. This indicates that as far as the treatment of female sterility due to ovulatory dysfunction is concerned, the effect of sweet basil can well match that of clomiphene, and abortion shortcoming because of the use of it is less than that of clomiphene. What's more, there are no any side effects. It's more convenient to use capsule preparation than to use decoction.

According to clinical observation, most of the patients with female sterility because of ovulatory dysfunction have symptoms of Kidney Deficiency to the varying degree. Among the 91 cases statistically collected and treated with sweet basil, clinically, Syndrome of Kidney Deficiency was

321

considered to be the main factor, 55 cases were diagnosed as Syndrome Kidney Deficiency; 23, Syndrome Blood Stasis; and 13, Syndrome of Cold Uterus. After the treatment, the total effective rates of Syndrome of Kidney Deficiency and Syndrome of Blood Stasis were close to each other, the former being 92.7%, and the latter being 91.3%. Syndrome Cold Uterus gained poor curative effect, with a total effective rate of 84.6%.

After the confirmation with clinical and basal research, sweet basil not only can cure female sterility due to functional ovulatory dysfunction, the decoction and capsules can also well treat dysmenorrhea. There once was a research on the use of sweet basil for 30 cases with dysmenorrhea. Among 30 cases, there was apparent effect on 21 cases (86. 7%). Basal research has confirmed that sweet basil can restrict the activity of PGF_2 and noticeably restrain the spastic contraction of Blood Vessels and the smooth muscles of uterus, lower the adhesiveness and aggregation of platelet, apparently regulate and improve blood rheology, and lower the specific viscosity of the whole blood and plasma. When it is used clinically, it can not only well regulate menstruation, that is, promote ovulation, cure hypermenorrhea and dysmenorrhea, but also cure sterility, and change the usual principle to treat dysmenorrhea, mostly, use medicines that can control ovulation (Jin Weixin, et al, 1991)

Pharmacological Experimental Study of Sweet Basil

This experiment, through uterogravimetry in rats, medication to the rats whose ovary were taken away, and vaginal smear observation, confirms that sweet basil capsule has estrogen activity. At normal state, estrogen is secreted by ovary. To the immature rat, it can improve the development of its uterus. The group of young rats was given sweet basil extract (no oil in it), and the next group was given basil capsules. Compared with the control group, the two groups had an obvious increase in weight ($P < 0.05$), but the increase of weight of the group given sweet basil capsule was not so apparent as the group given sweet basil extract. This indicates that sweet basil has noticeable estrogen activity, and though sweet basil oil can intensify the effect, it was not so apparent. After the rat with complete ovary was given the drug, after vaginal smear observation examinations, it was found that sweet basil extract capsule and E_2 all can stimulate vaginal epithelial cell differentiation—from deep basal cells to superficial cells gradually, and keratosis takes place. The more the estrogen is, the higher the degree of keratosis is, and it makes it display estrinization. However, the effect of sweet basil capsules is not so strong as that of E_2, and though sweet basil extract can make the rat display estrinization, and epithelial cells keratosis occurs, its effect was not so strong as sweet basil capsules. Experimental results also show that sweet basil capsules could not make ovary increase in weight; that is to say, it has no effect in the growth of development of ovary. This may be because that this drug only has estrogen activity and can not influence hypothalamus and adenohypophysis.

Through young rat ovulation test, plasma progesterone content measurement, and test of rabbit large follicle maturity, it has confirmed that sweet basil capsules promote follicle maturity and ovulation; furthermore, its action is stronger than that of sweet basil extract. Plasma progesterone contents of the two groups are higher than that of the control group, that is, the content reaches pro-ovulatory plasma progesterone level. The more the numbers of ovulation are, the higher the progesterone level is; that is, the ovulatory action of sweet basil capsules and progesterone level show a positive correlation. Rabbit follicle maturity test shows that sweet basil capsules can make increase the numbers of ovulation of large follicles of rabbit ovary; that is, they can make the follicles grow and develop rapidly to pre-ovulating state, and estrogen level is obviously higher than that of pre-administration level and that of control group. After sweet basil capsules were given to the young rats and the rabbits, E_2 level in blood increased rapidly. Under the effect of E_2, G_nRH neuron of hypothalamus releases G_nRH, and therefore, stimulates adenohypophysis to secrete LH and FSH. Especially, sweet basil capsules can make GTH

323

and LH release reach their peaks; therefore, ovulation takes place. Also, sweet basil capsules as an estrogen, which may be like the estrogen, changes to form catecholoestadiol or catecholamine under the effect of α-hydroxylase in hypothalamus that is, catechol estrogen. The estrogens of this kind have both the functions of catecholamine (CA) and estrogen. On one hand, it can strengthen the effect of noradrenaline in the brain through restricting the activity of tyrosine hydroxylase and COMT, and therefore, promote the release of G_nRH. On the other hand, because of the structural similarity with the estrogen, in hypothalamus and adenohyophysis, it may struggle for receptors with estrogen, and counteract against the negative feedback action of estrogen to hypothalamus and adenohypophysis, and build up the sensitivity of adenohyophysis to G_nRH.

That sweet basil capsules can promote ovulation and raise the levels of E_2 and P has been confirmed through experiments. It was found that, the pregnancy rate in sweet basil extract group and sweet basil capsule group was both strikingly higher than that in the control group. Furthermore, the effect of the sweet basil capsule is better than sweet basil extract ($P < 0.01$). Clomiphene group experiment was repeated 2 times, and the pregnancy rates were both lower than those of the control group.

After the study of the effect of promoting the circulation of blood and removing Blood Stasis of sweet basil, and its influence on the myoelectric activity of the smooth muscles of rabbit, the following conclusions have been got: ① When the smooth muscles of the uterus of the rabbit induced by hypophysis contract spasmodically, sweet basil has a strong effect in releasing spasm, reducing the contraction frequency of the muscle tendons of the uterus smooth muscles, and decreasing the spike potential value obviously. In control group, Tong Jing Ling (Magic Pill for Dysmenorrhea) could only reduce the frequency. So, as far as releasing the spasm of the smooth muscle of the uterus induced by hypophysis is concerned, sweet basil is better than Magic Pill for Dysmenorrhea. ② To painful spasm caused by oxytocin, sweet basil has a strong effect in releasing pain, which is stronger than that of Magic Pill for Dysmenorrhea. ③ Sweet basil can notably control platelet aggregation and raise the depolymerization rate, but the effect of Magic Pill for Dysmenorrhea is not as strong as sweet basil. ④ Sweet basil can lower the length, wet weight, dry weight of thrombus forming outside the body compared with those before medical administration, but Magic Pill for Dysmenorrhea has no effect. ⑤ Sweet basil can decrease the specific viscosity of rabbit plasma, but Magic Pill for Dysmenorrhea can remarkably decrease the specific viscosity of the whole blood, the specific viscosity of plasma, and compressed volume, but quicken blood sedimentation. So, it can be seen that sweet basil is effective in treating dysmenorrhea.

References

Cai Xiaosun. 1985. An Analysis of the Treatment of 110 Cases with Sterility. Shanghai Journal of TCM. (9): 18-20

Cao Kaiyong, et al. 1989. Huichun Zhuangyang Ling Yihao (Pill No. I for Youth-Restoring) Is Used to Treat Impotence—Analysis of 102 Cases. TCM and Western Medicine Combined Gynecology and Obstetrics Information Data. 1989-1990 (Totaled No. III): 69

Chen Deyong. 1984. Preliminary Report of Inducing Ovulation by Burying Thread in Sanyinjiao. The Journal of Integrated Chinese and Western Medicine. 4 (9): 521-522

Chen Runwen. 1990. Treatment Based on Syndrome Differentiation of Spermatorrhea. A Symposium of the First East China Area TCM Andrology Seminar. Series No. II

Chen Wenbo. 1989. A Clinical Observation of 100 Cases of Non-liquefaction of Seminal Fluid Treated According to TCM Theory and Syndrome Differentiation. TCM and Western Medicine Combined Gynecology and Obstetrics Information Data. 1989-1990 (Totaled No. III): 65

Chen Wenbo. 1987. A Clinical Analysis of 66 Cases of Male Sterility due to Azoospermia Treated with Shengjing Zanyu Wan (Pill for Sperm Formation and Pregnancy). A Symposium of the First National TCM Andrology Academic Seminar

Dai Deying, et al. 1988. Clinical Summary and Experimental Study of 40 Cases with Sterility due to Endometriosis. Shanghai Journal of TCM. (1): 14-16

Dmowski W P, et al. 1980. The Luteinized Unruptured Follicle Syndrome and Endometriosis. Fertil Steriol. 33 (1): 30

Fan Huaguang, et al. 1987. Treatment of 50 Cases with Endometriosis Complicated with Sterility. Practical Gynecology and Obstetrics Journal. 3 (4): 189-190

Gu Meili, et al. 1988. Serum Pregnendione Determination and Endometrium Biopsy Are Used to Evaluate Corpus Luteum Func-

326

tion, Practical Gynecology Journal. 4 (2): 85

Gui Suiqi. 1987. LUFS. Practical Gynecology and Obstetrics Journal. 3 (4): 211-212

Gui Suiqi, et al. 1990. An Evaluation of Ultrasonic Examination and Abdominoscopy in the Diagnosis of LUFS. A Symposium of the 3rd National TCM and Western Medicine Combined Gynecology and Obstetrics Academic Conference. 154-156

Guo Lianshu. 1988. Research in the Mechanism of the Drugs Restoring the Kidney and Invigorating Yang in the Treatment of Male Sterility. A Symposium of the Second National TCM Andrology Academic Seminar. 13-15

Hamilton C J G M, et al. 1985. Follicle Growth Curves and Normal Patterns in Patients with the Luteinized Unruptured Follicle Syndrome. Fertil Steriol. 43 (4): 541

Jia Kefu, et al. 1988. A Clinical Analysis of 121 Cases with Tubal Sterility Treated with TCM and Western Medicine in Combination. Clinical Medicine. 8 (7): 304-305

Jia Yanbo. 1987. My Views on the Method of Activating the Circulation of Blood and Removing Blood Stasis in Treating Impotence. Hebei Journal of Chinese Medicine. (2): 30

Jin Weixin, et al. 1988. Male Sterility Treated with Shengjing Tang (Decoction for Promoting Spermiogenesis) and Yiehua Tang (Decoction for Sperma Liquefaction)—A Clinical Analysis of 248 Cases. The Journal of Chinese Medicine, 29 (5): 43-45

Jin Weixin. 1984. Yiehua Tang (Decoction for Sperma Liquefaction) and Shengjing Tang (Decoction for Promoting Spermiogenesis) in the Treatment of 30 Cases of Male Sterility. Journal of Shandong TCM College. 8 (2): 29-30

Jin Weixin, et al. 1991. Decoction for Removing Obstruction in Oviduct Treats Sterility due to Obstruction in Oviduct—with a Report of 108 Cases. China Medicine Journal. (2): 32-34

Jin Weixin, et al. 1987. Research of Female Ovulatory Dysfunction Treated with Sweet Basil. Journal of Shandong TCM College. 11 (4): 25-26

Jin Weixin. 1991. A Clinical Observation of Sweet Basil Capsules Treating Sterility due to Ovulatory Dysfunction. The Journal of Medium Medicine. 32 (2): 43-44

Jin Weixin. 1989-1990. TCM Treatment of Hyperlactinemia. Combined TCM and Western Medicine Gynecology and Obstetrics

Information. Total No. 3: 40

Li Biao, et al. 1988. Analysis of the Progress of Syndrome Differentiation and Treatment of 8506 Cases of Male Sterility. A Symposium of the Second National TCM Andrology Academic Seminar. 34-37

Li Guangwen. 1990. Clinical Research on Shiying Yulin Tang (Decoction of Amethyst for Pregnancy) Treating Sterility. Study of Diagnosis of Male and Female Sterility and TCM Treatment (unpublicized data). 32-40

Li Laitian, et al. 1990. Clinical Research in "Do Not Forget to Treat Blood Stasis". A Symposium of the First East China Area Andrology Seminar. Series No. I

Li Shijie. 1989. A Clinical Observation of 41 Cases with Impotence Treated by Acupuncture. TCM and Western Medicine Combined, Gynecology and Obstetrics Information Data. 1989-1990 (Totaled No. III): 69-70

Li Xiangyun. 1989. An Analysis of 87 Cases with Obstructed Oviduct Treated with TCM Drugs. The Journal of Chinese Medicine. (7): 33-35

Li Xiangyun. 1987. Clinical Report of 257 Cases with Sterility Treated According to Syndrome Differentiation. Materia Medica. (10): 38-40

Li Xiangyun. 1989-1990. A Clinical Report of 40 Cases with Endometriosis Treated Mainly with Drugs Promoting the Circulation of Blood to Remove Blood Stasis. TCM and Western Medicine Combined Gynecological and Obstetrical Information. Total No. 3): 46-48

Li Xiangyun. 1989. TCM Drugs Treating 19 Cases with PCOS. Liaoning Journal of Chinese Medicine. 13 (1): 14-15

Lin Zhijun. 1987. A Summary of Treatment of 154 Cases with Ovulatory Sterility. Hubei Journal of Chinese Medicine. (3): 15-17

Liu Jizhang. 1987. Clinical Observation of Acupuncture Induced Ovulation. Beijing Journal of Chinese Medicine. (5): 42-43

Liu Minghan. 1987. A Preliminary Research on Removing Obstacle from the Uterine to Relieve Spermatorrhea in the Treatment of Functional Non-ejaculation. A Symposium of National TCM Andrology Academic Exchange Conference Material

328

Liu Minghan, et al. 1990. An Observation of Clinical Curative Effect of Functional Non-ejaculation Treated Mainly with Tong Jing Ling (Pill for Removing Obstruction in Spermatic Duct)— An Analysis of the Comparison of 130 Cases. A Symposium of the First East China Area Andrology Seminar. Series No. III

Liu Ping, et al. 1988. Enzyme Immunoassay of Urinary LH Combined with Ovulation prediction by Ultrasound and Its Clinical Application. China Gynecology Journal. 23 (2): 66-67

Lu Haonian. 1988. A Clinical Observation of Intrauterine Injection of TCM Drugs Treating Sterility due to Obstructive Fallopian Tube. TCM and Western Medicine Combined Gynecology and Obstetrics Information. Total No. 2: 49-50

Nan Zheng. 1989. Analysis of Curative Effect of 165 Cases of Impotence Treated with Yangling Changchun Dan (Long-Live Youth-Keeping Pill) and Experiment Studies. TCM and Western Medicine Combined Gynecology and Obstetrics Information Data. 1989-1990 (Totaled No. III): 68

Niu Dehui. 1990. Clinical and Laboratory Study of Materia Medica Treating 76 Cases with Hyperlactinemia. A Symposium of the 3rd National Gynecology and Obstetrics Academic Conference TCM and Western Medicine. 179-181

Ou Chun. 1990. A Clinical Observation of 182 Cases of Too Many Dead Spermia. Shanghai Journal of TCM. (5): 26

Qi Guangcong, et al. 1988. A Clinical Observation of 50 Cases with Non-ejaculation Treated by Electrical Massage Machine. A Symposium of the Second National TCM Andrology Academic Seminar. 119

Rice J P. 1986. Obstet Gynecol. 67: 718

Shi Lingyi, et al. 1984. An Analysis of 70 Cases with Polycystic Ovary Syndrome Treated Based on Syndrome Differentiation. The Journal of Chinese Medicine. (2): 111

Shui Houdi. 1990. An Observation of the Comparison of TCM and Western Medicine in the Treatment of Non-ejaculation. The Journal of Chinese Medicine. (4): 38-39

Shui Houdi. 1990. A Clinical Observation of 100 Cases of Non-ejaculation. A Symposium of the First East China Area Andrology Seminar. Series No. III

Su Yanhua, et al. 1989-1990. Animal Experimental Observation of Endometriosis Treated with the Drugs Promoting the Cir-

329

culation of Blood and Removing Blood Stasis. TCM and Western Medicine Combined Gynecological and Obstetrical Information. Total No. 3: 43-44

Sun Aida, et al. 1988. Diagnosis of Ovulatory Sterility (Comparison of Hysterosalpin Gography and Abdominoscopy). Beijing Medicine. 10 (1)

Sun Ce, et al. 1986. Immune Sterility Treated in Combination with TCM and Western Medicine. Shanghai Immunology Journal. (6): 364

Sun Huanming, et al. 1985. Shaofu Zhuyu Tang (Decoction for Removing Blood Stasis in the Lower Abdomen) in the Treatment of 20 Cases of Non-liquefaction of Seminal Fluid. Henan Journal of Chinese Medicine. (3): 29

Sun Yueli. 1981. Method of Restoring the Kidney to Remove Phlegm Treating 133 Cases with Polycystic Ovary Syndrome. Shanghai Journal of TCM. (6): 14-16

Tang Qingming, et al. 1989. A Clinical Observation of 117 Cases of Impotence Treated with Xianzi Dihuang Tang Jiawei (Modified Decoction of Curculigo and Rehmannia). TCM and Western Medicine Combined Gynecology and Obstetrics Information Data. 1989-1990 (Totaled No. III): 70-71

Wang Changyong, et al. 1987. A Report of A Research on Sweet Basil. Journal of Shandong TCM College. 11 (2): 50-51

Wang Mingxiang. 1990. Observation of the Clinical Curative Effect of Herbal Drugs in the Treatment of Non-liquefaction of Seminal Fluid. A Symposium of the First East China Area TCM Andrology Academic Seminar

Wang Qin, et al. 1989-1990. The Influence of TCM Artificial Cycle in Hypothalamus-Hyophysis-Ovary Axis. TCM and Western Medicine Combined Gynecol and Obstet Information Date. Total No. 3: 31-32

Wang Shurong, et al. 1990. Blood Flow Promoting Effect of Tongguan Tang (Decoction for Removing Obstruction from Oviduct) (Sterility No. IV) and Its Effect to Animal Reproductive System. TCM and Western Medicine Combined Diagnosis Treatment and Research of both Male and Female Sterility (unpublicized material). 124-126

Wang Shurong, et al. 1990. Ovulation Inducing Effect of Shiying Yulin Tang (Decoction of Amethyst for Pregnancy) and

330

Effect in Animal Reproductive System. Diagnosis of Sterility and TCM Treatment (unpublicized data). 49-69

Wang Zhaolun, et al. 1987. A Research of Chemical Composition of Sweet Basil (1). Journal of Shandong TCM College. 11 (2): 53

Wang Zhaolun, et al. 1990. Determination of the Trace Elements of Sweet Basil—Research of Chemical Composition of Sweet Basil (2). Journal of Shandong TCM College. 14 (6): 60-61

Wang Zhaolun, et al. 1990. Volatile Content of Sweet Basil Picked at Different Times and Determination of Volatile Composition—Research of Chemical Composition of Sweet Basil (3). Journal of Shandong TCM College. 14 (6): 62-64

Wang Zhongmin. 1990. A Clinical Report of 60 Cases of Spermatorrhea Treated by Baihui, Huiyin Acupoints. A Symposium of the First East China Area TCM Andrology Seminar. Series No. II

Xia Liying. 1989. Pharmacological Experimental Study of Sweet Basil. Research of Sweet Basil and Its Treatment in Sterility due to Ovulatory Dysfunction (unpublicized scientific data). 38-111

Wu Jinceng, et al. 1990. Clinical Research in Nux-vomica Seed Powder in Treating Functional Non-ejaculation—A Controlled Observation of 172 Cases. A Symposium of the First East China Area TCM Andrology Seminar. Series No. III

Wu Shuxi. 1987. Immune Factors of Female Sterility. Practical Gynecology and Obstetrics Journal. 3 (1): 8-9

Xu Fusong. 1989. Treatment Based on Syndrome Differentiation of Male Sterility. The Journal of Chinese Medicine, 30 (5): 5-6

Xu Fusong. 1990. The Treatment of Sexual Disorder in Male. The Journal of Chinese Medicine. 31 (12): 4

Xu Jingsheng. 1988. Experience of Applying TCM Cyclic Regulating Menstruation. Shanghai Journal of TCM. (3): 10-11

Xu Runsan. 1987. A Summary Report of 115 Cases with Obstruction in Fallopian Tube Treated with Sini San Jiawei (Modified Powder for Treating Cold Limbs. The Journal of Chinese Medicine. (9): 41-42

Zhang Liwei, et al. 1990. Approach to Diagnosis of Hypoluteoidism. Practical Gynecology Journal. 6 (2): 92

Zhang Qin, et al. 1984. A Report of 110 Cases of Non-ejaculation Treated by Acupuncture. The Journal of Chinese Medicine. 25 (4): 60

Zhao Songquan. 1985. An Observation of Pailuan Tang (Ovulatory Decoction) Treating 59 Cases with Various Ovulatory Disorders. Tianjin Journal of Chinese Medicine. (4): 8-9

Zhou Hong. 1990. Observation of the Curative Effect of Panicled Swallowwort Root (Radix Cynanchi Paniculati) in the Treatment of 300 Cases of Too Many Dead Spermia. A Symposium of the First East China Area TCM Andrology Seminar. Series No. III

Zhou Wenyu. 1989-1990. Combined TCM and Western Medicine Treating Hyperlactinemia. Combined TCM and Western Medicine Gynecology and Obstetrics Information. Total No. 3: 41-42

Zhu Guangyao. 1990. Spermatorrhea and Impotence Treated with both Acupuncture and Materia Medica. A Symposium of the First East China Area TCM Andrology Seminar. Series No. II

Zhu Wenxin, et al. 1989-1990. Preliminary Observation of Endometriosis Treated with the Drugs Promoting the Circulation of Blood and Removing Blood Stasis to Improve Blood Dynamic Indices of Uterine Artery. TCM and Western Medicine Combined Gynecology and Obstetrics Information. Total No. 3: 44-45

Zhu Xiudu, et al. 1987. An Observation of Acupuncture Combined with TCM Drugs Inducing Ovulation in 59 Cases. Shanghai Journal of TCM. (3): 12-13

Yang Wenlan, et al. 1990. Clinical Observation of TCM Yugong Pian (Uterus-Nourishing Tablet) Treating Dysfunctional Primary Sterility and Irregular Menstruation. A Collection of Papers on the 3rd National TCM and Medium Combined Gynecological and Obstetrical Academic Experience Exchange Conference. 123-130

Yu Jin, et al. 1990. Clinical Study of Electroacupuncture Promoting Ovulation. A Symposium of the 3rd National TCM and Western Medicine Combined Gynecological Academic Experience Exchange Meeting. 44-49

不孕症诊断与中医治疗

金维新　编著

聂文新
　　　　译
张　宇

白永泉　审校

英文编辑　陈　平

＊

山东科学技术出版社出版

中国济南市玉函路 16 号　邮政编码 250002

中国山东莱芜市印刷厂印刷

＊

1999 年(大 32 开)　1 版 1 次

ISBN 7 – 5331 – 2339 – 5

R·704

05400

14 – E – 2796P